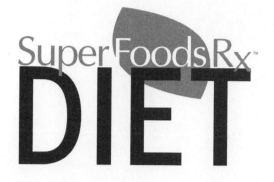

SuperFoodsRx™
DIET

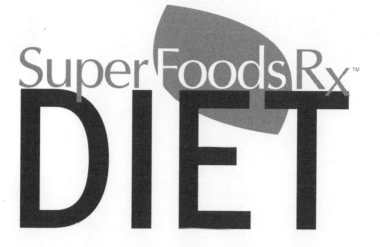

SuperFoodsRx™
DIET

Lose Weight with the
Power of **SuperNutrients**

Wendy Bazilian, DrPH, MA, RD
Steven Pratt, MD
Kathy Matthews

RODALE

© 2008 by Rodale Inc.

Rodale books may be purchased for business or promotional use or for special sales. For information, please write to:
Special Markets Department, Rodale Inc., 733 Third Avenue, New York, NY 10017

Printed in the United States of America
Rodale Inc. makes every effort to use acid-free ∞, recycled paper ♲.

Yogurt photo on cover by © John E. Kelly

Library of Congress Cataloging-in-Publication Data

Bazilian, Wendy.
    The superfoodsrx diet : lose weight with the power of supernutrients / Wendy Bazilian, Steven Pratt, and Kathy Matthews.
        p.   cm.
    Includes bibliographical references and index.
    ISBN-13 978–1–59486–740–8 hardcover
    ISBN-10 1–59486–740–2 hardcover
    1. Reducing diets.   2. Functional foods.   I. Pratt, Steven.   II. Matthews, Kathy, date   III. Title.
RM222.2.B3922 2008
613.2'5—dc22   2007042975

Distributed to the book trade by Macmillan

2 4 6 8 10 9 7 5 3 1   trade hardcover
2 4 6 8 10 9 7 5 3 1   direct marketing hardcover

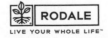

RODALE
LIVE YOUR WHOLE LIFE™

We inspire and enable people to improve their lives and the world around them
For more of our products visit **rodalestore.com** or call 800-848-4735

Contents

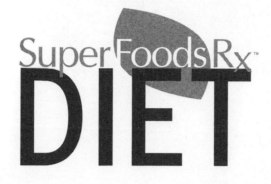

SuperFoodsRx™
DIET

The Promise of the SuperFoodsRx Diet

The SuperFoodsRx Diet will change your life. You are about to embark on a journey to lose excess weight but you will enjoy significant additional benefits. You'll gain vitality, reduce your risk of chronic disease, and live optimally at the weight and level of fitness you and your body deserve. You'll be adding as you're losing—adding SuperFoods, increasing your energy, and adding years to your life. That's the long-term promise of the SuperFoodsRx Diet program.

The SuperFoodsRx Diet is not a quick fix. It's not designed to be an eating plan that you follow for a few weeks to lose some weight and then abandon. It's truly a mind change and a life change.

....

Here's what some SuperFoodsRx dieters have to say:

- I've lost over 30 pounds and 7 inches from my waist after 16 weeks on the SuperFoodsRx Diet. My average weight loss was 3.75 pounds weekly in the first phase of the diet. I began the diet wearing a size 38 pants and XL shirts; I now wear 32 pants and medium shirts. These foods taste so much better to me now than the french fries and burgers I used to eat. —D. M., 51-year-old male insurance manager

- At 6 weeks on the diet I'd lost over 22 pounds. I was thrilled. And now at 16 weeks, I'm down over 40 pounds and 5 inches from my waist. I used to wear a size 20 or 22; I just bought a pair of size 14 jeans. I've never felt better about myself and the way I look. —S. A., 51-year-old single mom

🌿 I couldn't believe that I could keep up the steady weight loss I've enjoyed on this diet. So far I'm down 36 pounds with 4.25 inches off my waist and 6 inches off my hips! I've been on the diet for 16 weeks and I've found it easy to live with. I have a few more pounds to go and I have no doubt that I'll reach my goal soon. It's hard for me to believe that I've done this but the proof is in the mirror. —*C.C., 51-year-old female middle school librarian*

These people represent just a few of the many SuperFoodsRx Diet success stories. They lost weight when they thought they couldn't. They stuck to a diet when they'd failed in the past. The SuperFoodsRx Diet was their road map to success.

....

The SuperFoodsRx Diet literally will change your body. In just the first 2 weeks on the plan:

🌿 You will lose weight rapidly and safely.

🌿 The precise mix of foods will help control your appetite and actually boost your brain function so you can stick with your goals.

🌿 Your energy will improve.

🌿 You will lose inches, especially around your waist.

🌿 The appearance of your skin and hair will change within a week and you will look better than ever.

Wait a minute . . . look better than ever? How can you promise that?

Here's a story that may surprise you as much as it surprised us.

When we began to test our SuperFoodsRx Diet with various study groups, we were amazed and frankly perplexed when we listened to the comments of participants. Many of these people were obese and needed to lose a considerable amount of weight. Yet when we discussed their experiences with them—after only a week or two on the diet—we were thrilled to hear many of them say that they felt they looked better than ever. Their hair looked better, their nails were getting better and, most of all, they loved how great their skin looked. They described it time and again as a certain "glow." Yes, their clothes were looser—some had lost up to an inch in their waist measurement in a week—they loved the food (many were surprised they didn't experience any problems with hunger), and they felt calmer and more energetic. But what seemed to thrill them the most was the look of their skin and hair.

Frankly, we thought this was the power of positive thinking. But the comments were so enthusiastic and so convincing that we went to Dr. Hubert Greenway, the Chairman of Dermatologic Surgery at Scripps Clinic, to get his opinion. We showed him the tapes of the test subjects raving about their hair and skin after just over a week of eating the SuperFoodsRx Diet. Is it possible, we asked, that someone could experience such a change in such a short time or were these folks simply enjoying the added psychological benefits of seeing some real results while on a healthy diet?

Dr. Greenway explained that what these folks were reporting was real. He reminded us that the skin—the body's largest organ—responds remarkably quickly to any change in nutrition. You know how your face will sometimes break out if a certain food doesn't agree with you? Or how you'll get hives as an allergic reaction? Or how you may look pale just before you come down with an illness, or how even a bad night's sleep can show up on your face? These signals of your health, conveyed through your skin, emerge rapidly. The skin metabolizes nutrients quickly. Skin cells turn over rapidly and provide an effective window into health. It's not surprising, Dr. Greenway further explained, that when someone, particularly someone who has been following a fad diet, who's eating poorly, or who simply wasn't getting adequate nutrition, begins to enjoy the surge of nutrients and the hydration guaranteed by the SuperFoodsRx Diet, they'd see an immediate and significant improvement in their skin.

Well, that makes sense, we agreed. But how about a change in hair? Doesn't it take months for hair to grow? How could people see an improvement in their hair in only a few days? Dr. Greenway confirmed that while hair grows only about a quarter inch a month, the fast-acting cells of the sebaceous glands in the scalp—the same glands that affect the appearance of the skin—will have an immediate affect on the appearance of the hair when they get an infusion of nutrients, particularly healthy oils that promote growth and health. The proper balance of fatty acids in the diet has an immediate effect on the functioning of the sebaceous glands. So it's not the hair shaft itself that has changed in such a short time but rather the glands in the scalp that are responding to the nutrient surge. The healthy oil from these glands is affecting the appearance of the hair as it's distributed through brushing or combing.

This was very exciting news for us as well as our study participants. It's not just that we all like our skin to look great, although that's certainly true. The significant issue was that the improvements in skin tone and hair quality were signals to us that the SuperFoodsRx Diet was really effective, right from the first days.

This is very important. Why? Because when you're eager to lose weight you want to lose it any way you can. That's why fad diets, diet pills, exotic supplements, and weight loss surgery are so popular. But these methods can take a toll: on your energy levels, your appearance, your ability to stay trim and fit as well as your future health. We think the SuperFoodsRx Diet is a better way and you'll see immediate results in the mirror. *Your skin doesn't lie.* Your glowing, smoother, skin will show you like nothing else can that as your clothes get looser and your energy levels increase and your moods stabilize, your body is enjoying its best health ever. It's not just your skin and hair that are improving: *it's every organ system in your body* as you provide yourself with the most nutrient-dense foods on the planet. And that's how we want you to think about it: As you see your skin glow and your hair shine, think about every organ in your body—your heart, your lungs, your muscles, your intestines—getting stronger, more efficient, and healthier. They're glowing, too.

"Okay, big problem. Three weeks on this diet and my jeans are SO big and loose on me—they look horrible!!! Yahoo!!!"
—L .F., 43-year-young, stay-at-home mom

You, like our study participants, also will find the positive changes in your skin and hair powerfully motivating. Not to mention watching the measuring tape tighten around an ever more defined waistline and noticing the angle of your jaw becoming redefined. We've seen people thrilled to find that their rings are no longer impossibly tight, and joyful at being able to button their jackets. Such little changes mean quite a lot and keep you going. We have lots of built-in motivators in our plan—nutrient boosters, interchangeable meals, great snacks, and countless tips to help keep you on course. But perhaps the best motivator is going to be what you see in the mirror. And you don't have to wait until you reach your weight-loss goal to enjoy success: You'll see it in just days.

SuperFoods Are Forever

Most diets have a gimmick: high protein or high fiber or certain food combinations or timed eating. They all work for a while. Anyone who pays careful attention to what they eat and eliminates certain foods from their daily diet will inevitably lose some weight. But we know the end of this story. Diets like these are not lifestyles. They are a temporary fix. They're meant to be. They all tell you that you must follow a plan strictly for a few weeks, and then you can relax a bit, adding more foods and calories for a few more weeks, and then you go to "maintenance." You're typically left hanging with no plan save a few "tips" on what to do *later* when the goal is achieved. The problem is that the further you get from those initial weeks of commitment and success, the more the gimmick fades. In fact, the statistics on those who regain additional weight after trying to lose—yo-yo dieting—are utterly depressing.

People "fall off" diets because most diets are *designed* to be temporary and also because dieters lose focus. The process of going "on a diet" is usually immediate: You wake up and begin a new diet. The process of "falling off" a diet usually takes days or weeks. It happens because the diet is too restrictive to stick with, so unbalanced that you don't feel well on it, or you simply get tired of eating a limited palette of foods. You know the routine: You "cheat" because you're at a special event, you "modify" the diet because you're traveling, you "substitute" a favorite food for the diets required food. Before you know it, you're no longer on that diet and you're back to your other life, perhaps heavier than you were before and certainly more discouraged. The SuperFoodsRx Diet eliminates the whole issue of being "on" or "off" the diet. You make the SuperFoodsRx Diet fit you and your lifestyle and not the other way around.

SuperFoods rule forever! You focus on them when you start the diet and you'll be happily eating them years from now. Of course you have to watch your portions and learn a few strategies on how to incorporate these foods into your life, but once you understand and appreciate the benefits of the SuperFoods, you're armed for life—and for permanent weight loss.

We've found that the most powerful motivating factor of the SuperFoodsRx Diet is that it's not about eliminating foods; it's about including foods—Super-Foods—into your diet. You'll soon see that these are the foods you'll *want* to eat for the rest of your life.

There are two levels of the SuperFoodsRx Diet: the SlimDown and the FlexPlan. That's really all you'll ever need to know about the diet. It's very simple. You go on the SlimDown for 2 weeks, or longer if you like, and then you shift to the FlexPlan. The SlimDown promotes rapid weight loss; the FlexPlan is the eating plan you'll enjoy for the rest of your life. It's not restrictive. It encourages you to work treats and travel and special occasions into your eating plan. It's easy and it promotes a lifetime of successful weight management. We'll have lots more to say about the stages of the diet in the following chapters but you should know before you even begin that this diet is easy and flexible. Relieved? Most people are!

The Bonus of Plus Instead of Minus: You'll succeed on this diet because your focus will be on adding rather than subtracting foods. This simple shift is empowering. It's more fun, more satisfying, and more effective. Not only that, adding healthy foods rather than only trying to eliminate "fattening" foods could help you live longer. One study of nearly 60,000 women in Sweden found that those who ate a healthy, varied diet had a significantly lower mortality rate than women who consumed few healthy foods. The study concluded: "It appears more important to increase the number of healthy foods regularly consumed than to reduce the number of less healthy foods regularly consumed."[1]

SuperFoods Trump Willpower

What's the hardest thing about dieting? Most of us would agree: It's standing in front of the fridge or pantry at 10:00 p.m., starving, and giving in to a handful of cookies or a bowl of ice cream or a bag of chips. It's almost an out-of-body experience. You don't want to do it but you feel compelled to. Why? Because you're hungry. Or you think you're hungry. But it's really more than that. You may in fact be stressed or tired. One thing for sure: You're not feeling in control. The surprising fact is that you may be subverted by the very diet you're following. The way you feel—what we often refer to in relation to diets as willpower—is highly dependent on what you're eating. You'll find that the SuperFoodsRx Diet affects not only your waist but also your brain. It empowers you to choose healthy foods and has built-in and highly effective methods to convert you to the SuperFoods eating plan as a way of life.

SuperNutrient Power. Here's something that may surprise you: What you may think of as lack of willpower is often really lack of adequate, balanced nutrition. Most people don't realize the effect that chronic dieting has on their ability to make decisions. Most fad diets—or diets that are low in essential nutrients—make it nearly impossible for you to succeed in losing weight. That's because when you do not have a sustained and gradual release of blood glucose—which ideally comes from whole, nutrient dense, fiber-rich foods—your moods are affected such that you are extremely vulnerable to fuzzy thinking, mood swings, and impulsive behavior. Foods that are high in sugars and refined carbs and low in fiber lead to a rapid and extreme rise in glucose. This is inevitably followed by a surge in insulin. While the glucose is elevated and before the insulin has time to lower it you can actually experience a reduced ability to concentrate. Recent research has shown that chemicals found in the brain called orexins play a role in promoting mental alertness. High levels of glucose suppress orexin levels and interfere with your ability to concentrate *and* make you feel sleepy.[2] Indeed, one researcher at the U.S. National Institutes of Health found that the initial symptoms of depleted levels of Vitamin C are, surprisingly to

> "I love this diet because it works, I'm not starving, it is a long-term plan, and of course I will live longer and be healthier!"—Amateur golfer and tennis player, father of three

most people, irritability and fatigue.[3] In contrast, regular planned intake of fiber-rich, nutrient-rich foods balance your brain function and encourage the feelings of energy and control that ensure good food choices.

Obviously the emotional vulnerability that can result from less than optimum nutrient intake makes you far less likely to stick to your resolve and far more likely to munch a candy bar, down a coffee or grab any junk food that will instantly boost your blood sugar and "restore" your equilibrium. But the price of these "boosts" is increasing calories and increasing fat storage and ultimately a fatter body.

The SuperFoodsRx Diet manages blood sugar levels to increase your ability to focus and enhance your desire to eat foods that honor your body and promote weight loss. The careful composition of simple, delicious meals and the regular SuperNutrient Boosters—those delicious mid-morning drinks—act to stabilize your blood sugar and keep you feeling strong, optimistic, and committed.

The SuperFoodsRx Diet Overture

Most of us begin diets in a rush. We're eager, maybe even desperate, to get rid of that excess weight so we read something or hear something on TV that inspires us and the next day we're eating in a whole new way. We believe that the impulse to change a very important part of your life—your daily meals—without adequate preparation is, in fact, counterproductive.

"Since starting the SuperFoodsRx Diet I have more energy, sleep better, am less hungry, and have no more heartburn/acid reflux every night."
—Edna A, single mom with a purple belt in karate

In fact, for many people, it's the reason that their diet is unsuccessful. We know that we diet as much with our minds as our mouths. The SuperFoodsRx Diet takes full advantage of all we know of the psychology of dieting. That's why we've created our own "overture" to the actual diet program. The SuperFoodsRx Diet Prep & Practice Week is your warmup to a successful diet. It's the step you'll take that will make this diet different in that you'll be *mentally* prepared to lose weight. You'll learn a lot more about it in a forthcoming chapter. This initial week is critical to your success and also a fun and easy way to ease into your new lifestyle. During this week you do some prep—in your kitchen, in the market—and you do some practice. Choose a few SuperFoods meals you like, practice keeping track of your foods, and practice getting a little exercise. Your Prep & Practice Week is going to be a giant step on your road to a longer, healthier life.

The Super Flexible SuperFoodsRx Diet Meals

Have you ever looked at a diet plan, glanced at the menus, and said to yourself, "No way I can follow this…I don't like half of those meals." Or, perhaps

How practical is it really for a diet to prescribe specific meals for certain days for three or four weeks? Many diets will specify seven different breakfasts—one for each day of the week. Many diets require you to cook 21 different meals each week! Who eats like that? Who has time to prepare those meals? If you've been frustrated by other complicated diet plans, you will love the SuperFoodsRx Diet's interchangeable—mix and match—meal plans. You don't have to follow a rigid list of meal suggestions; you simply pick your favorite meals—lunch and dinner have been carefully calibrated so that they are interchangeable—and make *your own* menu! Don't you find you repeat certain breakfasts a few times a week if not daily? Aren't there certain surefire lunches or dinners that you could enjoy twice a week? The SuperFoodsRx Diet allows you to fully customize your eating plan to your tastes and your allotted prep time. You do have to plan ahead and fill out your weekly menus but there's tremendous flexibility within the suggested meals. As long as you follow the simple SuperFoods 1, 2, 3 guidelines you'll enjoy delicious, easy meals, increased energy, and steady, rapid weight loss that actually lasts. Super-FoodsRx dieters have often seen over 8 pounds lost and 2 inches off the waist in just 14 days, and some have even experienced 5 pounds and a whole inch gone in only the first week. After 6 weeks? As many as 22 pounds, and an *average* of nearly 16 pounds, 12 total inches off the body, 3½ off the waist alone—gone for good! And the weight continues to come off and stay off. *What about calories? Yes, calories do count. But on the SuperFoodsRx Diet, you don't have to count them! The meals and menus are designed for built-in calorie control.*

> "One of things that I love about this diet is that while there are recipes provided, there are no preset meals or recipes. The food is all food that I like. The whole plan is extremely 'portable.'"—Susan A, accountant

more frustrating, have you ever struggled to follow a diet plan by modifying it to your taste? So the dinner they suggest on Tuesday—one of the few you like—you substitute for the prescribed dinner on Friday and Saturday and so on. Once you begin to make these changes in an eating plan, you feel less and less committed to it. It's human nature. You're not really following Diet A: You're following your *version* of Diet A. But as you move farther and farther from the recommendations, your success rate probably plummets until you throw in the towel.

SuperFoodsRx Diet in a Nutshell

We've tried to make the SuperFoodsRx Diet the most effective, easy to follow, healthiest diet in the world. We've looked to gold-standard weight-loss research, cutting-edge data on the benefits of the SuperFoods to weight loss, behavioral studies that identify the most effective weight-loss techniques and, last and far from least, actual people like you trying to lose weight, in order to formulate a plan that can promise more than any other plan you may have tried: weight loss plus optimum health. If you follow this diet, you will lose weight. You'll also look great and feel great. We promise. But you do have to do your part.

Here's the SuperFoodsRx Diet in a nutshell so you can see what's ahead.

The Prep & Practice Week

This is your diet kickoff week. It's critical. During this week you'll:

- Shift to eating mainly SuperFoods and increase your fluid intake
- Revise your kitchen to make it a SuperFoods-friendly place to work and eat
- Shop for the SuperFoods
- Begin a very simple exercise plan

- Choose the SuperFoods menus that you'll follow next week in your SlimDown
- Begin your food diary

The SlimDown

This is your diet springboard. This is where you'll see the most weight and waist loss. You'll follow the SlimDown for at least 2 weeks. You may choose to follow it longer but that's up to you. During the SlimDown:

- You'll follow the SuperFoods SlimDown menu that you've created, choosing from the Super-Food meal selections.
- You'll choose from the SuperFoods 1, 2, 3 categories for all your meals.
- You'll amplify the exercise you began in the Prep Week.

The FlexPlan

This is real-life eating. You'll go on the FlexPlan when you've reached a certain weight-loss goal (it doesn't have to be your final goal!), when your life demands a more relaxed approach to dieting (travel, special events, and such), or just when you feel like it. The FlexPlan offers:

- Continued, but slower, weight loss
- Continued reliance on the SuperFoods 1, 2, 3 categories
- Flexibility to add extras such as wine, dessert, an extra snack, and so on, with specific guidelines and strategies

"I love that the foods on this diet can be ones that are really easy to prepare. I'm so tired when I get home that, for now, simple is the answer. I'll diversify and try more recipes eventually because this is a permanent change for me but I really like that I can still follow this diet right now without lots of time preparing different meals. I intend to make this diet plan a permanent change, so I will get more creative with time."—Pat B., 58-year-young, busy medical receptionist

The LifePlan

This is the chapter that ties it all together. Here you'll find the critical information you need to enjoy the most benefits of SuperFoods for the rest of your life. You'll find recommendations as well as information on how various aspects of your life affect continued, lifelong weight loss:

- Keys to Long-Term SuperFoodsRx Diet Success
- The Role of Stress
- The Importance of Sleep
- SuperFoods in Real World Scenarios

····································

So there you have it.

One last thing: Change isn't easy. We've provided a lifeline for you: a plan that is effective, safe, and practical. We won't pretend that changing your life, changing a big part of your life—what you eat—is an easy task. It's a challenge. But we've seen people succeed on this diet who have failed on others. You can do it, too. We'll even feature some of the tips and strategies that successful SuperFoodsRx dieters want to share with you. Each step you take on this plan is going to be rewarding. Each day you'll feel stronger. It's just one day, one delicious SuperFoods meal at a time.

Chapter 1

SuperNutrients for Super Weight Loss

I f only there were a magic bullet for weight loss, something you could take that would keep you satisfied *and* boost your body's ability to lose weight. It would have to be safe, and it would be nice if it tasted good, and also if you could get it without a doctor's prescription. Well, there is, or are, such substances: the SuperFoods! It sounds too good to be true but in fact the rich array of nutrients—SuperNutrients—in the SuperFoods actually can help you lose weight. How can this be? The SuperFoods are commonly known to be functional foods. This means that they provide benefits to the body beyond simple sustenance. We've long known that functional foods like the Super-Foods play a role in cancer prevention, reduction of risk for cardiovascular disease, stroke, diabetes, and a host of chronic ailments. But research is now demonstrating that many of these same foods can also *boost* your ability to burn calories and *reduce* excess weight accumulation.

When you think about it, doesn't it make sense, doesn't it seem natural, and isn't it an appealing notion that you could *lose* weight employing the very thing that created your excess weight—food? Of course, the critical issue here is *choice* of food. It's the *right* food, SuperFoods, that makes the difference and bolsters all your efforts to reduce weight and inches and increase health. So you don't have to have surgery or take a drug or adopt an extreme approach in order to manage your weight. You can turn to nature and the natural functioning of your body to choose foods that will promote weight loss in a variety of safe and effective ways. You can reach your weight-loss goals with the SuperNutrients in SuperFoods.

We've long known that the SuperNutrients promote overall health. If you analyze the healthiest diets in the world, these nutrients turn up time and again. Countless studies have shown that the higher your level of these nutrients, the slower you'll age and the less likely you will develop chronic disease. These are the SuperNutrients that make superstars of certain foods that contain abundant quantities of them—the SuperFoods:

Alpha-carotene	Folic acid	Resveratrol
Beta carotene	Lutein/zeaxanthin	Selenium
Beta cryptoxanthin	Lycopene	Vitamin C
Fiber	Omega-3 fatty acids	Vitamin D
Glutathione	Polyphenols	Vitamin E

The Synergy of SuperNutrients and SuperFoods

It's important to remember a crucial factor when looking at the weight-loss promoting abilities of SuperFoods: synergy. Synergy is the key to the effectiveness of the SuperFoodsRx Diet and, in fact, the key to the choice of the individual SuperFoods themselves.

When I was first studying the various properties of specific foods, it was a revolutionary notion that propelled me. The idea that intrigued me was that certain foods were actually better for you, better for your health, than others. This went beyond the obvious comparisons of, say, a steak and a salad. Most people would guess that a salad is more health-promoting than a steak and they'd be right. But what about the ingredients in that salad: the types of lettuce, the various vegetables? And what about the other choices that we make every day about which foods to include in our diet? I gradually ascertained, by studying volumes of research and discussing critical nutritional issues with the researchers themselves (many of them world-renowned scientists and colleagues), that certain foods like blueberries, spinach, salmon, and a number of others—14 in all—indeed deserved the distinction of being called Super-Foods. They are uniquely rich in an array of nutrients that have powerful health benefits and their nutrient profiles lift them above many other foods in their same category.

Let's take a look at the SuperFoods themselves. The original *SuperFoodsRx* book featured 14 original foods that research had demonstrated could help promote health in powerful ways. You've probably read about them as they're frequently mentioned in the media. Each of the 14 foods was chosen because of the strength of its nutrient profile: it featured nutrients—SuperNutrients—that are particularly powerful in promoting health and/or nutrients that are difficult to find elsewhere. In addition to the main flagship, SuperFood, each food has what we called "sidekicks." The sidekicks are foods with a nutrient profile that is similar to the flagship food and as such they are good alternative choices.

14 ORIGINAL SUPERFOODS & THEIR SIDEKICKS

Beans: all dried beans and low-sodium canned beans plus string beans, sugar snap peas, green peas

Blueberries: purple grapes, cranberries, boysenberries, raspberries, strawberries, fresh currants, blackberries, cherries, and all other varieties of fresh or frozen berries

Broccoli: brussels sprouts, cabbage, kale, turnips, cauliflower, collards, bok choy, mustard greens, Swiss chard

Oats: Super sidekicks: wheat germ, ground flaxseed; Sidekicks: brown rice, barley, wheat, buckwheat, rye, millet, bulgur wheat, amaranth, quinoa, triticale, kamut, yellow corn, wild rice, spelt, couscous

Oranges: lemons, white and pink grapefruit, kumquats, tangerines, limes

Pumpkin: carrots, butternut squash, sweet potatoes, orange bell peppers

Salmon: Alaskan halibut, chunk light tuna, sardines, herring, trout, bass, oysters, clams

Soy: tofu, soy milk, soy nuts, edamame, tempeh, miso

Spinach: kale, collards, Swiss chard, mustard greens, turnip greens, bok choy, romaine lettuce, orange bell peppers

Tea: green and black

Tomatoes: watermelon, pink grapefruit, Japanese persimmons, red-fleshed papaya, strawberry guava

Turkey: skinless chicken breast

Walnuts: almonds, pistachios, pumpkin, sesame and sunflower seeds, macadamia nuts, pecans, hazelnuts, cashews, peanuts, pine nuts, Brazil nuts

Yogurt: kefir

After the original SuperFoods book was published, research of course continued. By the time the second book, *HealthStyle*, was under way there were additional foods, and sidekicks, as well as some extraordinary spices—Super-Spices—that could be counted as SuperFoods.

ADDITIONAL SUPERFOODS, SIDEKICKS, and SUPERSPICES

Apples: pears

Avocado: asparagus, artichokes, extra virgin olive oil

Dark chocolate

Dried SuperFruits: raisins, dates, prunes, figs, apricots, blueberries, cranberries, cherries, currants

Extra virgin olive oil: canola oil

Honey

Kiwi: pineapple, guava

Onions: garlic, scallions, shallots, leeks, chives

Pomegranates: plums

SUPERSPICES

Cinnamon	Oregano
Cumin	Thyme
Garlic	Turmeric

What makes say, spinach, a SuperFood when compared to other green leafies? Spinach provides your body with a rich infusion of SuperNutrients including lutein/zeaxanthin, beta-carotene, plant-derived omega-3 fatty acids, glutathione, alpha lipoic acid, vitamins C and E, the B vitamins including thiamine, riboflavin, B6, and folate; minerals including calcium, iron, magnesium, manganese, and zinc; various polyphenols, and betaine. That's a pretty impressive array of nutrients for a simple, delicious leaf. And, in fact, it's only a *partial* list of the nutrients in spinach.

The SuperNutrients in most of the SuperFoods (with the exception of soy and yogurt) that particularly enhance their ability to promote health are a category of SuperNutrients called the phytonutrients. These phytonutrients (from the Greek word "phyto" for plant) are nonvitamin, nonmineral, and noncaloric components of plants foods that provide significant benefits to your health. In spinach, just as one example, the somewhat amazing array of phytonutrients includes the carotenoids lutein, zeaxanthin, and beta-carotene among many others.

We mentioned the concept of synergy earlier. Spinach is an excellent example of synergy in a particular SuperFood. It's the power of all the nutrients working in concert that makes spinach and the other SuperFoods such standouts in the world of nutrition. But there are actually two levels, if you will, of synergy that come into play when looking at these foods: the synergy of nutrients in the SuperFoods themselves and the synergy of the SuperFoods themselves eaten together on a regular basis in your daily diet—the Super-FoodsRx Diet.

In the foods themselves, the SuperNutrients they contain work together to amplify an effect that any of the single nutrients might not have if working alone. It's the synergy of the nutrients in whole foods that have sometimes caused consternation in the world of science when single-nutrient research projects have failed to prove a hypothesis that initially seemed inevitable. For example, most people associate calcium with preventing osteoporosis. But research employing a single factor, calcium, doesn't always prove this hypothesis. Why? Because building strong bones takes calcium working along with other constituents including vitamin D, boron, vitamin C, and magnesium, among others. And exercise figures into the equation as well since it's the weight-bearing exercise that stimulates bones to use those multiple nutrients to build, rebuild, repair, and preserve strong and healthy bones.

In the SuperFoodsRx Diet, synergy again is key to effectiveness but in this instance it's the synergy of all of the SuperFoods that you'll be eating together that will help you feel and look better than ever and of course lose weight. Your goal is a healthy, whole-foods diet that emphasizes the SuperFoods.

This synergy of SuperFoods eaten together and regularly is important. For example, though we know that oranges and green tea, to choose two Super-Foods, have special properties that will help you lose weight, we also know that these foods are most effective and powerful when eaten in concert. Here's a very specific example of this amplifying benefit: While we know that broccoli and tomatoes, both SuperFoods, are independently recognized for their ability to help prevent cancer, a study published in the journal *Cancer Research* reported that when both are included in the daily diet, the ultimate effect on prostate cancer is greater than when either vegetable is eaten alone. As the report noted, "The combination of tomato and broccoli was more effective at slowing tumor growth than either tomato or broccoli alone."[1] And we are convinced that this amplifying ability of the SuperFoods to create a health-promoting environment is even stronger when they're eaten together regularly as a major part of your daily diet.

While the SuperFoods themselves can go a long way to promoting health and preventing chronic ailments like heart disease, cancer, diabetes, and osteoporosis among others, they can't obliterate the effects of other, poor food choices. Which means that you can't eat steak, french fries, and a giant cinnamon roll and expect that a cup of green tea is going to bail you out. It just doesn't work that way. In order to achieve the best results in terms of short- and long-term health, you need to rely on a diet based primarily on the

SuperFoods and their many sidekicks working synergistically in concert to help you achieve your immediate weight-loss goals as well as your long-term health goals.

As noted earlier, the power of the SuperFoods isn't just relegated to reducing your risk for long-term disease. The exciting news is that these same foods also actually promote weight loss. Once again, it is the SuperNutrients that make significant contributions to the power of these foods to help get your body back in balance and shed pounds. Here's one way to look at it: You know how when you wash a load of heavy items like towels, sometimes the spin cycle becomes unbalanced? At first the machine spins normally but then after a few revolutions the unbalanced weight begins to take its toll and the washer begins to rock, the motor makes angry banging noises and eventually, if you don't stop the cycle, the washer will practically start walking across the floor and ultimately grind to a stop. This lack of balance takes a toll on the motor. Your body, like the washer, functions best when it's balanced. When it's unbalanced it's more prone to function poorly, which translates into increased risk for chronic ailments including obesity. The best way to get your body back in balance is with the best foods—the SuperFoods. You know you can almost force a washer to spin properly when it's unbalanced by wedging it into place, which will appear to solve the issue—for a while. It may continue to work but the toll on the motor working under these conditions becomes ever more disastrous. This is akin to what can happen when you try unhealthy fad diets to lose weight: You may get short-term results but in the end you'll be taking a toll on your "motor" that will be hard to recover from.

To place the weight-loss discussion in context, we should recognize that science is an evolving process and the research data on particular nutrients and their effect on weight are, in large part, preliminary. We would love to be able to tell you that if you eat salmon and spinach for a week you'll lose 10 pounds. But that's just not the case. However, the positive changes you'll see in your metabolism as a result of eating these foods in concert are real, though of course they will vary based on your own biochemistry and genetic heritage. Research is just beginning to reveal these subtle but powerful effects. Some of this very recent, emerging research has only been done on animals, not humans. With only one or two noted exceptions, the scientific research that inspired the original *SuperFoodsRx* and *SuperFoodsRx HealthStyle* was derived primarily from studies on humans in clinical trials. As you might imagine, it's quite a challenge for scientists to design a strong double-blind study on humans that would focus on a particular nutrient. It's complicated and, in some cases, irresponsible, to manipulate the diets of real people so as to exclude important nutrients. We point this out to you to make it clear that we're not making extravagant claims for the powers of these foods. When it comes to weight loss, people can feel desperate and can become vulnerable to false promises. But the peer-reviewed research we're citing here does suggest that we are on the verge of further important discoveries about how certain foods and their nutrients—the SuperNutrients—play important roles in the complex picture of weight loss. Our hope is that more research of its kind will be conducted in the coming years so that the extraordinary value of the SuperFoods will continue to be confirmed, both as health-promoters and welcome, powerful support to those trying to lose weight.

The SuperFoods/Weight Loss Connection

So let's take a look at what we do know about the SuperFoods and their SuperNutrients and how they can work in synergy to help you shed pounds. It's both exciting and motivating to learn about the special properties of the individual SuperFoods in relation to weight. Somehow when you think of a food as having a *positive* benefit, such a promoting the rate at which you burn calories, rather than just a *neutral* benefit, such as not being high in calories, say or saturated fat, it's inspiring. As one large study that investigated functional foods and weight control put it when discussing the value of adding foods like nuts and tea to the diet to help control weight, *"if the dietary components were combined, their effects could be significant."*[2] We're sure that you'll find when *you* combine these SuperFoods your results will indeed be significant.

The Secret Lives of Fat Cells

Let's take another look at fat and some of the fascinating properties of fat tissue that have only recently been discovered. We used to think that fat cells were simply cells that stored fat. We've always known that if you eat more calories than your body needs, your fat cells stretch to store those extra calories. But until fairly recently fat cells were basically viewed as simple storage units. What's new—and extremely useful and important information if you're trying to lose weight—is that we now know that fat cells are far more complicated than previously realized. Indeed, fat cells are little metabolic machines, actively churning out a variety of substances that can affect your weight, appetite, and how many calories you eat as well as how efficiently your body uses those calories for energy. These substances produced by your fat cells, known as adipocytes, include leptin, ghrelin, interleukin-6, tumor necrosis factor alpha, angiotensinogen, adiponectin, and resistin. In general, the more fat cells you have and the fatter those cells become, the more of these substances they can pump into your bloodstream. These enlarged fat cells that you have due to excess weight secrete the

Here's a comment from the author of one large research study about the American diet: "A large proportion of Americans are under-nourished in terms of vitamins and minerals. You can actually be obese and still be undernourished with regard to important nutrients. We shouldn't be telling people to eat less, we should be telling people to eat differently."[3]

aforementioned substances into the blood at levels that ultimately begin to damage the circulatory system and impair blood flow. This impairment can ultimately lead to developing diseases such as diabetes, hypertension, cardiovascular disease, and even certain types of cancer. It stands to reason, and research is now beginning to back up the notion, that the same foods that can have a protective effect against these diseases—the SuperFoods—can also play a welcome role in controlling weight gain and maintaining a healthy weight.

We don't need to go into great detail about these particular substances and their unique effects on your metabolism but you should know that scientists now recognize that the chemistry of weight gain and weight loss is far more subtle and complicated than first believed. And it's this complicated chemistry that opens the door to SuperNutrients having a real effect on weight gain and loss.

So let's take a look at some of the SuperFoods and their SuperNutrients that are going to help you shed pounds on the SuperFoodsRx Diet.

Green Tea and Your Weight

What if you could improve your insulin activity and thus help stabilize your blood sugar and balance your energy levels throughout the day? And what if, at the same time, you could boost the speed at which your body burns calories *and* stop your body from storing extra fat? Well emerging evidence suggests that you can do just that by regularly sipping a delicious cup of green tea. Green tea has always been a stellar SuperFood, foremost because of its SuperNutrients but also because it's readily available, virtually calorie free, tasty, inexpensive, and easy to incorporate into your daily diet. It's wonderful news to find that it also is of real benefit to those trying to lose weight.

We've known for a long time that polyphenols—the main active ingredients in green tea—have powerful effects on the body. The polyphenols act as antioxidants that protect the body from the negative effects of free radicals and help prevent oxidative damage. Polyphenols are antibacterial and antiviral, and also play a role in preventing cell mutation.[4] They are active agents in helping reduce the risk of cancer, osteoporosis, and stroke. At the same time, they can help lower blood pressure, promote heart health, and even play a role in preventing damage to your skin from the sun's ultraviolet rays. Polyphenols are also powerful anti-inflammatories and we know there's a strong connection between obesity and inflammation: If you are obese your body is inflamed. The polyphenols fight that inflammation. Other research has shown that the theanine in green tea may play a role in reducing stress,[5] which we are learning can be a powerful promoter of weight gain.

In addition to these extraordinary benefits, we now are seeing evidence that green tea can be a wonderful addition to the diet for those trying to lose weight. While there is still much to learn about the beneficial effects of green tea in relation to body weight, research findings point to two components of the tea: caffeine and the epigallocatechin gallate or EGCG, which is a plant compound known as a catechin found in green tea. Originally it was simply hypothesized that the caffeine was the compound most responsible for promoting weight loss but we are now learning that green tea—as well as many black teas—has mild "thermogenic properties" beyond what can be explained by its caffeine content.[6] In other words, tea can actually boost metabolism by creating heat or encourage calorie burning. In a 2001 Tufts study, people who drank five 10-ounce cups of Chinese oolong tea a day for 3 days increased their metabolism 3 percent more than folks who drank water.[7] In addition, tea has been shown in several studies to break down or oxidize more fat when individuals consume brewed tea when compared to water or a placebo.[8] What's more, an increasing body of evidence also shows that not only can tea enhance fat burning, but the SuperNutrient polyphenols actually inhibit the storage and accumulation of new fat.[9]

If mildly increasing metabolism, enhancing fat burning, and decreasing the tendency to store fat isn't compelling enough, another significant role that green tea can play in weight gain or loss is related to its effect on insulin regulation. Insulin is a hormone that in addition to being essential to the regulation and use of blood sugar for energy plays a critical role in fat storage. This powerful hormone plays an important role therefore in weight regulation and research has shown that green tea does in fact have an impact on insulin regulation.[10] In this case, it appears to be the EGCG in green and oolong tea and EGCG along with epicatechin gallate, tannins, and theaflavins in black tea, that play this insulin-enhancing role. This again underscores why the whole tea leaf itself and the synergy of the many nutrients are more effective than a single nutrient supplement.

What about black or oolong tea? While most of the studies on tea and weight loss have focused on green tea, there is evidence to support that, in addition to increasing metabolism as mentioned above in the study done at Tufts, oolong and black tea also have a beneficial effect on overweight and obesity.[11] One study that looked at whether tea prevented obesity in mice concluded that ". . . oolong tea may be an effective crude drug for the treatment of obesity . . . "[12] You'll therefore most certainly want to enjoy both green and black tea regularly, whether you're trying to lose weight or simply trying to maintain and promote good health.

Another finding concerning tea may suggest even greater benefits than usually recognized. You've surely noticed that many foods and drinks these days are advertised as being high in antioxidants. Antioxidants neutralize free radicals, the harmful substances produced in our bodies by our metabolism. A researcher in Pretoria, South Africa analyzed the antioxidant or "radical scavenging capacity" of a variety of fruits, vegetables, and teas. The study results showed that one or two cups of tea, made from green, black, or oolong tea, provide a similar antioxidant ability as five servings of fruits and vegetables or 400 milligrams of vitamin C.[13] Of course these results were in the laboratory: The author of the study urged caution in applying these results to humans because the bioavailability of the vitamin C would depend on a host of factors. But the finding is yet another compelling argument for the value of adding tea to your diet.

Orange Power

Oranges have long been one of the favorite SuperFoods. They're sweet and delicious, low in calories, high in fiber, and great traveling companions because they don't have to be washed before eating. Of course the "super" feature of oranges and their sidekicks as well as the new SuperFood, kiwi, is their extraordinarily high levels of vitamin C. We encourage most everyone to boost their intake of vitamin C because, despite the wealth of healthy food choices we have today, 20 to 30 percent of us in the United States have marginal blood levels of vitamin C and, amazingly, 16 percent of us are actually deficient in this critical nutrient.

Vitamin C is a truly powerful nutrient—one that helps promote overall health in countless ways. Research has shown that it has a positive influence on cardiovascular health, can help prevent certain cancers, and is even protective against risk of stroke.

But the compelling news about vitamin C for SuperFoodsRx dieters is the suggestion from a handful of studies that this nutrient may actually play a role in promoting weight loss. One large study found a relationship between vitamin C status and fat distribution. This study, reported in the *American Journal of Clinical Nutrition*, found that blood levels of vitamin C were negatively associated with body fat distribution. In other words, independent of body mass index (BMI), age, supplement use, socioeconomic levels, or smoking status, the higher the vitamin C in the study participants' blood, the lower their waist-to-hip ratio.[14] This held true for both men and women. Now this study didn't demonstrate a *causative* relationship between abdominal fat and vitamin C levels—one can't say the lack of vitamin C was directly responsible for the fat distribution—but clearly there is some relationship between maintaining optimal levels of this important nutrient and body composition.

Other researchers have found an even more interesting relationship between vitamin C levels and *efficiency* of weight loss. One review discussed several studies that have shown a relationship between vitamin C status and the body's ability to break down fat for fuel as well as multiple studies that show an association between low levels of vitamin C and increased degree of obesity. The author of that review commented that people with adequate vitamin C status oxidize 30 percent more fat during moderate exercise than those with low vitamin C status.[15] Given this preliminary evidence, people with low vitamin C intake—a very large percentage of the population as we've just seen—could be potentially resistant, or at least sluggish, when it comes to weight loss. Other research has shown that improving vitamin C status is associated with significantly more weight loss compared to a placebo.[16] The implications of this are obvious: Vitamin C is yet another piece of the puzzle the helps us maintain a healthy weight and the SuperFoods that contain rich supplies of this SuperNutrient, like the orange and its sidekicks, are useful weapons in the battle of the bulge.

Wild Salmon and the Power of Omega-3

The news that wild salmon can play a significant role in a weight reduction diet confirms the value of the primary SuperNutrient it contains—omega 3 fatty acids. While delicious salmon offers a host of healthy nutrients including B vitamins, selenium, vitamin D, potassium, and healthy protein, perhaps its most valuable contribution to your health is that it offers one of the richest whole food sources of omega-3 fatty acids. You've probably been hearing about omega-3 fatty acids recently. There's been much discussion about the importance of fish like salmon in the diet and in fact the American Heart

Association® recommends eating at least two servings of fish—particularly fatty fish like salmon and its sidekicks—weekly. The major benefit of these polyunsaturated fatty acids called omega-3s, in particular DHA (docosahexanenoic acid) and EPA (eicosapentaenoic acid), is that they make blood platelets less "sticky" thus protecting circulatory health, they may promote cognitive functioning, and there's also a growing body of evidence that they may reduce the inflammatory process in the entire body. It's this latter benefit—reducing inflammation—that seems to most benefit those trying to lose weight.

We now know that inflammation, while a useful and important bodily response to injury, can sometimes become a chronic condition in which the body continually produces chemicals that inflame tissues. This constant inflammation ultimately can significantly increase the risk of developing diseases like arthritis, asthma, cardiovascular disease, and stroke. Most interesting to people trying to lose weight, chronic inflammation can also disrupt the performance of leptin, a hormone that plays a critical role in hunger and appetite regulation. Fat actually produces leptin but chronic inflammation can promote leptin resistance in which leptin is being produced in ever-larger amounts but the body is not responding to it as it should. Ultimately this means the leptin is unable to completely fulfill its role of turning off the hunger signal and boosting your metabolism. We are beginning to see that the overall role of leptin along with this issue of leptin resistance could be a critical factor in the issue of weight management. Enter wild salmon, a top source of the omega-3 fatty acids.

Research studies are beginning to reveal the power of omega-3s to promote weight loss in a variety of complex ways. One study with mice found that fish oil affected body fat distribution among the subjects. In this study the mice were divided into three groups. Some were fed soybean oil, some lard, and others fish oil. Those who were fed fish oil developed less visceral fat, which refers to the fat surrounding the organs that is difficult to reduce and a major risk factor for cardiovascular disease[17]. These fish oil–fed mice also had lower leptin levels and, as we've seen, these lower levels of the hormone leptin would help regulate both appetite and metabolism.

Another study on mice found that the quality of dietary fat—in this case omega-3 fatty acids versus saturated fat—could actually affect the hormones that in turn affect the hypothalamic satiety center. In this study the omega-3 altered the brain's regulation of metabolism and limited the development of obesity.[18]

We also now know that the ratio of omega-6 to omega-3 fatty acids in our bodies plays a major role in how the central nervous system controls our metabolism and thus our weight. The wrong ratio primes you for weight gain because the wrong balance of these fatty acids makes you want to eat more. Since most Americans consume far more omega-6 than omega-3 fatty acids, the SuperFood wild salmon and its rich supply of omega-3 fatty acids can contribute significantly to weight-loss success.

There's another issue worth considering in regard to weight loss and dietary fat: Researchers have recently been learning that it's not just the amount of fat in the diet that affects weight loss or gain; it's also the type of fat. Studies have found that diets high in saturated fat promote weight gain beyond the simple mathematics of caloric intake. In one study on mice, researchers found that subjects fed varying types and amounts of fat benefited most from a diet of healthy fats. Indeed, in this study a high-saturated fat diet induced obesity, and the group fed omega-3 fats (after a period of eating saturated fats) *saw a complete reversal* of the weight gain that had been induced by the saturated fat, even though caloric intake was constant on both types of fat.[19] The group fed omega-3 fats experienced both reduced fat and reduced leptin levels. The take-away message, according to the researchers, was that "Equally high fat diets emphasizing PUFAs (polyunsaturated omega-3 fats) may even protect against obesity."

Another study with overweight adults in Australia found that those participants who had supplemented with fish oil and who had also followed an exercise program experienced more fat loss than those who had been given fish oil supplements alone but had not exercised or had been given a placebo with or without exercise.[20] The subjects were not on a calorie-restricted diet and so the loss of fat was not associated with a lower calorie intake. It's quite encouraging to know that both fish oil consumption along with exercise has been proven to be a more effective fat-loss strategy than either supplementation alone or exercise alone. The SuperFoodsRx Diet is the first diet to help you achieve weight loss by a careful combination of specific foods and exercise working in concert to maximize your body's ability to shed weight.

Yogurt for Your Waistline

It's been gratifying to see the explosive growth in the varieties of yogurt available in most every supermarket. It's almost hard to remember that there once was a time when it was difficult to find more than one or perhaps two brands. And you'll notice that many brands these days make prominent mention on their packaging of the "live active cultures" that their product contains. This is important because many of the benefits of yogurt are associated with these live active cultures. Yogurt is, quite simply, milk that via the work of friendly bacteria has had its naturally occurring lactose, or milk sugar, turned into lactic acid. The work of this transformation is done by those friendly bacteria—the "live active cultures."

The health benefits of nonfat or low-fat yogurt, our dairy SuperFood, are considerable. Yogurt has been favorably associated with helping to reduce the risk of the following conditions: certain cancers, allergies, lactose intolerance, inflammatory bowel disease, irritable bowel syndrome, hypertension, elevated cholesterol, certain kinds of ulcers, diarrhea, and vaginal and urinary tract infections. Obviously, making nonfat or low-fat yogurt a regular part of your diet is a smart decision. But there's even more reason for people trying to lose weight to include yogurt in their diet. Most of us know that yogurt, as a dairy product, is rich in calcium. Yogurt is an excellent source of calcium because, unlike whole milk, it's low in saturated fat. And of course the friendly bacteria, absent in milk, play a role in yogurt's health benefits, particularly those related to healthy digestion. But over and above the other benefits of yogurt, there is now some exciting evidence that people who have a rich supply of calcium in their diets are less likely to gain weight. There's still more research to be done on this subject but one study showed that women with the highest calcium intakes had the lowest risk of obesity and the slowest weight gain as they aged. As the researchers put it, "increasing calcium intake can be estimated to reduce the prevalence of overweight and obesity by perhaps as much as 60 to 80 percent."[21] In another small 2-year study of young women that investigated the relationship between nutrients and body composition among exercisers, researchers found that the young women with a high calcium intake gained less weight and body fat over the 2 years than those with the lower calcium intake.[22] Another study that received a great deal of attention found that over a period of 12 weeks, 34 obese adults on a calorie-reduced diet who consumed three servings of yogurt a day lost 22 percent more weight and 61 percent more body fat as well as 81 percent more fat from around their middles (and nearly four times the amount of inches lost around their waists) when compared to those consuming a diet low in dairy foods.[23]

While the above studies didn't show a *causative* relationship between calcium intake and weight status, animal studies *have* shown this solid relationship between calcium intake and body fat, body weight, and weight gain. One study on mice found that when calories were restricted, the mice on a high-calcium diet lost more fat than the mice on a low-calcium diet. The researchers speculated that the calcium could help in the breakdown of fat. While the low-calcium diet promoted fat storage, the high-calcium diet promoted fat usage and slowed fat storage.[24] Interestingly, the mice on the low-calcium diet also had lower core body temperatures than the high-calcium diet mice and this too resulted in increased fat storage. Additional research in animals and humans has shown that higher-calcium diets promote fat breakdown, inhibit the creation of new fat cells and fat storage, and may even preserve metabolism during calorie-reduced diets, which could potentially speed up weight and fat loss.[25]

Why would calcium have such an effect on weight? One possible reason is the relationship between calcium and your body's energy metabolism. Low calcium levels stimulate production of a hormone—parathyroid hormone or PTH. A food shortage also stimulates high levels of both these hormones and so there is speculation that your body "reads" low levels of calcium as a starvation situation and stores excess energy, or fat, for future energy needs.

It's more than the calcium in yogurt that seems to promote weight loss. Researchers have learned that healthy bacterial flora can make a difference in weight loss. The probiotics in yogurt enhance gastrointestinal health and a healthy GI system has a lot to do with how you metabolize calories.

Finally, while emerging evidence points to the power of foods like yogurt to actually enhance weight loss, long-established studies confirm that a rich supply of calcium in the diet, like that from yogurt, is a critical component of a weight reduction diet for other reasons: namely muscle and bone preservation. We've long known that one of the risks of weight loss is losing muscle and bone mass. Adding rich sources of calcium to a weight-reducing diet, along with a program of exercise—both features of the SuperFoodsRx Diet—is therefore adding insurance that muscle and bone loss as a result of general weight loss will be minimized, while your metabolism is preserved. [26, 27]

Walnuts: Fat-Busting Fat

No one can deny that walnuts and their sidekicks pack a nutritional wallop unmatched by most other foods. Their unique combination of vitamins, minerals, plant sterols, protein, polyphenols, and healthy fats make them an almost unbeatable ally in your efforts to promote both short- and long-term health. Nuts are also a rich source of fiber. And they are low in saturated fat (less than 7 percent) and high in unsaturated fat (from 40 to 60 percent).[28] The fat in nuts is particularly valuable because some of this fat is plant-derived omega-3 fat. This is the same kind of healthy fat discussed above as coming from fatty fish like the SuperFood wild salmon. And nuts also provide a version of this fat, and though it is different in some ways from the omega-3s in fish, it nonetheless provides many of the same benefits.

We have an impressive body of research demonstrating that regular consumption of nuts can reduce your risk of developing coronary heart disease as well as diabetes, certain cancers, and other chronic ailments. Regular nut consumption has also been associated with a reduction of all causes of mortality.[29]

But now we get to the question that's probably on your mind. How can we recommend nuts on a diet that's geared for weight reduction? It does seem counterintuitive. But the truth, perhaps amazingly, is that studies have shown that people who eat nuts regularly actually seem to have lower body weight than those who don't eat nuts.[30] How can this be explained? One study speculated that the beneficial effect that nuts seem to have on body weight could be related to the ability of nuts to suppress appetite as well as fat absorption.[31] It was noted in the study from the *American Journal of Clinical Nutrition*, cited above, that preliminary evidence showed that people who consumed nuts seemed to excrete more fat from their bodies.[32] Additional evidence? One large study of more than 8,865 adults showed that when eating patterns were assessed, even after adjusting for age, sex, smoking, leisure time physical activity, and other known risk factors for obesity, those who ate nuts two or more times weekly had a significantly lower risk of weight gain than those who rarely or never ate nuts.[33] Here's another point to consider: Nuts, when added to a weight-reduction diet like the SuperFoodsRx Diet, seem not only to promote more weight loss and more permanent weight loss but also seem to improve insulin sensitivity,[34] which could certainly be a factor in nuts' ability to help with appetite control and resulting weight loss.

So there's no question that walnuts and their sidekicks are excellent additions to your SuperFoodsRx Diet for two reasons: They'll help you maintain your good health and, believe it or not, they'll help you lose weight. There's one caveat: Portion control is absolutely essential! Nuts are high in calories. If you begin to munch handfuls of nuts a few times a day, you'll be undoing all the good that nuts could do for you. You'll read about portion control in the coming chapters and it's important to stress this issue regarding nuts. A portion of nuts is roughly 1 ounce and can range from 158 calories (pistachios) to 195 calories (pecans). So you obviously have to limit your nut consumption. We like to think of nuts as condiments, using small pieces to sprinkle on a bowl of yogurt or oatmeal. You'll see interesting ways to incorporate nuts into your diet—and reach your weight loss goals—when you read The SuperFoodsRx Menus, Meals, and Recipes (page 188).

Soy

Soy is an ancient food that contributes not only to overall health but also to efforts to control weight. Many studies have demonstrated soy's ability to promote health. Soy protein seems to boost heart health by contributing to lower blood pressure and playing a small role in lowering cholesterol in an overall cholesterol-reducing diet.[35] Soy has also been shown to possibly

If you have been diagnosed with breast or prostate cancer, discuss the role of soy in your diet with your health-care team.

contribute to reducing cancer risk, reducing risk of bone fracture or osteoporosis, and better managing diabetes.[36, 37, 38] A critical issue to consider when evaluating soy's health benefits is that all of the benefits seem to be linked to whole soy *foods*, not soy supplements. So please stick with soy foods: tofu, edamame, soymilk, soy nuts, tempeh, and miso. Many of the health benefits of soy are associated with its unique and rich source of the phytonutrients called isoflavones. Two of these isoflavones, genistein and daidzein, act as both antioxidants and estrogens that when consumed in foods may help contribute to reducing the risk of coronary heart disease as well as protecting against breast or prostate cancer as part of an overall healthy lifestyle.

Adding soy to your diet, as suggested in *The SuperFoodsRx Diet*, usually is a health plus if only because it provides a protein source—and a complete protein at that—that has a lower and healthier fat content than meat, the protein it usually replaces. We know due to overwhelming research that a largely plant-based diet can have tremendous health benefits.[39] Any shift in your diet toward increased plant consumption is good and the SuperFoodsRx Diet relies liberally on plant foods, even featuring a Veggie Day. (You'll notice that most of the SuperFoods are plant-based foods.)

So you can count on the fact that soy foods can be good for you. But can they help you lose weight? The emerging answer is yes. A study on overweight people showed that those following a low-fat, high-soy protein diet lost *more* fat while preserving *more* lean muscle than a control group that received only lifestyle education without the soy-enhanced diet.[42] And in a meta-analysis review of different styles of diets over a 24-week period, researchers found that weight loss was most rapid and significantly more weight was lost on a very low-calorie diet that specifically included soy when compared to three other dietary interventions that included meal replacements, energy restriction, or low-calorie programs.[43] One simple reason for these results is that we know that when you substitute vegetable protein, like soy, for animal protein you tend to consume fewer calories because plant-based protein is generally lower in calories than animal protein. And soy protein is the only plant protein that's considered a complete protein, containing all the essential amino acids.

We also know that soy can increase the production and thus the levels of glucagon in the body. Glucagon is a hormone that works to counteract the response of insulin in the body, and these increased glucagon levels may also contribute to soy's ability to help control weight as well as regulate blood sugar. Glucagon also helps slow the production of enzymes that are involved in making more fat cells.[44] We know from animal studies that soy protein can reduce body fat accumulation and improve insulin sensitivity.[45]

There's yet one more emerging area of study on soy that points to the possibility that it could play a role in promoting weight loss. In a study of rats, researchers found that soy isoflavones actually played a role in reducing inflammation, a condition that we've looked at as playing a role in exacerbating obesity and weight gain. The rats in this study that consumed soy isoflavones had improved insulin sensitivity, which seemed to be caused by a reduction in inflammation.[46]

If you're a postmenopausal woman who has metabolic syndrome, you could benefit from regular consumption of soy nuts. In a study published in the *American Journal of Clinical Nutrition*, postmenopausal women diagnosed with metabolic syndrome, also called Syndrome X, who ate soy nuts over a period of 8 weeks enjoyed better glycemic control and better lipid profiles when compared to a control group.[40] Metabolic syndrome is diagnosed when individuals have three or more of the following factors:

- Waist: 40 inches or greater for males, 35 inches or greater for females
- Serum triglycerides: equal to or greater than 150 mg/dL
- HDL cholesterol: less than 40 mg/dL for males and less than 50 mg/dL for females
- Blood pressure: equal to or greater than 130/85 or currently taking high blood pressure medication
- High fasting glucose, or blood sugar levels, of at least 100 mg/dL or currently taking diabetes medication[41]

Beans

Here's some information that will surely turn you into a bean convert: According to recent research, adults who eat beans weighed an average of 6.6

pounds less than those who don't eat beans even though the bean-eaters consume nearly 200 additional daily calories than those with a bean-free diet![47] They also had a significantly reduced risk of having an elevated waist circumference or becoming obese. How is this possible? Actually, this test result demonstrates a basic principle of the SuperFoodsRx Diet: If you substitute high-quality SuperNutrient SuperFoods for less-nutritious foods, weight loss can become automatic. Beans are star performers in any weight-loss program for a variety of reasons. Perhaps their most important characteristic for dieters is their high fiber content. You've probably heard about high-fiber diets. There's no question that increasing your fiber intake can help you lose weight and maintain a healthy weight. Adding beans to your diet can significantly improve your fiber intake. Various studies have demonstrated that fiber increase is associated with weight loss. One scientific review that examined a host of studies on the effects of low-calorie diets on hunger, weight loss, and manipulation of macronutrients, found that subjects experienced triple the weight loss when their diet was *both* low in fat *and* high in fiber. This result was found when those diets were compared with diets that were only low in fat.[48] The clear message is that diets that are both high in fiber with an appropriate amount of healthy fat—like the SuperFoodsRx Diet—are ultimately more effective for achieving permanent weight loss.

Beans supply a multitude of other benefits to those trying to lose weight in addition to boost their fiber. Beans are low in fat (only 2 to 3 percent), an excellent source of complex carbohydrates (the "good" carbs we're all looking for), and a terrific source of plant-based protein—again, the "good" protein that's free of cholesterol.

Another point to remember about beans: Sometimes in our search for low-calorie foods we tend to forget the most obvious; namely, that one of the biggest enemies of dieting is hunger. If you're hungry, you'll be tempted by the jelly beans on your co-workers desk, the breadbasket at a restaurant, and the cookies at a friend's get-together. Beans can be your weapon against hunger. Beans make a major contribution to satiety—they make you feel full. This is due again partly to their high fiber content but it's also because of their excellent mix of complex carbs and protein and their rich supply of vitamins, minerals, and phytonutrients. Beans give you a big fiber and protein bang with minimal calories. One-half cup of pinto beans or kidney beans has around 8 grams of fiber and 7 grams of protein, all for about 110 calories. Beans take a long time to digest and they provide an excellent source of long-lasting energy. Beans at lunch can make the difference between a 4:00 p.m. slump and a steady flow of energy to get you through the most trying afternoon.

Here's another issue that seems to point to how beans can benefit weight control. Increasingly, obesity is being recognized as a disease of inflammation. When you are obese, you are inflamed. Your cell walls are made up of fat and when you're inflamed these cell walls are more vulnerable to oxidation or damage by free radicals. Research has shown that beans help to protect cell walls from oxidation,[49] which protects your overall health and keeps your metabolism in balance.

Beans are one of the most ancient foods known to man and can still be considered an important cornerstone of our modern diet. In fact, the USDA lists beans in two food groups, beans being the *only* food to earn this distinction—the vegetable as well as the meat/bean category. They're included in the vegetable category because of course beans are a plant-based source of important vitamins, minerals and phytonutrients, and they're listed in the meat category because they are an excellent source of protein.

From a practical standpoint, there are few foods more versatile, inexpensive, and easy to incorporate into your diet. For those with little time and those trying to save money, as well as dieters simply working to reach their weight-loss goals, beans are the answer. If you have a can of beans in the pantry, you have a meal.

Turkey: The High-Protein/ High-Nutrient Solution

High protein, low protein. Most people who have paid any attention to dieting and weight-loss recommendations in recent years have been bombarded with advice about the pros and cons of high-protein diets. While there certainly is some evidence that some people do, in the short term, lose weight on a diet that favors high protein, there are a number of caveats to this approach to weight loss. For one thing, the operative notion here seems to be "short-term." Short-term weight loss is rarely anyone's goal. Few of us want to lose weight for a few weeks: We want to lose it forever! And many studies have shown that high-protein diets are only effective in the short term. Keep in mind that there's no magic formula for even the short-term success of a high-protein diet. Most any diet that heavily emphasizes one category of macronutrients like protein will probably be effective in the short term. As your food choices are substantially reduced, you naturally eat less. But there are additional and perhaps more significant dangers to a high-protein diet. These dangers are linked to two issues associated with common high-protein foods: too much saturated fat and too few nutrients. Among the most popular food choices in any high-protein diet are red meat and whole dairy foods like cheese. These foods tend to be high in saturated fat and any diet high in saturated fat will promote development of various health problems. Many studies have suggested that there is a relationship between saturated fat in the diet and colon cancer, coronary heart disease, and also Alzheimer's disease. Saturated fat is also known to increase serum cholesterol levels. So while a dieter on a high-protein diet is increasing his intake of saturated fat which has been linked to a range of health problems, he is also reducing his intake of high-quality whole foods like healthy carbohydrates and fruits and vegetables which are rich in the very nutrients that have been associated with reducing risks to the most common chronic causes of disease and death.

To step back for a moment, there's no question that evidence points to some association between high-protein foods and weight loss. In one study, people who had a higher protein intake experienced a decreased appetite and what the researchers termed "significant weight loss."[50] Those researchers speculated that the decreased caloric intake might have been caused by increased leptin sensitivity, which would have lessened appetite. Another study on mice gives some intriguing, if preliminary, indication that protein can exert an effect on metabolism. In this study, mice that were fed double the normal amount of leucine, an amino acid present in protein, had a significant reduction in obesity as well as an improved insulin response and improved total and LDL-cholesterol levels.[51] In another study with mice, leucine seemed to affect energy storage, reducing storage in the fat cells and favoring fatty acid utilization (using fat for fuel) by the muscle cells.[52] Clearly, if you're trying to lose weight you don't want to store much energy but instead burn it efficiently as fuel. Healthy, lean protein sources that provide important amino acids help you do just that.

So it can seem at times that you're stuck between a rock and a hard place, when it comes to protein: While protein can help you lose weight and maintain your muscles and energy, there are significant downsides to a high-protein diet. The solution? Skinless turkey is the answer to the quest for a high-quality protein that will support weight loss while, at the same time, promote health. The fact is that high-quality, low-fat sources of complete protein are hard to find. While animal protein is everywhere in our markets and restaurants, the available options tend to be very high in saturated fat. Turkey, which is also readily available, is low in saturated fat (3 ounces of ham has 5.5 grams of saturated fat; the same amount of skinless turkey breast has less than 0.2 gram of saturated fat). While low in saturated fat, turkey is also rich in the nutrients that promote health including niacin, vitamin B6, vitamin B12, iron, selenium, and zinc.

So when you're looking to lose weight, determined to prolong your health and eager to keep your metabolism humming along, choose the SuperFood turkey. You'll find lots of suggestions for turkey meals in the SuperFoodsRx Diet recipes.

Blueberries & Broccoli, Spinach & Tomatoes, *and introducing Onions, Apples, Kiwis, & Pomegranates: The Low-Cal Antioxidant Powerhouses*

While the research on SuperNutrients and their promotion of weight loss is fresh and encouraging news, perhaps it's time to remind ourselves that the basics are important, too. When you're trying to lose weight, calories do count. Blueberries, broccoli, spinach, and tomatoes and all their sidekicks are critical players in the SuperFoodsRx Diet because they all contain an impressive array of SuperNutrients that fight disease and prolong health. Indeed, blueberries pack an incredible amount of disease-fighting antioxidants into their little globes. And broccoli is generally recognized as a significant first line of defense against cancer. Spinach is a nutrition powerhouse that has been the subject of countless studies and has proven its worth as one of the best sources for a long list of vitamins, minerals, and phytonutrients. Tomatoes are a versatile and delicious source of lycopene, the carotenoid that is a powerful cancer fighter and friend to a healthy heart. Berries, broccoli, spinach, and tomatoes all provide antioxidants that are closely associated with preventing cardiovascular disease, diabetes, certain cancers, and degenerative eye diseases like cataracts and macular degeneration. Moreover, as we face an epidemic of cognitive decline and impairment among the aging populations, berries in particular, have been shown to lessen the risk of these dreaded conditions related to the brain and cognition. Tomatoes, a featured actor of the health-promoting Mediterranean diet, have demonstrated health benefits, particularly in relation to certain types of cancers as well as heart disease. For those reasons alone these SuperFoods would be critical additions to anyone's diet.

Given all these positive attributes, and the fact that these four foods are all widely available and delicious, it's easy to see why anyone would be eager to incorporate them into his or her regular diet. But if you're eager to lose weight, it's important to consider another benefit of these four SuperFoods: They all make a significant contribution to a weight-loss program simply because of what they *don't* provide—excess calories!

With all the new and occasionally conflicting information that appears regularly in the press about nutrition and weight control, we sometimes forget about the basics. The bottom line of all dieting is the calorie. A calorie is simply a unit of heat energy. It's a measure of how much energy a particular food provides to your body. You need energy, in the form of calories, to keep your bodily systems functioning, even if you do nothing but sit at a desk all day. Active people need more calories; inactive people need fewer. The basic equation of dieting is that any extra calories you consume are stored in your body as fat. To lose weight you need to burn more calories than you take in, either by reducing your caloric intake or by burning extra calories with physical activity. *The SuperFoodsRx Diet* includes strategies to achieve both these goals.

The challenge for today's dieter is to reduce calorie intake while *at the same time* boosting nutrient density. The reduced calorie intake will burn fat and encourage weight loss while the increased nutrient density diet will promote health and, as we've seen with the SuperFoods described above, contribute to the biochemistry of weight loss. The four SuperFoods— blueberries, broccoli, spinach, and tomatoes—all make major contributions to this dual goal.

Even though most people, and certainly most dieters, are familiar with the basic concept of calories and the need to reduce them in order to lose weight, many of us take in far more calories than we realize. We know that the rate of obesity has been climbing in the United States for the last 30 years. It's interesting to look at just one factor in this rising tide of obesity to get some perspective on how excess calories creep into our daily diet. Our consumption of liquid calories—soft drinks and fruit drinks—has increased to the point where they now comprise 21 percent of adults' total daily calorie intake.[53] Before the 1990s, sodas and fruit drinks were responsible for only about 5 percent of the average person's daily calorie intake.[54] (Ten years ago, the main calorie contributor to the diet in the United States was white bread, which was responsible for only 5 to 7 percent of caloric intake.) That's a huge jump in caloric intake from beverages. And one of the problems with those beverages is that the calories they contribute to your diet aren't even satisfying. Probably in part because drinks pass so quickly through the mouth, the stomach, and into the intestines, there's less time for your brain to receive a signal that you're feeling full. In fact in one study, subjects consumed three different beverages (cola, diet cola, or water) with the same meals on different occasions. The researchers observed that the subjects ate a similar amount of food whether the beverage had calories or not, which resulted in a significant increase in total meal calories when the regular cola was consumed. And when the portion of the meal was increased on another occasion, they consumed even more of the beverage regardless of the type.[55]

The previous is a clear example of how calories can creep up on us, literally making us fat. As few as 100 extra "hidden" calories on a daily basis like salad dressing on salads or drinkable calories with healthy meals can result in more than 10 extra pounds in a year's time. Recognizing the importance of calories offers an opportunity: Choose foods that are low in calories, satisfying, and also contributors to your overall health like the SuperFoods blueberries, tomatoes, broccoli, and spinach. These SuperFoods will fill you up while providing minimal calories and lots of SuperNutrients; in other words the maximum nutrient density bang for a minimal caloric buck. For example, you could eat all of the following

1 cup raw spinach	7 calories
1 cup cherry tomatoes	27 calories
1 cup broccoli	30 calories
1 cup blueberries	82 calories
Total:	146 calories rich in SuperNutrients.

Or

You could have a can of cola for 155–170 calories, a lot of sugar, and no nutrition.

You could guess that eating low-calorie foods would help you to lose weight. Many studies have demonstrated this. But it's important to recognize that losing weight isn't always about cutting back on food intake. For example, research has demonstrated that *adding* a simple low-calorie salad at a meal may contribute to lower overall calorie consumption in the meal. One study showed a naturally decreased intake of about 100 calories overall when women consumed a salad to start.[56] In another study, obese women who *added* more fruits and vegetables to their diet while cutting fat intake actually lost more weight over 12 months and felt less hungry than women who simply reduced their fat intake.[57] The fact that this group of women lost weight and experienced less hunger than the women who simply tried to cut fat is significant as hunger is one of the major reasons people are unable to stick with a diet. Another study showed that healthy-weight adults actually consume *more* fruits than their overweight or obese peers[58], putting to rest the diet myth born of the low-carb craze that "fruit can make you fat."

Finally, solid research has shown something that is both a bit surprising, but also very encouraging for experienced dieters with a long history of restricting intake: A major study examining the diet habits of 7,500 adults showed that individuals who consumed a lower-overall-calorie diet as their normal behavior actually consumed *more food* in terms of size and weight from most food groups than individuals who ate a high-calorie diet. This lower-calorie diet included more of the SuperNutrient SuperFoods as well as other foods that were high in fiber, high in water, and actually weighed more.[59]

So stick with the basics: Choose low-calorie SuperFoods like broccoli, spinach, tomatoes, and blueberries, as well as apples, kiwis, pomegranates, and onions, at every opportunity and you'll be satisfied, well nourished, and well on your way to weight loss.

Oats & Pumpkin: Fiber Forever

These two SuperFoods might seem like strange bedfellows. But they do have an important nutritional feature in common: They are both very high in fiber. Perhaps you've been hearing more about the importance of fiber in your food lately. We're gratified that there's more focus on fiber these days as I've always been a major proponent of increasing fiber intake. From the standpoint of health promotion, we know that people who consume the most high-fiber foods are the healthiest. And most of us don't get enough fiber. Our Paleolithic ancestors ate roughly 47 grams of fiber daily while our intake today in Western cultures hovers around 17 grams daily. The National Academy of Sciences has established an adequate intake level of total daily fiber at 38 grams for men and 25 grams for women. If you were focusing on increasing fiber alone, your preferred fiber recommendation is 45 grams daily for adult men and 32 grams daily for adult women. However, you need to increase your fiber intake over time and your efforts to do so can lead to increased calorie consumption if you are not careful about your choices. In any case, this diet is not based on a specific fiber count and if you follow the SuperFoodsRx Diet you will be consuming the healthiest fiber-containing foods and you won't have to worry about counting either calories or fiber grams.

Fiber is what we call the indigestible carbohydrates in food and it's found only in plant foods including fruits, vegetables, grains, and legumes. The old-fashioned view of fiber was that it was solely important for promoting "regularity." We now know that fiber plays a much more crucial role in metabolism and particularly in weight control. Many studies have shown that people who eat diets high in fiber tend to weigh less.[60] We know from the Nurse's Health Study, for example, that women with the highest fiber intake had nearly half the risk of major weight gain compared to women with the lowest fiber intake.[61]

But how do high-fiber foods promote weight loss? The first contribution that foods high in fiber make to a weight-loss plan is that fiber-rich foods tend to be low in calories. Eating these foods will satisfy you while adding few calories to your daily intake. That's simple math. A slightly more complicated issue concerning fiber's effect on weight is that fiber actually works to curb your appetite. A hormone produced by your small intestine called cholecystokinin stimulates a feeling of fullness that tells you to stop eating. The combination of nutrients and fiber in the foods you eat helps increase production of this hormone and fiber plays a particular role in prolonging its presence in your system, thus enhancing your satisfaction from food.[62] Indeed, research has shown that over the long term, in studies lasting over 6 months, weight loss was more than three times greater in individuals who consumed a lower-fat, high-fiber diet than those who consumed a low-fat diet alone.[63] So high-fiber foods like oats and pumpkin fill you up and keep you satisfied. When you include them in your meals, you'll struggle less with hunger and thus will find it much easier to stick with your weight-loss goals.

Fiber also plays a role in reducing the rate at which blood glucose rises following a meal. Fiber actually slows down the speed at which your body turns carbohydrates into blood sugar that you will use for energy. This enhances the overall stability of your blood glucose and can help favor your healthy sustained energy, while also playing a positive role in helping you lose weight.

The two SuperFoods pumpkin and oats are excellent examples of high-fiber foods that provide a host of nutritional benefits. People are often surprised that pumpkin is included as a SuperFood but it's one of the best sources of healthy carotenoids available. Carotenoids are the orange, red, or yellow fat-soluble compounds found in plants that protect the skin from sun damage. More than 600 carotenoids have been identified so far and they've been linked to a host of health-promoting and disease-fighting activities. But it's the fiber in pumpkin that makes a special contribution to weight control. A half-cup of canned pumpkin has 3.5 grams of dietary fiber for only about 40 calories. This is more fiber and fewer calories than any average slice of bread, even a whole grain variety. And canned pumpkin can be added to soups and casseroles and a host of delicious meals. You'll find recipes using canned as well as fresh pumpkin in the SuperFoodsRx Recipes. Remember too that canned pumpkin is available in every supermarket and can be kept on your pantry shelf ready for use anytime.

Oats: It's what's for breakfast! Oats, and their sidekicks, are excellent additions to a weight-reduction diet. Various studies on whole grain consumption such as those provided by oats have shown that they are associated with reduced weight gain. One research study looked at data on more than 17,000 men over an 8-year period and found that as whole grain consumption at breakfast went up, weight gain over time went down.[64] Not only do oats and their sidekicks help sustain weight loss, they also provide important nutrients that are critical to health but are sometimes squeezed out of some low-caloric diets.[65] The low-carb diet craze of recent years has confused many people about the role of grains in their weight-reducing plan. In fact, research shows that whole grains make a critical contribution to successful weight loss for all the reasons outlined above. Many people also have found that low-carb diets made them feel poorly and lacking in energy and, at least partly for these reasons, are difficult if not impossible to stick with in the long term. The SuperFoodsRx Diet includes all the healthy, whole grain foods that your body needs to stay healthy as you steadily and permanently lose weight and inches.

....

We think you will agree after learning about the power of these particular SuperFoods that losing weight is not necessarily about eating less; it's about eating smart. We hope we've inspired you to embark on the best and healthiest weight-reduction plan, the SuperFoodsRx Diet.

Chapter 2

Before You Begin . . . .

You're eager to begin your new SuperFoodsRx lifestyle. But before you actually dive in, I want to discuss two important points about eating and weight control: how to set your weight-loss goal and how to cope with portion control. I think you'll find this information extremely useful and perhaps surprising.

SuperFoodsRx Portion Control

You walk into a restaurant, sit down, and are greeted by a waiter who asks to take your order. You select carefully. A SuperFood, wild salmon, is on the menu, so you're happy to order that. You ask for some brown rice in place of the white rice. You're pleased to see that seasonal vegetables are listed and are happy to choose them. You order a shrimp cocktail as an appetizer because you've heard that it's a good lean protein. The waiter places your order and returns promptly with a beautiful meal. It looks delicious but it's not really yours. Not yet.

Whose is it then? It's a generic portion for a *generic customer* until you make it your own with portion control. Think about it—a *generic* portion. This same meal would be set before you if you were a 5-foot 3-inch female or 6-foot 6-inch NBA player—regardless of your weight or activity level.

Portion control is the key to personalizing the meals you eat, both at home and when dining out.

Portion control has nothing to do with deprivation. Portion control is an opportunity. Consider it your chance to customize the foods you choose to fit your size or the size you want to be.

Most people who need to lose weight live with some mixed feelings about food—feelings that often include some degree of guilt. It's your fault, right?

You didn't have enough self-control. You didn't push the plate away, put down the fork, and jump on the treadmill. Well, set aside the guilt and consider this: *If you live and eat in America today and you don't want to gain weight, then you are engaged in a constant, demanding and sometimes exhausting battle*—unless you learn the *simple basics of portion control*. Why? Because, unless you are a serious athlete or engage in daily physical labor, you may have become accustomed to eating quantities of food that are totally mismatched for your relatively sedentary or even in some cases moderately active lifestyle. You may be eating amounts appropriate to a lumberjack and living the lifestyle of a geisha. Those two facts are the rock and the hard place that you're between. You have to *make an effort* to burn calories and *make an effort* to eat reasonable amounts of healthy foods.

Of course we have to take personal responsibility for the aspects of our health that we can control. According to large-scale national research among adults ages 20–74 years, the prevalence of obesity increased from 15 percent in the late 1970s to 32.9 percent in the early 2000s. But pause and think for a minute: Why is it that we are seeing an obesity epidemic today, an epidemic that has more than *doubled* in a mere 3 decades?[1]

Could it be that people in recent years have lost all sense of self-control? Could it be that two-thirds of us have suddenly acquired a contagious weight-gain disorder? Is there something in the air or about the way we live that makes us absolutely ravenous day and night? No. No. And certainly no. The truth is that the food industry—restaurants, food producers, food packagers, and marketers—with clever strategies and alluring ad campaigns entice us to buy too much food for our needs and encourage us to eat too much of that food in countless situations. Their business success is based on their ability to get you to buy their food. Food marketers have helped make the absurd seem normal. You have been an easy target—unknowing and unarmed and without the strategies necessary when it comes to resisting the lure of buying and eating ever more fattening foods in ever growing amounts.

But it's not just about the food. Once upon a time people had to walk more, do more physical work and even expend energy to stay warm and cool. It actually requires calories to sweat or maintain body temperature in a cold environment, and central heating and air conditioning are relatively new developments. In those days people burned a lot of calories in the routine activities of their daily lives. And many of them ate fewer calories than we do. They stuck to local farm-fresh food, grass-fed meats and dairy foods from grass-fed cattle, natural fats, and minimal sweets. Remember those Christmas stories about children getting an orange as a gift? That really happened. An orange in fact was considered a special treat. No one had yet dreamed of Death by Chocolate or a fried Snickers bar. While our grandparents and great-grandparents' medical care was relatively primitive compared to the care available today, and while their vulnerability to infectious diseases made them less healthy than you in many ways, the quality of their diet and their physical activity levels were often far more health promoting than yours.

I want you to think about this confluence of too much food and too little activity to help you appreciate why it can be difficult to lose weight. *It's not about "willpower"—it's about outsmarting a culture that's trying to bulk you up.* If you don't pay attention to the obstacle course before you, you won't be prepared to succeed. You need to relearn what constitutes an appropriate amount of food for your body. *The SuperFoodsRx Diet* will introduce you to a host of techniques that will ease your path to weight loss. You'll get in touch with your hunger. You'll learn to link your moods to your food intake. You'll focus on what exactly you are eating. But perhaps among the most important tools you need to manage the world of endless choice and massive portions are a few simple rules of portion control. Once you apply those easy guidelines to the terrific SuperFoods that will form the backbone of your diet, you'll be on your way to lifetime success.

Many people have commented that learning about portion control on the SuperFoodsRx Diet has been key to their ultimate success. Time and again, people have remarked that they can't believe how much they used to eat and are amazed that following this diet keeps them satisfied. This never surprises me because research has shown it to be true. As one study reported, "Despite increases in intake, individuals presented with large portions generally do not report or respond to increased levels of fullness, suggesting that hunger and satiety signals are ignored or overridden."[2] It's really true. You will not miss the giant portions you may have been eating. One man on *The SuperFoodsRx Diet* told me that I would have been horrified to see the quantities of food he'd been eating before he began the diet. In fact his actual words were: *"If you could have seen how much extra I was eating before, you would have fallen down to the floor."* He had simply become accustomed to eating large amounts and thought he needed those massive quantities to feel satisfied.

The truth is that people often initially shy away from discussions about portion sizes. They flash back to a health class with a grainy film of carrots and cubes of cheese dancing with measuring spoons. I want you to wash all those associations away. We're going to use portion control as a *simple* tool and a mantra. It's another technique that you'll find invaluable in your efforts to honor your body. It will help you recognize what your body really needs. Portion control is an opportunity to make a choice that's right for you.

On the SuperFoodsRx Diet, *the two essentials to your success are the SuperFoods themselves and portion control.*

It's easy to manage those two—far easier than calorie counting. We told people in previous books that learning about the SuperFoods would change their lives and it was true. We're telling you now that the SuperFoods plus portion control will change your dieting life and ultimately, the quality of your whole life for good.

SuperFoodsRx Portion Control Basics

Here are the two game pieces you need to practice portion control:

A tennis ball

A deck of cards

These two very familiar shapes represent the amounts you should be eating of various foods. It's that easy.

🌿 Fruits, vegetables, grains and legumes should be the size of a tennis ball.

🌿 Protein foods (turkey, salmon, etc.) should be the size of a deck of cards.

Get a deck of cards and a tennis ball and put them right on the kitchen counter. Look at them regularly and hold them in your hands. Imprint them in your mind. One SuperFoodsRx dieter who was very successful in reaching her weight loss goals actually spray-painted both the deck of cards box and the tennis ball gold. You could pick a color that complements your kitchen décor. Another enthusiastic SuperFoodsRx dieter actually carries around her deck of cards and tennis ball in her purse. These visual cues help you and others in your family. And that mountain of pasta served to us in many restaurants is in fact the equivalent of three or four or more healthy servings.

Now it's quite true that the complete, unabridged story of portion sizes can be far more detailed and complicated than the SuperFoodsRx version. Many good references work with compact disk-sized pancakes and golf ball-sized servings of granola. You don't need to worry about these details on *The SuperFoodsRx Diet*. I've found that people can become confused and discouraged when their diet becomes too complicated or if they have too many new visuals to remember. I've had people confide to me that they've given up on a weight-loss plan because they knew they wouldn't use a food scale and they couldn't remember if they should be eating cubes of cheese the size of dice or the size of a matchbook or a slice of bread the size of a CD . . . or was that the checkbook? *Few people can successfully diet in the real world when the **details** of a healthy lifestyle overshadow the pleasure of eating.* The first step of The SuperFoodsRx Diet, the SlimDown, is very specific about what you'll be eating, and the recipes have been carefully measured and tested to take care of the portion sizes for you. You won't need to focus on portion control in the SlimDown.

You can eat all you want of . . . well, nothing. Some weight-loss programs will tell you that you can eat all you like of certain foods. I believe this just helps to more firmly establish patterns that make it ever more difficult to lose weight. A large component of successful weight loss is, after all, behavior change. Eating massive or even large amounts of any food simply reinforces behaviors that got us into trouble in the first place. This is one reason, by the way, that so many diets fail: They tell you what to eat but not how to change your life to eat well. The simple fact is you really need to learn to control the amounts of food you eat; to ignore this courts diet disaster. It's not a punishment; it's about being honest with yourself instead of playing tricks. It's not about deprivation, either. You'll find that you can be satisfied and leave the table contented when your body has become accustomed to eating healthy portions of foods.

The second step of the program, the FlexPlan, builds in flexibility by incorporating your SuperFoods and again, if you've got your tennis ball and your deck of cards, that's all you'll need to know.

Some Portion-Control Tips

Here are some general tips that will help guide you as you learn to observe, assess, and practice with appropriate portion sizes:

Eat Mindfully. Many of us find ourselves eating too much because we're simply not paying attention. Sometimes this is because we're doing something else—watching TV or reading—but sometimes it's because we're simply accustomed to eating on the run. Try to make your meals a relaxed, focused part of your day. Be aware. Pay attention to what you're about to eat. Notice how much food you have on your plate and make a decision about whether it's your amount or that NBA player's I mentioned earlier. Eat slowly and savor each bite by actually tasting what's in your mouth, exploring the flavor and texture, and enjoying the pleasure of the food. Remember that it takes up to 20 minutes for your brain to register that you're full and satisfied so don't rush. If you're eating with family or friends, put your fork down and pause for conversation. Enjoy the entire experience of your meal and you'll find that when you finish you'll feel refreshed rather than tired and overstuffed.

Read Food Labels. Many of the best foods don't have labels but those that do offer some important information along with some confusing information, too. It can be challenging to navigate these food labels. I'll just touch on the topic briefly here because the Shopping Lists (pages 112 and 342) will guide you to the healthiest shopping choices. The number of servings in the container is an important fact to consider, and is also often a shock. Perhaps you thought that little packaged "single-serving" bowl of ramen noodles or certain other common soup cups was one serving. Examine the label and you may well find that it contains two servings, which means the nutrition information for the whole container is actually *double* the amount listed on the bowl. So you either have to get a friend to share that one Styrofoam bowl or evaluate what amount you will eat and how many of those nutrients—and in this case I'm talking about the calories, fat, carbohydrates, and fiber—you'll be getting from your portion. You can almost hear the person in charge of label information laughing as he sent that to the printer envisioning perhaps the picture of Lady and the Tramp sharing the single strand of spaghetti. So make sure you have a realistic idea of how many servings the package contains.

Different foods have different details on their Nutrition Facts panel and ingredients list that become important depending on the type or category of food. What information you should pay particular attention to on these labels is not provided by food manufacturers or even many health-care professionals. On pages 331-341, I provide some specific "safe shopping" criteria organized by the type of commercial food (canned soups, sauces, and beans; commercial salad dressings; breakfast cereals; energy bars; other grain products including bread, pitas, and tortillas; seasonings; and more), along with some brand-name examples so you can review the criteria side-by-side with the product in question when considering if a food can go into your shopping basket.

Measure Magic. See page 116 of the Prep & Practice Week for a little exercise that will show in bold relief what amounts you're accustomed to eating.

Control Salad Dressing. Salads are a staple of *The SuperFoodsRx Diet*, and the dressing you use is important, so I'm going to give you some guidelines on this sometimes-overlooked aspect of portion control. Your dressing has got to be delicious and it's got to be in a reasonable amount. Most of us don't pay much attention to the amount of dressing on a salad. We just feel virtuous for having a salad in the first place! But did you know that 2 tablespoons of some dressings can add as much as 20 grams of fat and about 200 calories to an otherwise healthy salad? And, while 2 tablespoons is generally the right amount of dressing to use, many salads have much, much more. Here are some tips on how to dress a healthy salad:

- Use a measuring spoon—a tablespoon—to add 2 tablespoons of dressing to your salad. You'll soon get used to how much dressing 2 tablespoons really is.

- When serving your family, dress and toss the salad family-style rather than having each person add dressing. This uses less dressing.

- Make your own dressings. We've provided some terrific, flavorful choices. See page 307.

- If you use bottled dressings, don't immediately choose the nonfat ones. You need healthy fats to absorb the nutrients in a salad. "Light" dressings can be low fat or low calorie or both. Also check to be sure sodium levels and other ingredients in bottled dressings are within the guidelines on page 337.

- *Just add water.* Many dieters have told me that this simple tip is extremely useful. You'll find that adding just a bit of water to many healthy bottled dressings will have virtually no effect on flavor and will make the dressing go much farther with fewer calories.

Manage Restaurant Portions. Managing portions in restaurants can be a challenge. Serving sizes in fast-food restaurants have gone up two to five times in recent years. Many restaurants serve food in amounts that are sufficient for two or three meals. When you're accustomed to eating foods in these portions, they begin to seem normal to you and you also tend to eat that way at home. But once you grow accustomed to using the deck of cards and the tennis ball as your guides, you'll be better prepared to gauge how much of the food on your plate in a restaurant should be eaten and how much should be left or wrapped to take home for another meal. The key to managing portions in restaurants is to manage the menu. One man on *The SuperFoodsRx Diet* eats out frequently for business and travel. He has told me that it's so easy to eat out—a "no brainer" he called it—because he just looks for the SuperFoods on the menu and eats amounts equivalent to the tennis ball and deck of cards. Other restaurant strategies include ordering an appetizer and a salad and skipping the main course, splitting an entrée with a friend, or asking the waiter to wrap half the main course to take home before it's even served.

Rely on the SuperFoodsRx Recipes. One way we've tried to help you manage portions is to create lots of recipes that serve one or two people.

*E*at for the size you want to be. This is the simplest guideline imaginable. Most of us eat for the size we *are* and that's just fine if we want to stay that size. But if you want to weigh less, then *less* is your intake guideline.

These recipes can all be easily doubled or increased further if you're serving a larger group. Most people find it very difficult to sort out how much of a recipe they should eat when it serves, for example, six people. And every recipe, say with salmon or turkey, is based on one deck of cards of that particular SuperFood so it makes planning, shopping and preparing very easy for you. There's no guesswork when following a recipe. And recipes like soups that serve more people include notations that tell you what to eat now, refrigerate, or freeze for later. So our SuperFoodsRx recipes will make it simple for you to shift your notion of what portion sizes should be and eat for the size you want to be.

Here's a brief list of how much you should be eating of certain foods on a daily basis:

Daily SuperFoodsRx Guidelines for Successful Portion Control

FOOD CATEGORY	TOTAL DAILY DIET
Whole Grains: (Oats and sidekicks—and remember to include potatoes here)	3–4 tennis balls per day
Fruits: (Blueberries and Oranges and sidekicks and the balance of other fruits you include in your daily diet)	2–4 tennis balls per day
Vegetables: Broccoli, Spinach, Tomatoes, and sidekicks and the balance of other vegetables you include in your daily diet	3–5 tennis balls
Protein: Wild Salmon, Turkey, Tofu, Soy beans, Beans, Yogurt	2–3 decks of cards (Use the tennis ball to estimate beans and edamame [soybeans].) (Use 1 cup for yogurt)

How Much Should I Weigh? The SuperFoodsRx 10 Percent Solution

Some dieters get so focused on just "losing weight" that they never actually come up with a clear idea of what their final goal is. Other dieters set too ambitious a goal and become discouraged when they don't reach it or move toward it slowly. I think the simple solution to this dilemma is to set an interim goal. An excellent interim goal is 10 percent of your body weight. This may not be your final goal but it is a terrific starting point. We know that if you lose *just 10 percent* of your body weight you can decrease your risk for heart disease, improve your heart function, reduce your blood pressure, and even reduce harmful levels of blood cholesterol and triglycerides.

What's your personal interim goal? If, for example, you currently weigh 180, then 18 pounds is 10 percent of your current weight. If you subtract 18 from 180 you arrive at your interim weight loss goal of 162. Achieving that interim goal will give you lots of reason to celebrate and at that point you can establish another interim goal and so on until you reach your ultimate goal.

We'll take a look at some of the benefits of this very achievable interim goal and then we'll review the current standards of how to measure weight and set a final goal.

Goodbye Skinny, Hello Healthy!

Okay, you know that losing weight is going to make you healthier. As I mentioned earlier, the very good news is that losing even a relatively small amount of weight can substantially reduce your chances of developing heart disease, diabetes or having a stroke. I've seen many people reach halfway or even closer to their interim goal on *The SuperFoodsRx Diet* in as little as one month. That's 4 short weeks! So every effort you make on this program is going to be

> **What is overweight?** Approximately 10 percent above the upper end of a healthy weight range, depending on other measurements of health and fitness.
>
> **What is obese?** Approximately 15 percent or more above the upper end of a healthy weight range depending on other measurements of health and fitness.

rewarded. Even if it takes a while to fit into your skinny jeans, well, you'll be reaping benefits long before you get that zipper closed.

So How Much Should I Weigh?

Here's the single most important thing you need to know about assessing your weight: No single method will tell you what you need to know. Now you can ignore for a moment the science on weight assessment. Many people I've worked with are simply happy with very personal goals: feeling good in their clothes, having energy to walk up stairs and play with children or grandchildren, feeling like they're back in control of their eating and in charge of their health. All these are excellent goals. But some folks like to see the science, too.

Back in the day, people gauged their weight with the venerable Metropolitan Life Insurance Company standard height-weight tables for men and women. These tables were introduced in 1943 and then revised in 1983. But they were faulty. For one thing, most people didn't realize that the tables were based on people wearing 1-inch heels. Other and perhaps more significant flaws were that the charts didn't objectively account for age, frame size, or take into account body fat distribution or degree of obesity. Over time these tables gradually fell into disfavor. Now most professionals rely on a combination of assessments to arrive at a goal or ideal weight for an individual.

Here are my recommendations for those who would like to set an ideal weight that might serve as a long-term goal. One important point: No single measure is the answer. So review these assessments and see where you fit in:

The Scale. This is what most of us use to assess our weight. Some of us avoid it; others rely on it exclusively. The scale is important but it's not the

A quick way to figure your healthy weight range:

Women: count 100 pounds for the first 5 feet of your height. Add 5 pounds for each inch of height above 5 feet. Then, to get a range, add and subtract 10 percent of this number and you'll get a healthy, average range.

E.g.: 5-foot 5-inch woman = 125 pounds +/– 10% = 112–138 pounds range.

Men: Count 106 pounds for the first 5 feet of your height. Add 6 pounds for each inch of height above 5 feet. Then to get a healthy range, add and subtract 10% of this number.

E.g.: 5-foot 8-inch man = 154 pounds +/– 10% = 139–169 pounds range.

Note: Use the *range* as your healthy weight can fall anywhere in the range and occasionally beyond it.

only measure because what is healthy varies from one person to the next. Fit and healthy weights come in many sizes. Some researchers want you to throw out the scale but I think it performs an important function. It's inexpensive and easy to use. Moreover, research has shown that people who monitor their weight regularly are more successful at managing and maintaining their weight over time. In one study of people who had lost an average of 42 pounds in a year, only 26 percent of people who weighed daily ultimately gained more than 5 pounds back versus 58 percent of people who did not regularly weigh themselves.[3] And your scale is impartial. But don't allow yourself to be tortured by the scale. Use it as one of your tools. Remember that it's not uncommon for people to lose inches on their waist for a period of time without anything registering on the scale because muscle weighs more than fat. The bonus of course is that muscle takes up far less space. That's why it's important to consider the number on your scale in your overall assessment picture but not allow it to be the final word.

I recommend you weigh yourself and record the results in your Food Diary on Monday and Friday mornings. On Monday you're beginning a new week and you might need a checkup to see how you did over the weekend. On Friday you'll want to see how you've done during the week behind you. Some people are tempted to "let go" over the weekend if they've done well during the week. This is obviously counterproductive, so allow any success—in weight or inches—you've achieved during the week motivate you to stay committed over the weekend. Remember that people who have been successful at weight loss show a consistency in their behavior from one day to the next—including the weekend.

Here's a table that will give you a good idea of what your weight range should be. Your long-term goal should be to enter *into* this range. First, you use the 10 percent solution to set your initial goal. You continue working the 10 percent solution until you enter the healthy range noted below. And if you're reading this book looking for a way to just shake the last 5–10 pounds from your already fairly lean frame, *The SuperFoodsRx Diet* will work for you, too. Just be aware that your 10 percent solution goal should not go below the low end of the healthy range provided in this table.

HEIGHT	HEALTHY WEIGHT RANGE	HEIGHT
5' 0"	97–128 lbs.	60"
5' 1"	100–132 lbs.	61"
5' 2"	104–136 lbs.	62"
5' 3"	107–141 lbs.	63"
5' 4"	110–145 lbs.	64"
5' 5"	114–150 lbs.	65"
5' 6"	118–155 lbs.	66"
5' 7"	121–159 lbs.	67"
5' 8"	125–164 lbs.	68"
5' 9"	128–169 lbs.	69"
5' 10"	132–174 lbs.	70"
5' 11"	136–179 lbs.	71"
6' 0"	140–184 lbs.	72"
6' 1"	144–189 lbs.	73"
6' 2"	148–194 lbs.	74"
6' 3"	152–200 lbs.	75"
6' 4"	156–205 lbs.	76"

NOTE:

- Healthy Weight Range is based on BMIs to establish a general range of healthy weight.

- Healthy Weight range is one of the measures to use in context with waist, Waist to Hip Ratio (WHR), BMI, and the mirror.

- Work within realistic guidelines for you. If you are well above the upper end of the range, aim to "enter" the range as your goal. If your weight is in the upper end of the healthy range, set a goal weight somewhere in the middle of the range as your goal.

Waist Measurement. Your waist measurement is at least as important as the scale in gauging your overall health. That's why we talk about losing weight *and* waist on the SuperFoodsRx Diet. It's interesting and important to recognize that people who can rank in a healthy range on the BMI chart (*see page 50*) can still be at high risk, particularly for heart disease, if their waist measurement is too high. The simple goal here is for your waist measurement to be smaller than your hip measurement. Too much fat around the waist presents an even greater health risk than excess fat in the hips and thighs. So if your waist is bigger than your hips, that's a clear indication that you need to lose. Ideally women should have a waist measurement below 35 inches and men below 40 inches. Here's how to check: Measure your waist circumference by drawing a plastic or cloth measuring tape snugly around your waist—at the narrowest part between your belly button and the bone on the midline of your chest that connects your ribs. Use a mirror to make sure you pull the measuring tape straight around.

A good, simple, healthy goal is to aim for your waist circumference to be

Good news for women: If you're postmenopausal and have a BMI of 30 or above, losing just 5 percent of your body weight can make your cells less resistant to insulin and thus lower your risk for chronic conditions including diabetes, high blood pressure, high cholesterol, and heart attacks.[4]

Your easy first goal is a waist measure less than your hip measure. Too much fat around the waist is a greater health risk than excess fat on the hips and thighs, which is considered to be protective. If your waist is bigger than your hips you need to lose "waist."

roughly half of your height in inches. Women can add up to 2 inches to the result; men, up to 3 inches. So if you're a woman who's 5-foot-6, or 66 inches tall, half of that is 33 inches, plus 2 inches equals 35 inches so you could have a waist measurement of roughly 35 inches or lower. A 6-foot man is 72 inches. Therefore, he could have a healthy waist measurement of roughly 36 plus 3 inches or 39 inches or less.

WHR. Waist to Hip Ratio is a good gauge of body weight distribution, particularly in terms of health. To figure out your WHR, measure the circumference of your hips at the widest part of your buttocks. Then measure your waist at the smallest circumference of your waist just above your belly button. Divide your waist measurement by your hip measurement and that's your WHR. Use the simple table below to determine if you are within a healthy range with your WHR. There are also a number of Web sites that can give you your exact ratio (search: waist to hip calculator) or take the opportunity to practice your math by simply dividing your hip circumference into your waist circumference. Your WHR goal is less than 0.8 for women and 0.9 for men for healthy weight distribution and lower heart disease risk.

MEN		WOMEN	
GOAL < 0.9		GOAL < 0.8	
WAIST LESS THAN	HIPS GREATER THAN	HIPS GREATER THAN	WAIST LESS THAN
20	22	25	20
22	24.5	28	22
24	27	30	24
26	29	33	26
28	31	35	28
30	33	38	30

(continued on page 48)

| | MEN | WOMEN | |
| | GOAL < 0.9 | GOAL < 0.8 | |
WAIST LESS THAN	HIPS GREATER THAN	HIPS GREATER THAN	WAIST LESS THAN
32	36	40	32
34	38	44	34
36	40	47	36
38	42	48	38
40	44	50	40
42	46	53	42
44	49	55	44
46	51	57	46
48	53	60	48

Measure your waist and hip circumferences and compare your numbers with the chart. Look first at your waist measurement and then look across to the corresponding hip measurement that would put you at or below risk.

Remember if you're male you should ultimately aim to get your waist circumference below 40 inches. Thirty-seven or fewer inches at the waist in men has been associated with even further disease risk reduction. If you're a woman, your ultimate goal is to work toward a waist circumference below 35 or even more aggressively to 32 or fewer inches over time.

The Mirror. Numbers will only tell part of the story. It's important to look at yourself realistically and judge your overall appearance in terms of health. Too many people become obsessed with a number—usually the one of the

You have to visualize your success in order to achieve it. You have to commit to identifying yourself immediately as a person who strives to improve your health and make efforts—no matter how small—every day to get there. This is what the "mirror" test is. If you don't like the way you look, then you have to change how you look at yourself and gradually you will look and feel differently!

scale—but this can be discouraging and counterproductive. If you look at yourself in the mirror, with an accepting and positive attitude, you will be able to appreciate signs of health that will become apparent after a short time on this diet. Go ahead, take a look. Are you eyes bright, is your hair glossy, is your skin clear and smooth? Do you radiate energy? The mirror tells the truth and these are all-important measures of success and are not to be discounted.

Are You at a Healthy BMI?

These are not exact ranges of healthy and unhealthy weights. However, they show that health risk increases at higher levels of overweight and obesity. Even within the healthy BMI range, weight gains can carry health risks for adults.

Healthy Weight: BMI from 18.5 up to 25 refers to healthy weight.

Overweight: BMI from 25 up to 30 refers to overweight.

Obese: BMI 30 or higher refers to obesity. Obese persons are also considered overweight.

BMI. Body Mass Index is an indicator of body fat based on your height and weight. BMI has been used for years as a good guide because it takes into account your frame size. The downside of BMI, which has been reported recently, is that it may overestimate body fat if you're an athlete or if you're very muscular and it may underestimate body fat if you're older and have lost muscle mass. It is important to remember that although BMI correlates with the amount of body fat, BMI does not directly *measure* body fat. Even though BMI is not considered the gold standard assessment tool that it once was, many doctors and medical tests still use it to assess weight and so I'm providing a table so you can see where you might fit in. Again, don't rely on this as your *only* weight assessment tool. I actually think the measuring tape, the scale, and the mirror are the most helpful tools.

Determining Your Body Mass Index (BMI)

The table below has already done the math and metric conversions. To use the table, find the appropriate height in the left-hand column. Move across the row to the given weight. The number at the top of the column is the BMI for that height and weight.

BMI (KG/M²)

HEIGHT (IN.)	19	20	21	22	23	24	25	26	27	28	29	30	35	40
58	91	96	100	105	110	115	119	124	129	134	138	143	167	191
59	94	99	104	109	114	119	124	128	133	138	143	148	173	198
60	97	102	107	112	118	123	128	133	138	143	148	153	179	204
61	100	106	111	116	122	127	132	137	143	148	153	158	185	211
62	104	109	115	120	126	131	136	142	147	153	158	164	191	218
63	107	113	118	124	130	135	141	146	152	158	163	169	197	225
64	110	116	122	128	134	140	145	151	157	163	169	174	204	232
65	114	120	126	132	138	144	150	156	162	168	174	180	210	240
66	118	124	130	136	142	148	155	161	167	173	179	186	216	247
67	121	127	134	140	146	153	159	166	172	178	185	191	223	255
68	125	131	138	144	151	158	164	171	177	184	190	197	230	262
69	128	135	142	149	155	162	169	176	182	189	196	203	236	270
70	132	139	146	153	160	167	174	181	188	195	202	207	243	278
71	136	143	150	157	165	172	179	186	193	200	208	215	250	286
72	140	147	154	162	169	177	184	191	199	206	213	221	258	294
73	144	151	159	166	174	182	189	197	204	212	219	227	265	302
74	148	155	163	171	179	186	194	202	210	218	225	233	272	311
75	152	160	168	176	184	192	200	208	216	224	232	240	279	319
76	156	164	172	180	189	197	205	213	221	230	238	246	287	328

WEIGHT (LB.)

Monitoring Your Progress

🌿 It's important to have a system to monitor your progress from week to week for the rest of your long, healthy SuperFoods lifestyle life. Here's a chart that will help you track all aspects of your changing body.

🌿 Your week-to-week success is defined by more than one criteria—and success is also defined as *moving* in the right direction.

At a minimum, record your weight and waist measurements on Monday and your weight on Friday.

🌿 The most important way to use these tools is to see how things *change* over time and how you play a key role in making change happen. Look to see *movement* in one or more areas—preferably down but *any shift* is a sign that something is happening. Stick with it and you will make progress—guaranteed!

Remember: Don't let ONE number define you.

Tracking Your Progress

Date	WEEK #		WEEK #		WEEK #		WEEK #		WEEK #		WEEK #		GOAL (DIRECTION) WEEK-TO-WEEK
	1		2		3		4		5		6		
	M	F	M	F	M	F	M	F	M	F	M	F	
Weight													↓
Waist													↓
Hips													↓
WHR													↓
BMI													↓
Mirror													↑
Other													

These could include blood pressure readings, blood glucose readings *or* occasional readings like cholesterol, triglycerides, etc. after a doctors visit.

- ↓ Looking for a downward trend over time.
- ↑ Looking to see improvements from week to week—subjective: energy, fitness, emotions, etc.

MY GOALS:	ME	WOMEN	MEN
Healthy weight range for me:		[from table]	[from table]
Waist circumference goal:		<35 inches	<40 inches
WHR		<0.8	<0.9
BMI		<25	<25
Mirror		Improve	Improve

My 10% weight loss goal is _____.

You're now ready to begin your new SuperFoodsRx Diet.

Chapter 3

The SuperFoodsRx SlimDown

Welcome to your SuperFoodsRx SlimDown. This chapter outlines the basic concepts of the diet. In Chapter 4, The Prep and Practice Week, you'll see how to prepare for the SlimDown and have a practice week that will help you ease into the diet. In this chapter we will first open your eyes to the concepts of the SuperFoodsRx Diet. So read this chapter first and then go to the next chapter, the Prep and Practice Week, to learn how to actually begin your SuperFoodsRx Diet. The SlimDown is the phase of the diet where your weight will begin to drop and inches around your waist will shrink. SuperFoodsRx dieters have often lost over 8 pounds and 2 inches from their waist in just 14 days. Some have even experienced a 5-pound loss as well as a whole inch lost from the waist in just 7 days. Whatever your rate of success, I can promise that after only 1 week you'll see and feel changes that will delight you and carry you swiftly into the next! The foods you're going to eat are delicious and filling and there's enough flexibility so that you can make selections you really like. In just one week you're going to feel like a new you! So take a deep breath and make a real commitment. Remember, it's only 2 weeks; make them a turning point in your life.

....

How long should you stay on the SlimDown? The SlimDown is geared to prime your body for the *safe, rapid loss of weight* and inches. You *could* stay on this phase as long as you like. But I actually think it's most practical to say on it for an initial 2 weeks and then evaluate your progress. You might choose to stay on it until you reach an interim weight goal or you might cycle between the phases every

2 weeks (see "How Much Should I Weigh?," page 42). Most people find that it's most efficient to go back and forth between the SlimDown and the Flex Plan on 2-week cycles. Remember, there are only two phases on this plan: You may want to be on one or the other—cycling back and forth—for the rest of your life!

Here's a typical day on the SlimDown. Remember, this diet is personal; your day will reflect *your* tastes, available prep time and daily work and family demands. But this will give you a clear picture of how a SlimDown day shapes up.

Breakfast
Oatmeal with Blueberries and Walnuts

Morning SuperNutrient Booster
Red 6–8 oz Knudsen's Low Sodium Very Veggie Juice

Lunch *Without*
Marvelous Mediterranean Salad with Feta (see recipe page 231)

Afternoon Snack
Almonds and raisins (1 heaping tablespoon of each)

Dinner *With*
Grilled Salmon with Yogurt Dill Drizzle (see recipe page 284)
Broccoli
Brown Rice
Salad

> "I would have bet my mortgage on my belief that my weight was due to a thyroid problem, hormone issue, or just a slow metabolism. But when I started eating according to the SuperFoodsRx guidelines, the weight loss was easy and rapid. I also had peace of mind, knowing that for once I was dieting in a healthy way. I could really feel that I was giving my body what it wanted."
> —Lynn M., mother of three

The SlimDown Guidelines Explained

Now let's explore some of the basic guidelines of the SlimDown and why they're important:

The SuperFoodsRx Food Categories. On the SlimDown and as you proceed to the FlexPlan when you're ready, you'll be working with the Super-FoodsRx categories. We've divided the SuperFoods into three categories to show you how to work them into your diet. Your ultimate daily goal is to choose from each of these categories at every meal, every day. Knowing the categories allows you to structure an excellent, healthy weight-loss diet wherever you find yourself. It's our shorthand to healthy weight loss. Remember that each of the 14 SuperFoods has sidekicks (page 3) so you're not limited to these specific foods, just one from say, the beans group which could include garbanzo beans or kidney beans, or say, the blueberry group which could include grapes, strawberries, cherries, etc.

Here are the categories:

Category 1: 1 serving of *each* most days
> Pumpkin, Oats, Walnuts, and all of their sidekicks

Category 2: 2 of these daily
> Beans, Salmon, Soy, Turkey, Yogurt, and all of their sidekicks

Category 3: 3 of these daily
> Blueberries, Broccoli, Oranges, Spinach, Tomatoes, and all of their sidekicks

Or, here's another way to look at it:

Category 3 at every meal

Category 2 at at least 2 meals

Category 1 at least 1 serving of each, every or most days

Category 1, in general, represents our **premium** foods that can be relatively higher in calories but are also rich in B and/or other vitamins, fiber, healthy fats, and powerful phytochemicals. Because of the calories in some of these foods, we need to keep a close eye on them. Pumpkin and its sidekick, sweet potato, are rather arbitrarily placed in this category, partly because of their nutrient profiles which include high levels of beta carotene and partly because they are consumed less frequently by most of us on a day to day basis. **You need to get a serving of *each* of the three selections in Category 1 on most, if not all, days.** That would mean, say, **oatmeal** for breakfast (or one of the recommended cereals of whole grain breads, etc.), a **sweet potato** for dinner (or a pumpkin/yogurt snack, or some orange bell peppers on your salad, etc.), and perhaps a small handful of **walnuts** (or almonds or pistachios, etc.) as a snack.

Category 2 is, essentially, our **protein** category. **You need to eat something from Category 2 at two meals each day.** This could mean a **yogurt** breakfast and a **salmon** (or tuna or halibut, and so on) dinner. That's the minimum goal for you to aim for.

Category 3 is the *"abbondanza"* or **plentiful** category. In general, it includes vegetables and fruits. **Try to get something from Category 3 at every single meal.** That could mean **blueberries** (or cherries, grapes, strawberries, etc.) for breakfast, a **spinach** salad (or romaine salad or bok choy) for lunch, and **broccoli** (or brussels sprouts, cauliflower, Swiss chard, etc.) for dinner. Ideally, you could choose something from every Category 3 group every day so that if you had **tomatoes** on your spinach salad and a sliced orange after dinner, you'd hit a SuperFoods Category 3 home run with every base covered. The foods in Category 3 are especially rich in micronutrients as well as low in calories and so they're you're "go-to" foods when you want something extra on your plate.

Portion Practice. As with the SuperFoods Categories, if you follow the SlimDown menus and recipes, you don't need to agonize over the exact portion sizes if you just follow the instructions for menus that you create. But you do need to familiarize yourself with the *amounts*—the portions—of food you're actually eating so that when you switch to the FlexPlan or when you're eating out or dealing with a host of real-life situations, you'll be able to accurately eyeball the amount of food on your

SuperFoods Categories:

Category 1 "premium": Pumpkin, Oats, Walnuts

Category 2 "protein": Beans, Salmon, Soy, Turkey, Yogurt

Category 3 "plentiful": Blueberries, Broccoli, Oranges, Spinach, Tomatoes

plate and know how much is just right for you and what's too much. Remember, restaurant portions are generally quite large and it's very helpful to be able to glance at a plate and know how much you should eat and how much you should leave or have wrapped for another meal. Use your power of observation as a way to *practice* portion control.

The portion control basics look like this. Try to really visualize these to get going on your *practice* with portions through observation:

- A tennis ball for the premium foods in **Category 1**, except for walnuts.
- A deck of cards for protein for the protein foods in **Category 2.**
- A tennis ball for the plentiful foods in **Category 3.**

Learn these two simple visual cues and that's really all you need to know. And if you really use them, they will help keep you on track for the rest of your life! Of course foods break down more precisely into differing amounts, so to be scrupulous I'll give you the exact portion sizes for each of the foods so you can be sure that you're "eyeballing" the right amount:

Here's the SuperFoods Category Serving Shorthand:

Category 3: every meal
Category 2: at least 2 meals
Category 1: once a day most days

And here's another way to look at it:

Category 1 most days
1 serving of each of the 3 SuperFoods (or their sidekicks) on most or every day of the week.

- Pumpkin—1 serving most days
- Oats/Grains—Maximum 3-4 servings daily

- Walnuts—Minimum ½, maximum 1 serving daily.

Category 2 in at least 2 meals
2-3 servings total from at least 2 of the Category 2 SuperFoods or sidekicks daily.

Category 3 at all meals
4-6 cups of at least 3 of the Category 3 SuperFoods or sidekicks daily.

Beverages:
- 1 or more cups brewed tea daily.
- 6+ cups water daily.

Category 1: *A tennis ball*

- Pumpkin & sidekicks except sweet potato: $\frac{1}{2}$ cup, also approximately 15 baby carrots, 1 large orange bell pepper
    - Sweet potato: $\frac{1}{3}$–$\frac{1}{2}$ cup or one, 2-inch diameter x 5-inch length raw sweet potato
- Oats and grain sidekicks: $\frac{1}{3}$–$\frac{1}{2}$ cup cooked
    - Bread, pita, tortilla: 1 slice
    - Grains: $\frac{1}{3}$–$\frac{1}{2}$ cup is approximately 5 tablespoons dry
        - Pasta: 1 ounce
- Walnuts & sidekicks: 2 tablespoons

Category 2: *A deck of cards*

- Beans: $\frac{1}{2}$ cup cooked
- Turkey, salmon & sidekicks: 3 ounces
- Yogurt: $\frac{1}{2}$–$\frac{3}{4}$ cup
- Tofu: 4–5 ounces
- Edamame: $\frac{1}{2}$ cup
- Soy milk: $\frac{3}{4}$–1 cup

Category 3:

Generally that "tennis ball" should be $\frac{1}{2}$–1 cup for all the Category 3 SuperFoods— lots of nutrient density (micronutrient bang) for low-energy density (calories). A serving is what "fits in your hand" for this category—that's important in terms of eyeballing and your ultimate success, but exact measurements here are less important.

Your goal: 4–6 cups (roughly 4–6 tennis balls) from **Category 3**: 1 "cup"—1 cup raw or cooked vegetables; 2 cups leafy greens; 6–8 ounces SuperNutrient Booster (vegetable juice); 1 cup fruit; 2 heaping tablespoons dried fruit.

"I've been surprised that the portion controls are much easier to deal with than I thought. I'm not hungry most of the time; in fact, I have to make sure I get all my meals in every day. I'm eating more often—but less food overall—to lose weight."—Susan A, mother of one and proud dog owner ("I've also put my dog on a SuperFoods plan. His energy and digestion have improved too!")

1 serving:

- Blueberries & sidekicks: ½–1 cup, ¾ cup blueberries, 10 strawberries, 15 grapes (½ cup), 1 cup sliced strawberries, 1 cup raspberries
- Broccoli: ½ cup (cooked), 1 cup (raw)
- Oranges & sidekicks: 1 medium (approximately 3-inch diameter) or ¾ cup cut or sections
- Spinach: 1 cup raw; ½ cup cooked
- Tomatoes: 1 medium (3" diameter) or 1 cup or 9–10 cherry tomatoes or ½–1 cup raw sliced or diced, ½ cup cooked

Beverages

- Tea: 1 serving is 1 cup (8 ounces).
- Water: 1 serving is 1 cup (8 ounces).

Mandatory Breakfast. A popular "dieting" technique employed by many people is the old "skip breakfast" routine. The idea—which seems reasonable at first blush—is that you'll consume fewer calories and get a head start on losing weight each morning by avoiding any caloric intake. And for some folks, it's relatively easy to skip breakfast because they're not very hungry first thing in the morning. Well it turns out this is counterproductive. The habit of making breakfast a regular practice plays an important role in losing weight and keeping it off. The National Weight Control Registry, a listing of "successful losers" who have maintained a 30-pound (or more) weight loss for at least a year reports that most—78 percent—eat breakfast every day and almost 90 percent eat breakfast at least 5 days a week. For one thing, as we've discussed, breakfast provides an infusion of nutrients that maintain consistent blood sugar and keep energy levels high. It ensures your ability to maintain mental focus and optimism and it actually boosts your metabolism. Breakfast really does "break your fast" from the night before: Your body actually requires some fuel after a night's sleep. For another, when you skip breakfast, you tend to rebound at lunch and dinner and consume more calories than you might otherwise. It's much harder to control your food intake when you're truly starving. One study published in the *Journal of the American Dietetic Association*[1] found that women who ate breakfast regularly tended to eat fewer calories overall throughout the day. When you enjoy the high-fiber, low-energy-density foods—such as oatmeal, strawberries, walnuts, and low-fat yogurt—that are featured in the Super-FoodsRx Diet, you'll become a breakfast convert as your energy levels stabilize and you feel the power of the SuperFoods at work all day long. Check out the full list of breakfast options starting on page 188.

Choose only two breakfasts. In the first weeks of a new diet, people are often excited and enthusiastic about trying new things, reading through the options and making a beautiful, varied menu plan for the week. STOP right there. I want you to keep your *level* of enthusiasm high, but don't sprint out of the gate only to find yourself running out of steam from the planning, the shopping, and the thinking of it all. Sometimes too many choices can make us lose our center. Make it simple and painless and delicious and interesting all at the same time. Just choose two breakfasts from the list and *practice* them. Rotate them or have one for a few days in a row, it doesn't matter. What does matter is that your two breakfasts will become part of your own permanent SuperFoods lifestyle collection. Vary your choices after you've gotten a few under your belt —and a few inches off your belt. You'll naturally change over time, shifting with the seasons or as your mood for a certain style of breakfast changes. Ultimately, you'll choose two or three breakfasts that you'll rotate on 2-week cycles. This makes planning *and* shopping so much easier!

Learn how to throw out food. It's very hard for many of us to toss food. But that little bit of food on your child's or your partner's plate is better off in the waste than on your waist. If there's enough left for another meal, package it up for the fridge or freezer. If you have leftovers after a party, freeze them or bring them to work to give to others or share with your neighbors. Make use of those small plastic or glass containers you have on hand. Don't let a good impulse—frugality—turn against you.

Veggie Wednesday. One day a week on the SuperFoodsRx Diet—both the SlimDown and the FlexPlan—you're going to enjoy Veggie Day—a day in which your food choices will be mostly from plants. What's the point of Veggie Day? Vegetables, fruits, legumes, nuts, seeds, and whole grains are our superheroes. They're delicious, filling and they taste great. They're terrific choices for those trying to lose weight because they provide important nutrients that will help spur weight loss. They also strengthen your conviction to make smart choices: They're so rich in fiber that they are filling and satisfying. Research has demonstrated that a plant-based diet can help manage weight. You'll be getting plenty of protein from yogurt, soy, beans, and eggs and enjoying the powerful benefits of vegetarian-style nutrition one day a week.[1] We have lots of delicious Veggie Day recipes such as Fresh and Light Tacos or Four Bean Chili or Asian Broccoli Salad with Asian Inspired Red Pepper Dressing and Quinoa, or a simple Veggie Burger with a whole grain dinner roll piled high with SuperFoods Vegetables and a side soup or salad. Wednesday is the perfect day for this: It's in the middle of the week, it's a good reminder that you're on a particular eating plan and it's a practice that will help to reinforce your new, healthy habits. If Wednesday isn't good for you, pick another day. But try to keep it the same day each week so it becomes your regular practice. It will anchor you and will be a lifelong practice that will remind you *every* week—even after you reach your goals that you're still living the lifestyle making sure not to ever turn back to where you were before—both physically *and* mentally. There are other reasons to rely on vegetables: for one, they protect against a host of diseases including cancer. One study found that a review of the data on all cancer sites strongly suggests that vegetables have preventive potential. That study reported that people who ate more of the following had lower incidences of cancer: raw and fresh vegetables, leafy green vegetables, Cruciferae, carrots, broccoli, cabbage, lettuce, and raw and fresh fruit (including tomatoes and citrus fruit).[2] Vegetables and legumes can also substitute for meats that can be high in saturated fat and calories and also contain substances that can promote diseases like cancer. In general, a plant-based diet, or at least one that is largely centered on vegetables, is a super way to manage your hunger and your weight as well as promote your long-term health. Every conscious step you take to eating healthy foods is a plus and helps you to feel in control. When you're in control, you succeed!

The SuperFoodsRx Salads.

Salads can be a terrific selection to promote weight loss. The trick is to choose the right kind of salads and, most especially, the right kind of salad dressings. The SuperFoodsRx Salads and dressings are perfect choices and, indeed, they're mandatory on the Slim-Down. I recommend that you have a salad and/or soup every day. A salad is a reminder that you're honoring your body with a nutrient punch daily. A salad is rich in SuperNutrients, high in volume, low in calories and, because the nutrient-rich vegetables are eaten in concert, you enjoy the synergy of multiple SuperNutrients working together. Making salads a regular part of your daily diet will pay off in the long term. Research has shown that a eating a low-calorie salad as a first course can actually reduce the number of calories consumed at that meal and improve your feeling of satisfaction. In one study researchers gave women low-calorie salads for lunch before serving the remainder of the meal. Those women ate about 100 calories less at the meals preceded by salad when compared to the calories they consumed at other meals.[3] Just how low-calorie can a green salad be? Consider that 2 cups of fresh spinach leaves, 10 slices of cucumber, 1 medium tomato, and ¼ cup of grated carrot has a grand total of 62 calories (along with a hefty 4 grams of fiber). When you add a healthy dressing like some of those on page 307, you're still way ahead of the game.

Salads not only help you control your calorie intake, they also make a significant contribution to your overall nutrient levels and thus help you prevent long- and short-term disease. Salad intake really boosts your nutrient levels as it helps promote weight loss. In one study published in the *Journal of the American Dietetic Association,* more than 9,000 women and more than 8,000 men were asked to report on their salad and raw vegetable consumption. Those who consumed the most salads enjoyed above-median blood levels of folic acid, vitamins C and E, lycopene, and alpha- and beta-carotene. And each serving of salad eaten was associated with a 165 percent higher likelihood of subjects meeting the Recommended Dietary Allowance for vitamin C in women and a 119 percent greater likelihood in men.[4] Keep in mind that the rich supply of nutrients in those salads is also acting to help promote weight loss. So enjoy your SuperFoods salad daily and recognize that it's helping you reach your goals. You'll see many terrific SuperFoods salad options, salad ingredient pairing suggestions, and simple dressings starting on page 230.

The SuperFoodsRx Soups. We love soups! They're delicious, filling, low in calories, and a great way to pack a ton of nutrients into a busy day. With soups, you can cook once and eat two or three or even four times. Soups are a great opportunity to boost your vegetable consumption. And they can serve as a meal or an appetizer. Soups provide not only great taste and satisfaction but also a synergistic combination of several SuperFoods from one or more categories in a single bowl. A SuperFoods soup is a virtual guarantee that you're on your way toward fulfilling your daily SuperNutrient needs. Most soups straddle one or more of the SuperFood categories, depending on the primary ingredients in that soup. During your SlimDown I want you to enjoy a soup and/or salad *every day,* and the SuperFoodsRx Kitchen has created some terrific soup recipes for you to enjoy. In fact, with a single SuperFoods soup base you can make up to 12 interesting soups that are SuperFoods SuperNutrient powerhouses, delicious *and* very easy (page 284). If you don't want to cook or simply want to have a soup supply in your pantry, ready to eat in a jiffy, I have a list of healthy soups to look for in your supermarket (page 332).

There's so much research to indicate that soups promote weight loss that it seems almost foolish not to rely on this great food daily. One study reveals the simple value of soup. As the researchers put it, "Eating soup as part of lunch or dinner led to both decreased consumption of calories and a slower rate of eating."[5] One study divided overweight and obese people into three groups and instructed them to eat either two daily snacks, or a daily serving of soup or else no special addition to their diets for one year. All of these folks were on a calorie-restricted diet, the only difference being the soup, snack or "nothing" addition. After one year, all of the participants had lost weight but, most interestingly, those who had enjoyed the daily soup lost 50 percent more weight than those consuming the snack.[6] Another revealing study at Purdue University found that when participants were fed 300-calorie servings of various soups before their lunches—which were not calorie restricted—the participants tended to eat fewer daily calories on days when they enjoyed the soup. Remember that these subjects had no restrictions on their other food intake and were allowed to eat freely throughout the day.[7] So check out our terrific and delicious soup recipes beginning on page 284 and make soup a part of your daily SlimDown.

Soup and Salad Monday.

Monday is your Soup & Salad Day. Monday is a great choice for this mealtime practice because it gets your SlimDown week off to a great start and it can help to get you back on track after your weekend, which is sometimes a difficult time for dieters. During the SlimDown, I recommend

"I really like that this diet isn't about gimmicks. No artificial tricks. No 'diet' foods. Just real tools for a successful lifestyle change. I like the Soup & Salad Mondays, which are good after the weekend. This is a real diet for real life."— C. M., active mom

you stick with Monday as your day to have a soup and salad together for lunch or dinner. It will get you into the practice and Monday is the perfect day to commit to your plan, even if it takes some forethought to do so. In the Flex-Plan, you will find that you can choose any consistent day you like if for some reason Monday is not convenient for you. But generally, Monday is a good "forever" Soup & Salad day—one that you might have to alter occasionally, but always come back to—from today forward.

On this day, you're going to enjoy the delicious and healthy benefits of both a soup and a salad together. Most people enjoy their Soup & Salad at lunch but you can have it at dinner if you prefer. Slot your Soup & Salad Day in on your menu plan and make a selection from the delicious soup and salad suggestions on page 198.

Carb Guidelines. We're talking about those grains now! Many people these days are in a state of total confusion about carbs. We're eating less of the kind our bodies need—whole grains—and too much of the kinds that are making us fat—refined grains in the form of bread, cookies, cakes, pastries, and such. According to the USDA's 1996 *Continuing Survey of Food Intakes by Individuals* only 7 percent of Americans were then reaching the federal recommendations of three or more servings of *whole grains* daily. And the average daily consumption was just a single serving of whole grains. This minimal intake of whole grains takes a toll on our health and also on our ability to lose weight. In fact, in a study looking at more than 74,000 nurses' fiber and grain consumption patterns over more than a decade, women who ate more whole

grains consistently weighed less than the women who ate less.[8] And the women with the highest intake of dietary fiber had nearly 50 percent lower risk of major weight gain than the lowest intake. Another compelling study confirmed yet again the fact that, contrary to popular belief, carbs don't make you fat. This study showed that overweight and obese women actually consumed fewer carbohydrates, complex carbs, and dietary fiber than their healthy-weight peers, again highlighting the importance of getting *whole* grains in the diet whenever possible if your goal is to lose weight.

What's often forgotten in a discussion of carbs is that they are in fact, the "master fuel" of nutrition, providing a steady flow of blood sugar to the body machine so that our cells can make energy for our bodies to perform. Under healthy conditions, the only nutrient that fuels the brain cells is blood sugar—for which carbohydrates really are essential. Additionally, in biochemistry, we say that "fats burn in the fire of carbohydrates" because in order to break down fat, you need important chemicals that are produced from burning those carbohydrates. So you need to get your carbs but you need to get the right kind of whole grain carbs and you need to get them in appropriate portion controlled amounts.

Lunch or Dinner: *With* or *Without*.

While whole grains are essential and you need to consume them frequently in your diet, I find that many people who are new clients or attend my classes do the swing on a pendulum between *all* or *none* when it comes to the grains. First and foremost, you *need* the nutrients that whole grains provide you. However, you *don't* need all the refined white flour products that the population is still inclined to eat nor do you need *as many servings* as we've become accustomed to. In fact, as of 2000, Americans were consuming two to three more *daily* servings of grains than just a few short decades before!

This is the grains rule: **Either/Or: With or Without.**

You will have a whole grain *either* at lunch *or* dinner but not both. Which will it be? You choose. One meal **with** and one **without**.

I've made it simple for you: You're going to eat your daily three to four whole grain servings in portions that occur strategically once or twice a day at meals, and also if you choose at snacks.

Rather than thinking about "carbs," you're going to focus on whole grains. You'll have them sometimes at breakfast in cereal or oatmeal for example, and then at either lunch or dinner but not both. So you'll be enjoying a lunch *with* grains (sandwich, thin-crust turkey pizza, wrap) and a dinner *without* grains (orange sesame salmon with broccoli, ginger grilled turkey tenderloin with a SuperFoodsRx side salad). Or alternately, you'll choose to have your grains at dinner and skip them at lunch. It's very simple and easy to remember. You can also think of the *without* grains meal as "lean and green" though of course your veggies don't always have to be green! And keep in mind that all the Super-FoodsRx lunch and dinner entrees are interchangeable. You'll also sometimes be enjoying a portion of whole grains in your afternoon snack.

Here are the grains all from SuperFoods **Category 1 (Oats)** (with the addition of potatoes) you'll be choosing from:

- Bread
- Pasta
- Rice
- Corn
- Cereal
- Sweet Potato and other kinds of potatoes*

Simple Carb Guidelines: Great news! The SuperFoodsRx Diet will have you eating only or mostly whole grains again—easily and without the confusion or nonsense that "carbs are bad." The question is therefore not *whether* to eat grains, but *what kind, how much,* and *when*.

What kind: SuperFoods grains—Oats, brown rice, barley, whole wheat, buckwheat, rye, millet, bulgur wheat, amaranth, quinoa, triticale, kamut, yellow corn, wild rice, spelt, whole wheat couscous and whole wheat pasta, wheat germ and ground flaxseed.

How much: 3-4 servings daily (1 serving is tennis ball sized, ½-⅔ cup, or one 80-100 calorie slice of whole grain bread)

When: Breakfast (often), _either_ Lunch _or_ Dinner, some snacks—and as a FlexPlan option when the time comes.

* Isn't a potato a vegetable? Yes, while not technically a grain, it has some nutritional similarities to whole grains and is similar calorically, too. So, for the purposes of your SuperFoodsRx Diet, potatoes—sweet and white—count as grains.

A glance at the SuperFoodsRx Diet meal suggestions on page 53 will give you an idea of the broad range of choices you'll have in selecting your **with** and **without** grain meals.

Afternoon Snacks. Your afternoon snack is mandatory. Why? Snacks have a valuable function in any weight-loss plan. The first is most obvious: They keep your hunger at bay. A SuperFoods snack with some healthy carb energy in whole grains or fruit, lean protein, and a bit of healthy fat. The healthy fat—like that from nuts, for example—also helps to activate leptin, a hormone that tells you you're full. Most of us find that the time between lunch and dinner is the longest period we go without food. This stretch can create havoc with your blood sugar levels and can make even your firmest resolutions harder to stick by. The last thing you want to do is arrive at dinnertime so hungry that you've become mentally fuzzy and feeling as if you have lost control. Many of us find ourselves eating half our dinner while we cook, or snacking randomly in the late afternoon until we've eaten more calories than we'd find in a typical meal. We get used to feeling "starving" at this time of day and never stop to think that we don't *have* to feel that way. If you have a balanced snack in the late afternoon, you give a little boost to your metabolism, you tamp down your hunger and you actually improve your mood. In fact, one study reported that those who enjoyed a snack also enjoyed an improved mood as well as better recall on a simple memory test.[9] (So you'll be able to *remember* to eat a healthy dinner!)

I suggest you choose two to four snacks from the lists on page 68. Having two to four snacks slotted into your 2-week cycles makes it easier to plan, shop and to have them prepped and ready in advance. Snack time is not for "thinking": You want to just grab and go. Pick two (no more than four) and you're set. You can change your choices in a short 2 weeks' time. I'll list some typical snacks here but don't forget to check out the complete list on page 213 and slot them into your weekly menu plan. Bear in mind that these snacks amount to about 120–150 calories each. If you don't have access to one of the suggested SuperFoods snacks, you can select a snack of that equivalent in calories.

Sample SuperFoods Snacks

15 baby carrots + 7–8 almonds or walnuts

Medium (tennis ball) apple with 1 tablespoon peanut or almond butter

½ cup blueberries with ½ cup cottage cheese or 1 ounce other cheese

2 whole grain crackers (AkMak or Wasa) with 1 ounce cheese

2 whole grain crackers (AkMak or Wasa) with 1 tablespoon peanut/nut butter

8 almonds + 1 mini box of raisins

15 baby carrots with ¼ cup hummus

SuperNutrient Boosters. The SuperNutrient Boosters are low-calorie, nutrient-dense drinks—almost like *shooters*—that are delicious, readily available little jolts in your diet day. They are important components of the SuperFoodsRx Diet and serve a few crucial roles in ensuring your weight-loss success: For one thing, the SuperNutrient Boosters are your insurance, increasing your ability to pack in all the nutrition that will promote weight loss. By enjoying a 6–8-ounce SuperNutrient Booster mid-morning, you'll keep your metabolism sparked. The process of digestion itself actually speeds up your metabolism and the SuperNutrient Boosters help keep your body's engines revved. Here's another, more subtle reason why I insist on the SuperNutrient Boosters: They're an easy, guaranteed daily diet *success* that will help keep you motivated and on track. No matter what happens in your day, you'll feel good that you took that positive step and sipped a SuperNutrient Booster. While you take the minute or two necessary to enjoy your SuperNutrient Booster, think about your weight-loss goals and about how this delicious boost of nutrition is helping you honor your body, put a zip in your step, and achieve success. Here are commercial examples of the SuperNutrient Boosters:

"I like that if you are hungry that you can have a snack or a SuperNutrient Booster. I do not feel I have to 'go without.' I have more energy and the first time I walked over 10,000 steps I was so thrilled and proud of myself! It was a really good feeling. I am happy I am finally doing something for myself!"—Carla A, 52-year-old administrative assistant

Red SuperNutrient Booster: low-sodium V8, Knudsen low-sodium Very Veggie®, and Trader Joe's low-sodium Garden Medley.

Green SuperNutrient Booster: Evolution™ Essential Greens or Evolution™ Organic V

There are also SuperNutrient Booster recipes so you can also make your very own. See page 321.

The Food Diary

Want a simple, easy, inexpensive way to virtually ensure that you'll lose weight? Keep a food diary! The research is true and I've seen it happen with clients time and again: *People who keep a food diary are more likely to lose weight*, no matter how much they have to lose, and no matter what their exercise habits or their age. Your food diary is your "insurance policy": There are so many things that can go wrong in your diet day, but taking a few minutes to write down what you've eaten is always one thing that's under your control. It doesn't even take a great deal of energy or time. Finally, the surprising benefit of a food diary is that it amplifies all the good choices you make during the week and strengthens your resolve. If you've never kept a food diary before, you're going to be amazed at how this simple tool will supercharge your efforts at weight loss.

If you skip the food diary, you will probably lose weight on this plan but I can nearly guarantee that won't lose as consistently and steadily. A food diary is that important. So make your mind up now that you're just going to do it. You don't have to do it forever but you should do it for at least a few weeks. After that, you can use your diary as a

Here are the healthy, metabolism-boosting fluids you'll be enjoying in your SlimDown:

- Water: at least 6 cups daily
- Green and black tea: 1 or more cups daily
- SuperNutrient Booster at mid-morning

. . . and don't forget:

- No caloric drinks
- No alcohol
- No "diet" drinks

> "I've been surprised that I am not hungry between meals and snacks on this plan. I was also surprised that I do not crave sweets and chocolate anymore and that the SuperNutrient Booster helps with any hunger."
> —C. J., mother of four grown children

tune-up when necessary. And don't rule out the possibility that it may become so helpful in your planning and long-term success that you use it as a meal and exercise planning tool for your healthy lifestyle.

Here is why a food diary works: You know the vows one makes in a marriage? Sickness and health? Richer or poorer? At the moment those vows are made, no one knows what they'll come to mean as the future unfolds. They're an act of faith. If you're not willing to make those promises, you may not be willing to weather the storms ahead. Same with a food diary: If you're not willing to commit to a simple act of writing down what you eat, then you're more likely to stumble at the first Twinkie or bucket of KFC. Keeping your food log is an act of commitment. It's part of the process. You decide to keep the diary. You feel a sense of purpose. You get your notebook. You reinforce your decision to reach your goals. You feel stronger, in control. You're paying attention! We all have good intentions but life gets in the way. Paying attention makes all the difference. A food diary is the best technique to keep life at bay and your diet on track. Really; that is the way it works. So don't even think of skipping this step.

Here's an interesting aspect of the power of food diaries: Studies have found that even though a food diary is not 100 percent accurate—even if you forget to log a mint or misjudge what was in that salad you had—just the act of keeping the diary has "considerable power as a predictor of success in achieving weight loss."[10] This is a revelation to many folks who might otherwise feel overwhelmed by the thought of tracking their food intake. Relax. Do your best. Your food diary will help you even if it's not perfect.

Your SuperFoodsRx Food Diary will serve 3 purposes in the phases of your diet:

⬛ During the **Prep Week** it will alert you to your own personal food patterns—both the strong points and diet dilemmas.

- During the **SlimDown** it will help keep you keep score on how well you're adhering to the plan.
- During the **FlexPlan** it will be a powerful reminder to help you keep track of your choices and a planning tool to keep you focused on your goals.

Find a Method. It's really simple: All you need to do is jot down what you eat in a handy place—usually a small notebook that you keep in your purse or briefcase. I'll detail some of the varying methods people have used, but don't get bogged down in details; just choose a method and use it.

The most important aspect of keeping a food diary is that it has to work for you. It has to be simple. Some of my clients have had difficulty with their food diaries because the method they thought would be best for them just didn't fit. Some people have to try two or three methods before they find one that sticks. Don't be discouraged if your first efforts don't meet with success. If you find yourself making excuses like "I left it in the car" or "I forgot my password" more than once or twice, then it could be that you've picked the wrong system for you and need to choose an alternative.

Many of my clients find the most time-honored method of keeping track of their choices is the simple pocket-size notebook. This method has obvious advantages: It's cheap, it's low-tech, and it's portable. And if you lose it or leave it home you don't have to give up. You can simply use a scrap of paper until you get your hands on another notebook, or find your original. But any notebook that will fit in your purse or briefcase will work. A few clients have told me that they keep an index card in their pocket and jot down their food diary notes there. At the end of the day or during their train commute or any convenient regular time, they transfer these notes into their Food Diary notebook. Some of my clients create abbreviations to record their mood (at a meal) as well as any exercise for the day, beverages they drank, and so on. Some folks like to record a week on a page; others prefer a day on a page. See pages 74 and 94 for samples of both these styles.

Some folks find that a portable PDA is an efficient way to keep their food diary. If this suits you, there are tracking methods and software programs that you can use to help you in logging your intake—high-tech style.

If you're at the computer frequently you might find that it works for you to keep your records there. The potential challenge with this method, however, is that you have to feel 100 percent confident that you'll be able to record every day. Some clients have told me that they began their food diary on their computer but then went on vacation or simply didn't have access to their computer for a day or two and this stopped them in their tracks.

Find a time to record. The ideal pattern is to make your food notes soon after you eat each meal or snack. For some people, this simply isn't realistic. In any event, you should try to record at least twice a day. Some folks find that it's bedtime before they get to their diary and the obvious problem here is that you often forget what you've eaten. It's been my experience that people most commonly forget those little bits that can make a big difference in their efforts at weight loss. The chips they took off their friend's plate at lunch, the half a doughnut they grabbed at that meeting. If you make a plan to record at regular intervals, it's easier to remember exactly what you've eaten and easier to resist something you really don't want to eat!

Food Diary/Health History. Here's another long-term benefit to your food diary: Every day we learn more about the effects of foods on health. The whole basis of the SuperFoodsRx movement is that certain foods are better choices for promoting health—as well as losing weight. A food diary can serve as a record that could be useful in your future health care. Not only can you pick up patterns that can be useful (You suffered from frequent migraines last spring until you stopped eating, say, chocolate. You never had gastrointestinal problems until you started eating [blank].) but knowing your eating patterns at certain times in your life could have implications for future health care.

It Takes Too Much Time!
Here's the Truth: It's very hard to spend more than 10 minutes a day keeping track of what you eat. Can you afford 10 minutes? How about 5 minutes, twice a day? How about 3 minutes in the afternoon and 7 minutes at bedtime? You know you have 10 minutes to give toward a slimmer, healthier you.

Food Diary Tools

🌿 **Your Mood.** What mood were you in when you sat down to dinner? Were you feeling stressed about a family or work issue? Were you distracted because you had to rush out to fulfill some obligation that evening? Were you feeling down because you hadn't accomplished something you'd hoped? Your moods can affect how much you eat. By noting in your SuperFoodsRx food diary your moods, you'll have an extremely useful tool for discovering your own personal links to eating and moods. If you know that you tend to eat more when you're rushed, for example, you can take that into consideration on days when time is short.

🌿 **Your Hunger Level.** How hungry were you when you ate that lunch or snack? Starving? Kind of half full? Don't really know? Many of us have actually lost track of what hunger actually feels like. We eat reflexively—it's lunchtime, it's dinnertime—but appreciating hunger and satiety is the bedrock of a healthy diet. Learning to eat until satisfied but not stuffed is a critical tool in long-term weight management. By noting in your food diary your actual feelings of hunger, you'll get in touch with how much food you need to be satisfied. This will help you get back in touch with real feelings of hunger. Here's a simple way to gauge your hunger level. Simply assign a number to the level of hunger you feel. Note this number in your food diary. It will give you useful clues to your eating patterns.

0 1 2 3 4 5 6 7 8 9 10

ravenous   utterly stuffed

Here is a sample of a blank food diary that you can copy and use. Here also is a sample of a filled-in food diary that will give you a good idea of what you should be aiming for as you create your own version. Remember, in the end, what works for you is what matters.

Daily Food Diary

Day/Date

	Hunger (0—10)	Mood ☹ 😐 🙂
BREAKFAST (TIME, WHAT, HOW MUCH)		
LUNCH (TIME, WHAT, HOW MUCH)		
DINNER (TIME, WHAT, HOW MUCH)		
SNACK (TIME, WHAT, HOW MUCH)		
SNACK (TIME, WHAT, HOW MUCH)		
OTHER (TIME, WHAT, HOW MUCH)		
OTHER (TIME, WHAT, DURATION)		

WATER (GOAL=6+ CUPS)

Circle   1 1 1 1 1 1 1 1 1 1 1 1

OTHER BEVERAGES

Tea (type, time, amount):

Other:

EXERCISE:

My daily steps today:

Other exercise (type, time, duration):

Where are the SuperFoods in your day? Go back and circle any SuperFoods that you ate today!

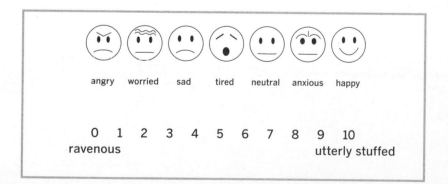

| angry | worried | sad | tired | neutral | anxious | happy |

0   1   2   3   4   5   6   7   8   9   10

ravenous   utterly stuffed

	Hunger (0—10)	Mood
BREAKFAST (TIME, WHAT, HOW MUCH)		
6:30 a.m. *Cup of coffee* 7:30 a.m. *Piece of toast with 1 tablespoon peanut butter* *Apple*	*3*	*content*
LUNCH (TIME, WHAT, HOW MUCH)		

12:30 p.m.   *Tuna salad sandwich (tomato, lettuce, 2 slices of bread, mayo and mustard)*
             Red grapes
             Cookie (Choc. chip from conference room)
	4	*drowsy/ anxious*

DINNER (TIME, WHAT, HOW MUCH)		

7:30 p.m.   *Out to dinner: 2 pieces bread*
             Cocktail shrimp
             Grilled salmon, asparagus
             Baked potato
 	
             2 bites of Mike's mousse
	1	*neutral, but starving*

SNACK (TIME, WHAT, HOW MUCH)		
Missed afternoon snack—forgot to bring something.		
SNACK (TIME, WHAT, HOW MUCH)		
9:00 p.m. *Piece of toast with jam*	*6*	*bored, drowsy*
OTHER (TIME, WHAT, HOW MUCH)		

ACTIVITY (TIME, WHAT, DURATION)

WATER (GOAL=6+ CUPS)

CIRCLE   ①①①①① 1 1 1 1 1 1

OTHER BEVERAGES

TEA (TYPE, TIME, AMOUNT):
cup of green tea mid-morning; cup of green tea after lunch

OTHER:
1 cup coffee at 6:30 a.m.

EXERCISE:

MY DAILY STEPS TODAY:
5,868

OTHER EXERCISE (TYPE, TIME, DURATION):
none

Where are the SuperFoods in your day? Go back and circle any SuperFoods that you ate today!

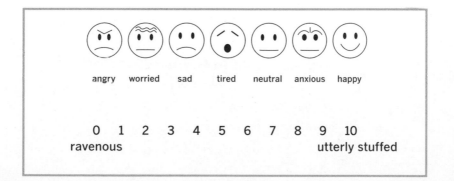

angry worried sad tired neutral anxious happy

0 1 2 3 4 5 6 7 8 9 10
ravenous   utterly stuffed

Sometimes clients complain that they seemed to have reached a diet plateau. No matter what they do, they can't budge the numbers on the scale. A food diary can be an extremely useful tool for those in this frustrating situation. The calculus of weight loss is not always simple. For example, if you lost 10 pounds it stands to reason that it takes fewer calories to maintain your smaller body. If you've been exercising a lot you may find that your clothes are looser but your weight hasn't changed. This is because muscle weighs more than fat—but takes up far less space—so you may be trimmer while maintaining your weight. An obvious piece of this puzzle is what you're eating. A food diary can help you assess your situation and recognize when a certain piece of the puzzle needs modification. A little more exercise? Perhaps fewer calories for your smaller body?

Sleep. I have provided some useful information about sleep in the LifePlan (page 175). For now it's enough to know that you will help to ensure your diet success if you work a full night's sleep into your SlimDown. Adequate sleep has a measurable effect on your ability to lose weight and to maintain a healthy weight. So don't neglect this critical health habit. Eight hours is ideal but at least 7 hours should be mandatory for your best SuperFoodsRx Diet success.

Exercise: Your Marching Orders

You can't just sit there; you've got to move! That's right. Every bit of research points to the fact that exercise is a critical part of weight loss. You've got to get moving! Where? Right out the door and down the block. That's right: Walk. I've found that walking really is the simplest way to get your exercise program off the ground. Or rather off the sofa. It's easy, it's inexpensive, and it's measurable. The extraordinary physical benefits of regular daily exercise are well documented. We know that exercisers can reduce heart disease risk as well as risk of diabetes, osteoporosis, colon cancer, and high blood pressure as well as other disease risks. The very good news is that these benefits can be enjoyed with a regular, moderate physical activity such as walking. It's easy to set and achieve goals when you exercise-walk, particularly with the help of a pedometer. In fact, research has demonstrated that walking is the chosen exercise among people who lose weight and subsequently maintain their healthy weight.[11] Your goal on the SlimDown is to walk 30 minutes a day. (If you already do some form of exercise, terrific! Keep it up. Just make sure that you get in at least 30 minutes of whatever exercise you choose daily.) I recommend that you get a pedometer to gauge your progress. They're readily available and inexpensive. If you don't have one, add that to your shopping list and get one.

How to Set Up Your Walking Program:

The overall goal of your walking program is to log lots and lots of steps on your pedometer. How many is lots and lots? For your Prep Week, you're not going to worry too much about how much you walk, you're just going to figure out *your* walking style. (But I should tell you, I've rarely had a client who wasn't eager to begin logging those steps to ever higher numbers!) You'll enjoy using a pedometer to record your steps, and walking is going to become a welcome part of your day—whether you do it in one long walk or smaller walks throughout the day.

Here are three steps you can take to get your walking program set up. You can do each step on a separate day or do them all at once; it depends on your schedule. But make sure you complete these exercises during the Prep Week so you'll be ready for regular, daily exercise during your SlimDown.

Your Pedometer. Your pedometer will be your new best friend. You'll attach it to your waistband (it's quite inconspicuous) in the morning and take

Take some time to organize yourself for exercise. Make sure you have comfortable walking shoes. Find an exercise outfit that's comfortable and appropriate to the weather. Women should make sure they have a supportive exercise bra. If you like to listen to music or books on tape, get a portable player and headphones. There are lots of options for radios and MP3 players that are appropriate for using during exercise. If possible, find a special drawer, plastic bin, or small gym bag to store your exercise things. It's so much easier and inspiring to have a "no-excuses, go-to" place where your equipment is ready and waiting.

> Your ultimate exercise-walking goal is 10,000 steps daily but as Lao Tzu said, "The journey of a thousand miles begins with a single step."

it off when you tumble into bed. (I've actually had SuperFoodsRx dieters tell me that they put it back on the waistband of their pj's if they get up at night for a glass of water. You don't need to go this far!) You'll be surprised by how much your pedometer will inspire you to move and help you keep track of your progress. One of your tasks this week is to get a pedometer. There are many good pedometers out there but one I like is the Digiwalker by New Life-styles SW-651. It's basic—no bells or whistles—inexpensive and accurate. Others by the same company have some other nice features, as well. I suggest you steer clear of pedometers that claim to record "calories burned." This is the least accurate feature of pedometers since they don't consider your height, weight, and gender, whether you're walking up hills or flat, heart-rate response, arms swinging, and so on.

To be sure your pedometer is recording properly, pay attention to how you set it up. It should be clipped onto your waistband or the belt of your pants or front pocket—parallel to the floor. It should rest flat against your body (don't let it tip forward). You may have to adjust it more toward your hip (away from the belly button) to get it to read properly. Set the pedometer to "zero" and walk around for 20 to 30 steps (counting the steps as you go.) Check the pedometer reading to make sure it's picking up the steps. If it's off a few steps don't worry, but if it is way off, readjust it on your waist, reset, and try again. Sometimes if you carry extra weight on your body or wear elastic-banded pants that fold over, the pedometer may tip forward or be slightly and not give a proper measurement. However, after you adjust it and try this procedure a few times, chances are good you'll find the right placement for your body.

How Often?

- 5–6 days weekly for a minimum of 30 minutes each day; 45 minutes is the goal.

- If you can build toward 60 minutes a day, your odds of achieving long-term success will greatly increase!

How Hard Do I Have to Work?

- You can spread your exercise and steps out throughout your day, which is one of the great appeals of walking as your chosen exercise. A hundred steps here, another hundred there; they all count. A thousand steps should take you approximately 8–12 minutes at a brisk (between 2.8 mph (12 minutes) and 3.8 mph (8 minutes) walking pace).

- But you should at one time during each day, move for **at least 20 minutes straight** at an intensity where you can still carry on a light conversation, but not sing. This is considered moderate intensity and at this level of exertion you should feel your breathing rate increase and your body start to warm up, but you should be able to maintain this pace without difficulty for a full 20 minutes.

- If you're already more experienced in your fitness routine, you can extend the duration or change the type of activity to aim for 30–45 minutes of continuous activity.

Step One: A Day's Walk

This one is easy. It's going to give you a reference point for all the days to come. Put on your pedometer when you get out of bed in the morning and wear it all day. That's right: all day. You simply want to have a gauge of how many steps you take in a typical day. I'll warn you: Most people are somewhat horrified at how

"I wanted to share a milestone I reached this weekend. I committed to be on track this past week, both with my eating and more importantly with my walking. Since last Tuesday I have walked each and every day for at least 20–30 minutes. But yesterday, I went to the gym, then worked around the house, then in the afternoon took the dogs for a walk to the park and to my amazement, when I got home and read my pedometer I had walked 10,105 steps...that is a first for me and it feels great!"—Danette S., 43-year-old, single parent of two

sedentary they are. But don't worry: This is just your beginning. You're going to be inspired to boost that number. For many people, just the act of wearing the pedometer gets them to seize more opportunities to walk. You'll probably be one of them. Record your daily steps and log it in your Food Diary.

Step Two: Timing Your Steps.

The walking goal—a well-accepted goal supported by research and many practitioners—is 10,000 steps. Some people are totally overwhelmed by this number. How can they possibly walk that much? Well here's an exercise that will shift your focus from a BIG number to the small possibilities in your day. Let's see how long it takes you to walk 500 steps. Walk around the block, the neighborhood track—wherever you can easily and safely walk. Use a stopwatch or the minute hand of a watch or clock. Jot down the answer. Does it take 5 minutes, 7 minutes, 10 minutes? Now take your 500-step figure and multiply it by 20. Record this number. This is how long it's going to take you to reach your goal of 10,000 daily steps. Knowing how many minutes it takes to cover 500 steps can help you insert small activity sessions in throughout your day. If you have just 10 or 15 minutes, you can add how many steps to your daily tally? Take a few minutes to think about when you might log in extra steps. Perhaps you could walk the dog? Take a walk around the block after dinner? Or simply walk while chatting on the phone? It all adds up and *it all counts*.

Some walking facts:

- 10,000 steps = approximately 4.5–5 miles
- 2,000 steps = approximately 1 mile
- 1 mile = approximately 100 calories burned
- 10,000 steps per day = approximately 500 calories burned per day
- 70,000 steps in one week (10,000 per day) burns approximately 3,500 calories

Step Three: Setting Your Goal

It's time to figure out how many steps are a good realistic beginning goal for your personal walking program. You'll do this by first figuring out a daily average of what how many steps you currently take. Put on your pedometer first thing in the morning. Set it to "zero" and leave it on for the entire day. Check it a couple of times to be sure it's recording properly. And the end of the day, remove the pedometer and record the number but don't reset it. Do this for 2 more days so you now have the number of steps you've walked in 3 days. Divide this number by 3 and you have your average daily walking count. This is going to be your baseline. You'll use it to set your SlimDown goal. Here are your guidelines:

- If you're at 3,000 or less daily steps average, aim to start your program with a goal of 4,000–4,500 daily steps and increase by 1,000 daily steps on a weekly basis until you reach 10,000.

- If your daily steps are between 3,000–5,000 steps, aim for 1,500–2,000 additional daily steps on top of your average and increase by 1,000 daily steps weekly until you reach 10,000.

- If your daily steps are 5,001–7,000—aim for 2,000 additional daily steps on top of your average and increase by 1,000 daily steps on a weekly basis until you reach 10,000.

- If your daily steps are at 7,001–9,000—aim for 2,000 additional daily steps on top of your average and increase by 1,000 daily steps on a weekly basis until you reach 10,000.

- If your daily steps are at 10,000 already as an average, increase your daily steps to 12,500–14,000 and be consistent with this number over time.

Strategies for getting those extra steps:

- Park in the farthest space from your destination.
- Get off public transportation a stop or two early and walk the rest of your way (plan ahead so you leave enough time!).
- Walk, run, and play actively with your children or grandchildren.
- Walk over to talk to a colleague instead of e-mailing.
- Take a walking break instead of a coffee break.
- Use part of your lunch hour to walk for 10–20 minutes.

- Unless you are on an upper floor in a high-rise building, take the stairs instead of the elevator—if this is hard at first, take the elevator part way and climb the remaining flights of stairs until you build up your stamina.
- Wear a headset or use a speaker phone so you can walk and talk while on the telephone.
- Take a lap in the mall before you begin your actual shopping.
- Hide your remote and change channels the old-fashioned way.
- Catch up with a friend or colleague with a walk-and-talk instead of over coffee.
- March in place while filing or making copies (this tip comes directly from one of our successful SuperFoodsRx dieters).
- Take up dancing.
- Walk laps in your home using stairs and other pathways, inside and out.
- Walk your dog.
- Join a community team for a new sport—or one you haven't done since you were a child.
- Take lessons—tennis, golf, bowling, dance—anything new that you've always wanted to try.
- Garden—including raking and mowing.
- Walk after your meals.

Exercise Alternatives. While the backbone of the SuperFoodsRx Diet exercise program is walking, you may want to choose another option. Perhaps you already have some form of regular exercise. If you are so inclined, now is the time to investigate a gym membership, a personal trainer, or an exercise class. Choose any opportunity for exercise that will be regular and will fit into your daily routine. Work out details during Prep Week if you'd like to choose one of these options. Note on your calendar when you'll participate. Make sure it's at least 5 days weekly beginning in your SlimDown. If you do join a gym or employ a trainer, your Prep week offers a good opportunity to schedule a training session. Nothing boosts your determination and energy levels like a good gym session.

Here's a chart that will help you stay on track:

DAY/DATE	GOAL	PLANNED EXERCISE TIME AND LENGTH	TOTAL DAILY STEPS (includes planned exercise time and daily steps)
e.g.: Tuesday, Jan. 1	*10,000*	*7:00 a.m. walk 30 minutes*	*8,106*
WEEKLY TOTAL			

D on't forget, no alcohol on the SlimDown. You will be able to enjoy a glass of wine or beer when you cycle to the FlexPlan but to promote maximum weight loss on the SlimDown, alcohol doesn't fit the equation. Remember, the work you do on the SlimDown will be rewarded and the results will show. If you're in the mood for a bit of bubbly while on the SlimDown, choose sparkling water!

Weekly Weight/Measure Check. We looked at the issue of your actual weight and waist goals in Chapter 2. Now is the time to start following those recommendations. Don't forget your twice-weekly weight check and once-weekly waist measurement. You should weigh yourself on Monday morning and on Friday morning and record your weight in your Food Diary. Don't worry if your weight sometimes jumps a half-pound or so higher than you'd expected. These fluctuations are normal. Also, measure your waist once weekly, on Monday. Record that figure, too.

2 More Important Tips

You now know the basics of the SlimDown and you're well prepared to actually begin to work with your menus. But I wanted to share two more thoughts with you that will help prime you for successful weight loss. They are:

- Pay attention when you eat!
- Manage hunger.

Pay Attention When You Eat. Have you ever sat down to watch TV with a bag of cookies or chips only to realize after a half-hour or hour that the bag is empty? You hardly realized you ate them and you certainly didn't savor them. This is a powerful example of mindless eating. You might think that when you're distracted by some activity you wouldn't eat as much but the converse is true. A relevant study found that women who ate snack cakes while they played a video game wanted to eat *more* than the women who ate the cakes with no other distractions.[13] So use this knowledge: Focus on your food. Don't try to accomplish other tasks while eating and that includes reading or even watching television. Savor every delicious bite and chew your food well. And you'll enjoy the meal more and feel fuller faster.

Manage Hunger. Sometimes we think we're hungry but we are in fact experiencing another distracting feeling that could range from boredom to anxiety. If your tendency is to immediately grab something to eat at the first sign of hunger, here's your proactive SuperFoods approach. Follow these steps:

- Take your emotional pulse: Are you bored? Stressed? Angry? Tired? See if you can identify something that may have triggered your feeling. Sometimes a brisk walk around the block, 5 minutes of meditation, or a phone

---

What's Wrong with a Nonfat Diet? Not Enough Fat! Remember when nonfat was all the rage? People avoided fat like the plague. We now know this is counterproductive in terms of both nutrition and weight loss. We need fats—the healthy kind. They play a crucial role in transporting nutrients through every one of our cells as well as keeping our blood vessels in good shape and a host of other important functions. Every cell wall is made up of fat so healthy fat equals a healthy cell wall. As I mentioned earlier, if you don't have some fat in your salad dressing, you won't get the most nutritional bang for your buck from those great green leafies or luscious lycopene tomatoes. And healthy fats also help you lose weight. In one study people were divided into two groups. One group ate a Mediterranean diet that included a moderate fat content of 35 percent. The other group was on a low-fat diet with only 20 percent of calories from fat. After 6 months both groups lost about the same amount of weight. But the real change came after 18 months. By then the average weight loss on the higher-fat diet was roughly 10 pounds compared to the low-fat dieters' loss of about 6 pounds. And after 1 more year the higher-fat diet group had been able to maintain almost all of their weight loss.[12] Of course the critical issue here is the *type* of fat. The SuperFoodsRx Diet includes healthy fats delivered through the your foods themselves such as in nuts, beans, lean turkey, and wild salmon and also only small, but powerfully healthy amount of added fats like olive oil. They're important to the diet. They make things taste good and they'll ensure you're getting maximal nutrients and maximum long-term success.

chat with a friend will steady and satisfy you. Make a list of 5-minute activities you can refer to for similar future sensations. It's incredibly empowering.

- Take a look at the time—is it nearing a mealtime? Have you remembered to have your snack? If it's within 30 minutes, drink a glass of water or a hot or cold glass of green tea and that will hold you. If it's time to eat, *eat*.

- If it's not a mealtime, have that glass of water and wait 10 minutes to reassess. The body's thirst signal can cross paths and create interference with your sense of hunger!

- Hunger hasn't passed? Have another 6–8 ounces of your SuperNutrient Booster and wait 10 minutes. Get some of the little cans of low-sodium V8 to have readily available in your car or office for occasions like these. See if the boost satisfies you.

Vexed by Variety

I once created a full week of healthy, calorie-controlled, menus and recipes for a magazine. My directions from the editor were to use a wide variety of foods and make each meal and snack delicious and appealing, but also unique. When the article was published, my mom called me and said, "Wendy, it looks lovely but if I actually made those foods I'd need over 280 ingredients and I'd be shopping for a full day!" While the menus were what the editor wanted, I knew that they were not altogether practical. It was interesting reading, but the probable execution of the week was highly unlikely! *And the* **execution** *of a plan is the key to success for achieving a healthy goal like losing weight.*

My mom's call reminded me yet again of something that many nutritionists and diet books ignore: You do not have to vary your diet as widely as you're often led to believe. Most people do not eat a different breakfast every day of the week. Most people repeat their favorite lunches a few times a week. This is perfectly fine and can be perfectly nutritious, too. If you follow the overall SuperFoodsRx Diet recommendations you'll be eating an extraordinarily healthy diet and you'll be losing weight, too—without spending all your spare time shopping and cooking.

- Still hungry? Have a handful of vegetables—baby carrots or cherry tomatoes or celery sticks. You can bring these to the office or cut them and keep them in baggies in a cooler in the car or in a container in the fridge. Wait 10 minutes. Reassess.

- Reevaluate the time in relation to your next meal or snack. By now 30 minutes have passed. If you still feel hungry, try a piece of fruit: an apple can be particularly convenient. Wait 10 minutes after the 5–10 minutes it takes to eat it and reassess again.

- Once more and finally, reevaluate the time and whether a meal or snack is near (you've passed some 40–50 minutes by now). If not, have a Super-Foods-friendly snack and call it quits.

This is such an effective strategy that my clients swear by it. It gives you a specific *strategy* with actual steps for evaluating your hunger and honoring your body by paying attention to what it is or is not saying. The body is that incredible, but many of us walk around without paying attention—or worse, having the desire but not the tools to explore sensations perceived as hunger. The end result is either overeating and feeling guilty or punishing yourself through *deprivation* when in fact there may be a reason for the feelings. And if you're worried about the caloric damage done by going through each of these steps—all told it's an absolute maximum of 250—but I guarantee you won't even get near this since meals or snacks on the SuperFoods diet are always just around the corner. You're likely to forget your hunger long before you get through the steps.

Let's review the SlimDown Guidelines:

SlimDown Guidelines:

The Food:

- Breakfast is mandatory.

- Carbohydrates in the form of grain and fruit or just fruit at breakfast.

- Grain carbohydrates at lunch or dinner *but not both*. You'll refer to these as *with* and *without* (grains, that is).
- SuperNutrient Booster every day at mid-morning.
- Afternoon snack every day.
- Use your SuperFoodsRx 1, 2, 3 categories.
- Eat from your SuperFoodsRx Meal Lists.
- SuperFoods salad or soup or both every day.
- Monday is Soup & Salad Day.
- Wednesday is Veggie Day.
- No food after dinner.
- Beverages: Water and Tea.
  - No alcohol.
  - No caloric beverages.
  - Up to 1 cup coffee daily (try to shift to tea).
  - Low-fat or nonfat milk or soy milk is okay as a snack or as part of a meal.
  - Green or black tea—one or more brewed cups daily.
  - 6+ cups water daily—*throughout* your day.

The Behaviors:

- Plan your week in advance selecting from the SuperFoodsRx Meal Lists.
  - 3 meals, 1 SuperNutrient Booster, 1 snack daily.
  - Breakfast variety: minimum 2 different breakfasts weekly.
  - Lunch variety: minimum 2–3 different lunches weekly.
  - Dinner variety: minimum 3–4 different dinners weekly.
  - Lunches and dinners are *interchangeable*.
- Daily recording in your Food Diary.
- Do not skip meals or snacks. Eat to boost your metabolism.
- Stop eating within 2, preferably 3 hours of bedtime.
- Monday & Friday weight checks.
- Monday waist measure check.

🌿 Exercise *minimum* 30 minutes daily, at least 5 days a week.

🌿 Sleep—aim for a minimum of 7 hours nightly.

Create Your Menu Plan

This is the fun part. If you didn't create your menu plan as suggested in the Prep & Practice Week detailed in the next chapter, now's the time to do it. Check out the list of SlimDown guidelines previously mentioned and the suggested Breakfast choices (page 188) and Lunch/Dinner choices (page 193) and use them to help you fill out your personalized SlimDown Menu plan. You can't go wrong on this system. All the calories and nutrients have been figured out for you. Just select the meals you prefer and slot them into your plan. When you choose from the specific meal options starting on page 188, you practically eliminate the need for any counting since virtually every meal option includes two or more SuperFoods in the appropriate amounts. This is really the easiest way to see rapid results on the SlimDown. Still, if you decide to create your own meal options, just look to the guidelines for building a SuperFoods meal on the fly, follow your portion control tips and you really can't miss.

🌿 Choose minimum 2, not more than 3 breakfasts to rotate in SlimDown and slot them in.

🌿 Choose 2–3 lunches to rotate for variety and slot them in

If you're a male, very active, or have 20 or more pounds to lose, here are some extra guidelines for you:

- Add one snack from the list (page 214) daily either with your morning SuperNutrient Booster or at another time in the afternoon. Space the snack at least 2 hours apart from another snack or meal. So for example, you might have a snack at 3:30, another snack at 5:30, dinner at 7:30 or 8:00.

- Add one tennis ball of additional fruit—a SuperFoods fruit or any other choice as long as you're meeting your other SuperFoodsRx Diet goals. This can be added to a meal or stand alone.

- Choose 3–4 dinners to rotate variety and slot them in.

- Choose your snacks in 2–3 varieties and slot them in.

- Choose your SuperFoodsRx Nutrient Booster and slot it in.

Take a look and reconfigure things a bit if neces-sary. Is there a place where you could have one of your meals as a leftover the next day? Or will you make a soup recipe that you can repeat another one or two days? Or perhaps you'd like to take the vegetables for one meal, cook a bit extra and enjoy it the next day as well. Some of my clients rotate the same lunches every other or every third day—or for a few days in a row and then shift. Same with dinner—do what feels good to you. Just remember—Soup & Salad Monday, Veggie Wednesday, your SuperNutrient boosters and snacks AND *with/without* grains lunch and dinner. *Voilà!* Allow enough time to think through your SlimDown week. The bit of effort you put into planning now will pay off in a big way as you move through the week. It's easy to succeed when it's all spelled out for you!

Do you have your meals and snacks all logged in? You're looking at a great week. Now make up your shopping list, get your fridge and pantry stocked, fire up your pedometer, and start losing!

Here's your checklist of top priorities while on the SlimDown:

- Use your Food Diary daily.

- Eat your SuperFoodsRx meals and snacks.

- Drink your green or black tea and water.

- Don't forget to exercise.

- Weigh yourself on Monday and Friday.

- Measure your waist on Monday.

- Get enough sleep!

In case you need a reminder:

The SuperFoods:

Category 1: Pumpkin, Oats, Walnuts

Category 2: Beans, Salmon, Soy, Turkey, Yogurt

Category 3: Blueberries, Broccoli, Oranges, Spinach, Tomatoes

Beverages: Tea (black or green), Water

The SuperFoodsRx Categories

Choose from the lists and check yourself on the guidelines:

Category 1:

- Minimum 1 serving of **each** on most or every day of the week.
- Maximum 3–4 servings from combined Oats/Pumpkin SuperFoods daily.
- Minimum $\frac{1}{2}$, maximum 1 serving Walnuts SuperFood group daily.

Category 2 in at least 2 meals.

- 2–3 servings total from 2 of the Category 2 SuperFoods or sidekicks daily.

Category 3 at all meals.

- 3–5 cups of 3 of the Category 3 SuperFoods or sidekicks daily.

Beverages:

- 1 or more cups brewed tea daily; 6+ cups water daily.

Suggestion: Circle category 1 SuperFoods in your day, outline with a square any category 2 SuperFoods in your day, use a highlighter pen to mark category 3 SuperFoods in your day. Count your totals and compare to your goals!

Weekly Plan/Food Diary for SlimDown

	MONDAY	TUESDAY	WEDNESDAY
Date			
Breakfast			
SuperNutrient Booster	SuperNutrient Booster	SuperNutrient Booster	SuperNutrient Booster
Lunch	*With* *Without*	*With* *Without*	*With* *Without*
Snack			
Dinner	*With* *Without*	*With* *Without*	*With* *Without*
Special Notes	Soup & Salad Monday		Veggie Wednesday

Comments...
 	
Exercise
  Activity:
  Duration:
  Steps:
 	
How are you feeling?			

THURSDAY	FRIDAY	SATURDAY	SUNDAY
SuperNutrient Booster	SuperNutrient Booster	SuperNutrient Booster	SuperNutrient Booster
With *Without*	*With* *Without*	*With* *Without*	*With* *Without*
With *Without*	*With* *Without*	*With* *Without*	*With* *Without*
	Don't forget— lunch and dinner are ALWAYS interchangeable!		Prepare for the Week Ahead!

Chapter 4

The SuperFoodsRx Prep and Practice Week

Now that you have a good snapshot of the SuperFoodsRx SlimDown, you'll find it useful to step back and take a look at how you can prime yourself for diet success. Here are some tips and suggestions to get you off on the right foot in this "pre-diet" practice week.

What's Your Diet Speed?

If you're like many people, you have a history of "RPM Dieting." That is, it sometimes seems like you make a *Resolution Per Minute*. It's so tempting to leap onto a diet bandwagon. You hear about a "hot" diet and suddenly you're totally eliminating all white foods or you're only eating a certain type of soup. I've seen too many people—clients and friends—begin to try and lose weight with a burst of admirable enthusiasm that fades as real life interferes and a dinner party or a trip or an empty cupboard or a deadline derails their efforts. RPM dieting rarely works. Obviously you *must eat*—every day—and eating takes preparation. But in order to successfully change your eating patterns, it's much better to begin by laying the emotional and physical groundwork. My guess is that any efforts at weight reduction that you've made in the past have neglected these crucial steps.

This time will be different. You're going to create an environment that will ensure success. You're going to take some simple steps that will help you make your new eating pattern as easy as opening the fridge. *You probably don't even realize how hard it is to stick to a new lifestyle when your environment is fighting every step of the way!* Most folks blame willpower. I've heard clients say, "Well, I just couldn't stick with that diet. I got too hungry and then I broke down and ate a whole sleeve of Oreos. At that point I just gave up." Well, of course you gave up! You opened the pantry and that giant box of cookies pleaded with you like a puppy at the pound to "pick me, pick me."

The SuperFoodsRx Diet Prep & Practice Week is useful because it helps you recognize the environmental traps that may have thrown you off course in the past. Since most of us do most of our eating at home, you'll take stock of the booby traps that can make losing weight such a challenge. You're starving? There's a terrific SuperFoods snack waiting for you right in the fridge. Is it dinnertime? Would it be so much easier to just order a pizza? Well, you've got the makings of a quick, really delicious SuperFoods "Fifteen Minute SuperFast" meal right there in the cupboard. Not only that, but you'll also be boosting your metabolism with green tea and a bit of simple exercise and generally tuning up your lifestyle. You're doing all the groundwork this week, and you're practicing eating the foods that will be the healthy mainstays of your new eating pattern.

Here's something else to keep in mind: *Half of successful weight loss is what's on your plate; the other half is what's in your head.* Motivation doesn't just come from wishing. It comes from changing your mindset and your environment: taking concrete steps to reach your goal. Each step you take confirms your resolve and strengthens your ability to stick to your plan. That's why the Prep & Practice week is not just about buying food; it's also about giving you an opportunity to feel strong. Every step you take this week is a bit more insurance that you will reach your goal.

At the Starting Gate: You're eager to begin your SuperFoods plan but before you do scan your calendar. Do you have a major business trip coming up? A family reunion? A stressful project that's nearing completion? You know yourself best but most people find their eating patterns are easier to change when their life is relatively stable. I tell clients that it's best to begin their SuperFoods SlimDown when they have at least 2 weeks that won't throw too many challenges at them. Once the SuperFoods lifestyle becomes your own, it will be easy to manage the routine obstacles that life throws at you.

Something to think about as you begin your Prep and then your SlimDown: You can live with giving something up for now—on the Prep and SlimDown—because you'll have strategies for including it later—on the FlexPlan. It's never a free-for-all because that's how most people got in trouble in the first place. But again, remember the promise that you'll never feel hungry when you follow the plan. Once you've completed at least a week of the SlimDown you'll know that's true. And you can see from the many comments from SuperFoodsRx Diet veterans that hunger is not an issue. So don't feel anxious about "giving up" something because later, when you come to the FlexPlan, you'll see that the issue isn't deprivation it's planning— planning to include things you enjoy.

The Prep & Practice Week—think of it as the SuperFoodsRx Diet with training wheels—is the week that sets you up for success.

Here's a preview of what you're going to accomplish this week.

Prep & Practice Week Tasks:

- Take Stock: Assess the foods that currently fill your fridge and pantry.

- SuperFoodsRx Shopathon: Purchase the SuperFoods that you prefer.

- SuperFoodsRx Kitchen SlimDown: Organize your kitchen into a SuperKitchen.

- SuperFoodsRx Practice: Select three menus/recipes to try from the SlimDown (page 52) for your Prep & Practice Week and select menus/ recipes from the SlimDown that you'll use next week when you begin the SlimDown.

- Review the three SuperFoods categories.

- Begin your SuperFoodsRx Food Diary.

- Focus on upgrading your diet all week with SuperFoods.

- Hydrate the SuperFoodsRx way with water and tea.

- Set Your Weight and Waist Loss Goals (page 42).

- Get started on your SuperFoodsRx walking routine.

Step 1: Take Stock

Certain foods bring us down. They contribute too much of the bad—sodium, trans fat, calories—and too little of the good—nutrients, fiber, polyphenols. Unfortunately, these foods are like the Sirens luring Odysseus to the rocks: They're always calling out to us. Ice cream . . . chips . . . cookies! It's very hard to resist them, especially at those low points in the day when you're most vulnerable. You know yourself: Are you really going to ignore the doughnuts at 10:00 p.m. and you're in the mood for some mindless munching? I suggest that if you have certain foods in your kitchen that you know are difficult for you to resist, you either dispose of them, or, alternatively, store them in a relatively inaccessible spot—a drawer or cupboard that puts them out of easy reach.

Here are the items that you need to take a look at:

Foods that contain trans fats. You can recognize trans fats by checking the labels of foods for "hydrogenated" or "partially hydrogenated" fats. You'll find these in many commercially prepared foods such as chips, crackers, cakes, doughnuts, pastries, peanut butter, frozen meals, and margarines and shortenings. You'll also find trans fats in cake, pancake, biscuit and muffin mixes, as well as dips, toppings, nondairy coffee creamers, gravy mixes, and even salad dressings. Trans fats are a health disaster: They boost bad cholesterol and lower good cholesterol, encourage inflammation and thus increase your risk of heart disease and stroke. There are two bits of good news when it comes to trans fats: There has been so much negative attention

Does it feel wasteful to toss that cereal and those bottles of salad dressing? Here are two points that should soothe your conscience: Many of the foods that we store in the fridge and the pantry that contain trans fats and high fructose corn syrup are those that might be past their prime anyhow. Take a look at the expiration dates on the containers. I'm willing to bet that as you collect these foods on the table, you'll find that a number of them are past, maybe way past, their expiration dates.

Here's another point: While you may be tossing out a few dollars worth of food, think for a minute of what you are willing to invest in your own health.

drawn to them recently that trans fats are being banished from many foods by restaurants and food manufacturers. (Cities like New York are leading the charge and banning trans fats in restaurants. Other cities and states are following the Big Apple's example.) So it is becoming easier to avoid trans fats when you eat out. The even better news about trans fats in terms of SuperFoods is that if you're following the SuperFoods plan you don't need to even think about trans fats. All of the SuperFoods are whole foods; none contain artificial trans fats.

Foods that contain high-fructose corn syrup. This includes soft drinks, candy, cookies, pies, fruit drinks, ice cream, pastries, and sweet baked goods like cinnamon rolls. You'll also find HFCS in places where you might not expect them like condiments, frozen desserts, peanut butters, salad dressings, and even ketchup. A friend recently asked me about a recipe she followed for a simple pasta sauce that called for a can of diced tomatoes. When she tasted the sauce she was puzzled by its sweetness. I suggested she check the label on the can of diced tomatoes. Sure enough, she found that it contained high-fructose corn syrup listed in the ingredients just below the Nutrition Facts panel. Many canned goods that you might not expect contain this sweetener, so as you scour your pantry (and of course when you shop), please read labels carefully and avoid buying foods with this ingredient.

High-fructose corn syrup has invaded your kitchen for a reason. It's a bit sweeter and much, much cheaper than cane sugar and for many people it has gradually corrupted their sense of taste until they've become virtually addicted to sweets. We love sweet foods. From infancy we humans are drawn to sweet like bees to the nectar. While this tendency may have been an evolutionary trait that led us to the benefits of the nutrients in certain berries and fruits, it's long outlived its usefulness. Manufacturers have capitalized on our lust for sweetness by lacing our foods with a sweet taste that, for many of us, becomes virtually addictive. Unfortunately, these days high-fructose corn syrup (HFCS) and regular corn syrup substitutes for real sugar. HFCS, a thick liquid sweetener made from cornstarch, first appeared around 1967 and now can be found in countless prepared foods. Intake of HFCS increased 100 percent between '67 and 1990 and its consumption exceeds the changes in intake of any other food or food group.[1]

While there's no documented causal link between HFCS and obesity, we do know that, for example, the metabolism of HFCS differs from the metabolism

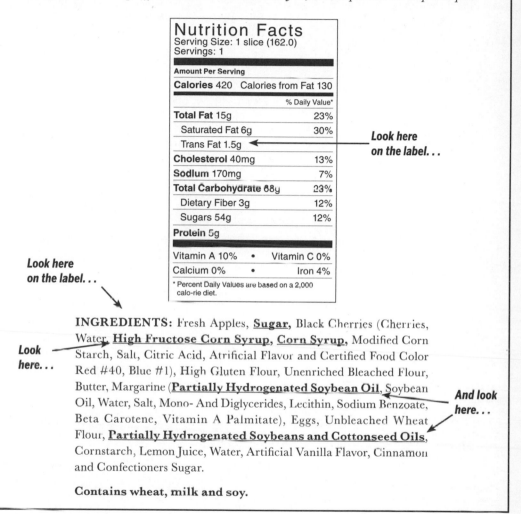

One commercial version of Cherry and Apple Pie

Don't let the enticing ingredients in the name deceive you, look deeper into the deep dish pie!

Nutrition Facts
Serving Size: 1 slice (162.0)
Servings: 1

Amount Per Serving

Calories 420   Calories from Fat 130

	% Daily Value*
Total Fat 15g	23%
Saturated Fat 6g	30%
Trans Fat 1.5g	
Cholesterol 40mg	13%
Sodium 170mg	7%
Total Carbohydrate 68g	23%
Dietary Fiber 3g	12%
Sugars 54g	12%
Protein 5g	

Vitamin A 10%	•	Vitamin C 0%
Calcium 0%	•	Iron 4%

* Percent Daily Values are based on a 2,000 calo-rie diet.

Look here on the label...

Look here on the label...

Look here...

And look here...

INGREDIENTS: Fresh Apples, **Sugar,** Black Cherries (Cherries, Water, **High Fructose Corn Syrup, Corn Syrup,** Modified Corn Starch, Salt, Citric Acid, Atrificial Flavor and Certified Food Color Red #40, Blue #1), High Gluten Flour, Unenriched Bleached Flour, Butter, Margarine (**Partially Hydrogenated Soybean Oil,** Soybean Oil, Water, Salt, Mono- And Diglycerides, Lecithin, Sodium Benzoate, Beta Carotene, Vitamin A Palmitate), Eggs, Unbleached Wheat Flour, **Partially Hydrogenated Soybeans and Cottonseed Oils,** Cornstarch, Lemon Juice, Water, Artificial Vanilla Flavor, Cinnamon and Confectioners Sugar.

Contains wheat, milk and soy.

of glucose. When consumed in large amounts, say by folks who routinely drink regular soda, HFCS seems to favor the creation of fat cells and fat storage. In addition, there is evidence that there may be some disruption of satiation (i.e., the feelings of fullness, of having had enough to eat) signals associated with regular consumption of HFCS. Obviously these two associations are not positive for people who are trying to lose weight.

High-sodium foods. This includes many canned foods particularly soups and some beans, crackers, ramen noodles, many condiments, and many prepared foods. Our appetite for salt is almost as voracious as our appetite for sugar. Salt can mask the lack of real flavor in many manufactured foods. We've become so accustomed to salty foods that we've almost forgotten that real, whole foods—SuperFoods—don't need salt to taste good. It's easy to find sodium on a food label listed in milligrams right on the Nutrition Facts panel, though it can be a bit tricky sometimes to figure out how much is too much.

Remember too that a high-sodium diet, in addition to being implicated in soaring rates of hypertension, can throw a monkey wrench into your efforts at weight control. Sodium makes you retain water and can make you feel bloated and discouraged. It can also, *duh!*, make you thirsty and, if in the past you've relied on sugary drinks to quench your thirst, you can see how sodium can encourage you to consume way too many calories.

Foods that contain added sugars or artificial sweeteners. You know that ice cream and cake have lots of sugar and you're probably well aware that these are not foods that are going to help you lose weight. While sugar is not the enemy, the amount we consume these days is a significant problem. The average American consumes 142 pounds of sugar a year, which is the average healthy weight of a woman standing 5-foot-8! To break it down to a small measure, on a daily basis most of us eat roughly 42 teaspoons of sugar. It's not all in our coffee. Countless packaged foods from sodas to fruit drinks to baked goods and even salad dressings, soups and packaged meal "helpers" contain a version of sugar whether it's called sucrose, dextrose, or maltose on the label. If you're trying to lose weight the added calories of these sweeteners will make your job harder.

Foods that contain artificial sweeteners are the stealth bombers of healthy eating. Food manufacturers have led us to believe that "low cal" is king. How

The Case Against Soft Drinks

Many of us sip them constantly. With meals, with snacks, day and night. But the soft drinks—even the diet drinks—are wreaking havoc with your weight and maybe even your health. For one thing those soft drinks are going right to your hips! They go down fast and they're not even really foods so you may ask, what's the problem? Soft drinks (and sugary juices and other sweetened drinks as well) can create a serious bulge in your total daily calorie intake without much reward in terms of satisfaction. It's pretty shocking to learn that calories from beverages on average account for 1 of every 5 calories in the American diet.[2] Worse news: Soft drinks alone are the source of 33 percent[3] of all added sugars and 7.1 percent of total calories in the American diet.[4] In teens, it's even higher pushing over 12 percent of total calories! Indeed, soft drinks are making a major contribution to our added poundage. Of course, if you cut out the 150 calories—all from sugar—you get in each can of soda from other places in your diet, you'd wind up even in terms of calories (except for the nutrients missed, which is a major minus!) but most people don't do this. Keep in mind that just one soda a day that's not compensated for by some other reduction in your diet can add up to 15 pounds in just 1 year. One interesting study of 15 young adults gave each participant an extra 450 calories a day: For 4 weeks those calories came from soft drinks; for another 4 weeks they came from jelly beans. When the volunteers were on the jelly bean regime they unconsciously cut calories from other sources from their diet. While on the soft drinks, they continued to consume their normal calorie intake and gained an average of $2\frac{1}{2}$ pounds each.[5] Some researchers think that the HFCS—the cheap sweetener used in most sodas—even stimulates appetite. While this link has not been proven, one thing we know for sure: Drink excess calories and you'll gain weight!

People just don't seem to notice calories from soft drinks. Researchers speculate that because the drink travels so quickly through your mouth, there's little time for a signal to get to the brain and alert it that you're consuming calories. Solid food provides more of the feeling of fullness that tells our brain we're full and it's time to stop eating.

Colas may pose their own particular health threats. The Framingham Osteoporosis Study found that women who drank one cola a day—diet or regular—had about a 4 to 5 percent lower hip-bone density than those who drank fewer than one cola a month.[6] We know that cola contains phosphoric acid, which leaches calcium from the bones and this no doubt explains in part this negative outcome associated with excessive, regular soda consumption.

do you achieve low cal? You take out the sugar or HFCS and replace it with an artificial sweetener. Then you can have ice cream or soda or candy or cookies that are "good" for dieters because they satisfy your need for a sweet without adding too many calories. Right? Wrong! In fact, some fascinating studies have concluded that folks who consumed diet soda (sweetened with aspartame in this study) were *more likely to gain weight* over time than those who consumed regular sugar sweetened soda. Indeed, the risk of overweight for those consuming one to two cans of *diet* soda a day was 54.5 percent versus the risk for those consuming *regular* soda which was 32.8 percent. *In fact, for each can of diet soft drink consumed each day, a person's risk of obesity went up 41 percent.*[7] Researchers are not suggesting that drinking diet soda causes obesity but there is no doubt that some connection exists. An interesting study with rats showed that those who were fed artificially sweetened drink along with their food ate more calories and food than another group of rats that had been fed real sugar.[8] We know for sure that since the widespread introduction of artificial sweeteners especially during the low-fat, "low-cal" diet days of the 1980s, the rate of obesity has skyrocketed. While studies linking artificial sweeteners to cancer such as bladder, leukemia, and lymphomas or migraines or other adverse health effects have never been conclusive and although the FDA tells us that artificial sweeteners are generally considered safe (other countries ban them because of their demonstrated health risk in animal studies), my own feeling is that there is enough evidence associating the use of artificially sweetened foods to weight gain and enough unanswered questions about the effects of these chemical substances on our long-term health that they're best avoided.

Aside from any health risk associated with artificial sweeteners there's also the issue of the overall sweetness quotient in the foods you eat. Artificial sweeteners are 200 to 600 times sweeter than sugar. When you regularly consume

It's not just about the calories when it comes to excess sugar in the diet. One recent alarming study showed that the effect of a diet filled with sugary foods can make you up to 70 percent more vulnerable to pancreatic cancer.[9]

Researchers believe this is because a constant flood of sugar puts your pancreas into overdrive as it struggles to produce the insulin your body needs to control elevated sugar in your blood.

foods that are extraordinarily sweet, your taste buds grow accustomed to this extraordinary level of sweetness and then crave it. So take a deep breath and remove the saccharin (Sweet'N Low®—pink); aspartame (Equal®—blue); and sucralose (Splenda®—yellow) from your home and from your daily routine.

Here's one more thought on artificial sweeteners versus sugar: Since the latter has only 16 calories per teaspoon, if you want to use an occasional teaspoon of sugar in a drink or a recipe, go ahead.

Unhealthy oils.
This includes corn oil in particular and most "vegetable" oils. While corn oil is better in some ways that butter or shortening, it still has a less desirable profile in terms of health promotion when compared to olive, canola, and other nut and seed derived oils, for example.

Refined flour and its spawn.
Refined is good in people; bad in flour. Refined white flour (enriched, bleached flour) is not just "lacking the fiber" as many people believe, but it has been stripped of nutrients—by some estimates a full 80 to 90 percent of all the micronutrients that were originally there! When refined, the fiber, antioxidants including vitamin E and selenium, as well as a slew of other key micronutrients like magnesium, zinc, potassium and the B vitamins are stripped right off. More than 50 percent of the thiamin, riboflavin, niacin, pantothenic acid, B6, folate, and vitamin E are lost. By law flour manufacturers have to fortify their refined flour with some of the same nutrients that were milled away. And those fortifications don't include important phytochemicals like lignans, phenolic acids, phytoestrogens, and other key nutrients.

Refined white flour products have no place in your SuperFoods weight loss plan. You'll find it in the flour sack you've got in the pantry and in many common foods like cookies, crackers, baked goods, doughnuts, and so on. You'll be delighted to find that these days there are excellent tasty alternatives to products containing refined white flour. If you bake, *whole grain* pastry or regular flour combined in the appropriate amounts with King Authur's unbleached flour are excellent alternatives. If it's the white color you're going for try "white" whole wheat flour. And the SuperFoods menus and recipes will suggest some delicious options when you're craving a baked treat.

Have you tossed some foods that might have ambushed you? Have you moved out of sight some foods that might be too tempting to avoid? Doesn't

Quickly Distinguish Your Whole Grains from Refined Grains

If the first ingredient listed is "enriched flour" or "enriched wheat," you've got a refined wheat product. Pass these products by and look further for your SuperFoods health.

Identify refined bread labels that will look like one of these two examples:

INGREDIENTS: enriched unbleached flour (flour, malted barley flour, niacin, reduced iron, thiamine mononitrate. . .), corn syrup, salt, . . .
   OR

INGREDIENTS: enriched wheat flour (flour, barley malt, ferrous sulfate. . .),

sweetener (high-fructose corn syrup or sugar), yeast,. . .

If the first ingredient (or second—only if it follows "water" as an ingredient) listed is "whole grain" or "whole wheat," you have a tasty and nutritious whole grain, SuperFoods sidekick. The word "whole" has designer label status in the bread and cracker aisles of your market. Accept no substitutes. Choose these.

Identify whole grain breads that have a label that may resemble this example:

INGREDIENTS: whole wheat flour, water, . . .whole oats. . . yeast,. .

your fresh start feel good? Studies really do show that taking positive steps toward health promotion is reinforcing. Each box of salty, sugary food you toss or tuck away on a high shelf is boosting your motivation and confirming your desire to stick to your goals. And you haven't even come to the fun part yet: restocking your kitchen with the SuperFoods that are going to be the foundation of your whole new fit, trim, and healthy lifestyle.

Step 2: Your SuperFoodsRx Shopathon

It's time to hit the market for the best and most delicious foods that will be the staples of your SuperFoodsRx Diet. These foods are going to be the powerful, delicious tools that help you achieve your weight loss goals without any sense of deprivation. I'm going to list them in two groups for the sake of convenience—pantry staples and fresh/frozen foods. I'm arranging the lists this way because many people find that they do "destination" marketing: They shop for canned goods, for example, at their local supermarket and fresh fruits and vegetables at a farmer's market or other local source.

Obviously, you won't be buying everything you need to eat for the duration of your SuperFoods Diet in one shopping trip! Some of the SuperFoods are fresh foods that should be purchased on a regular basis. But don't think you must be running to the market constantly. If it's difficult to get fresh produce, or if certain choices are out of season in your area, in many instances you'll be able to substitute frozen and canned foods. And of course you'll be buying foods you like! One of the great appeals of the SuperFoods concept is that each SuperFood has sidekicks that give you a range of choices. Unlike many diets, you aren't locked in to particular foods; you'll have a delicious range of choices.

STOP: Choose Your SuperFoodsRx Meal Selections

You're going to be heading to the supermarket but before you do take a moment to check out the SuperFoodsRx Meals on page 188. Your assignment is easy: Choose ONE breakfast, ONE lunch, and ONE dinner that you like as your selections. You're going to eat each of these choices at least once this week. Maybe you'll want to eat them more than once. That's fine. So maybe you'll have the Yogurt with Strawberries breakfast a couple of times (page 189), the Poached Salmon in Spinach Tortilla Wrap lunch twice (page 197) and the Ginger Grilled Turkey Tenderloin dinner once (page 269).

A Note on Coffee. Coffee, like so many foods, can be a healthy choice if you drink it in moderation. That's a big "if" with coffee because so many people use coffee as more of a drug than a food. Here's how I advise clients about coffee: If you drink one cup of coffee a day and it's a part of a satisfying ritual for you and it doesn't have any negative effect on your ability to sleep, then that's fine. If, on the other hand, you grab your first cup running out the door in the morning, your second cup in the car, your third cup mid-afternoon . . . well, you get the picture. If you use coffee as more of a jolt than a pleasure, then it's time to at least cut down if not stop. Some people who quit coffee cold turkey can notice some symptoms, including headaches and irritability, that actually signal caffeine withdrawal. These symptoms will disappear in a few days. If you've been a coffee "addict," try substituting tea—green or black.

Write *your* personal selections here and any ingredients you'll need to add to your Shopathon List:

	Selection	**Ingredients**
Breakfast	_____	_____
	_____	_____
	_____	_____
Lunch	_____	_____
	_____	_____
	_____	_____
Dinner	_____	_____
	_____	_____
	_____	_____

SuperFoodsRx Pantry Staples

Check the SuperFoodsRx Shopping Lists and Guidelines starting on page 331 for specific brand-name suggestions and guidelines for many of the choices below.

- **Plastic storage bags.** These are a dieter's best friend. You'll find they'll save you many, many calories over the coming weeks. If you don't already have some, I recommend you buy three sizes: the snack size, the sandwich size, and the gallon size. The resealable ones keep food fresher.

- **Plastic containers such as Tupperware or glass storage containers with lids.** These are widely available in a variety of sizes. You'll need some relatively small ones for nuts, for example, and some larger ones for fresh cut vegetables like red pepper slices.

- **Beans.** Choose two types of beans you like—kidney, garbanzo, or black beans. You can buy dried beans if you know you'll have time to cook them. If you're buying dried, make sure you patronize a store with good turnover. Old beans can take forever to cook and sometimes never really get tender. If you're choosing canned beans, look for low or no-salt-added varieties.

- **Tea.** Choose green and/or black tea. Try a brand that's new to you. It's nice to have a selection of two or three types of teas to choose from as

D id you know that SuperFoods are a nutritional bargain? Research has demonstrated that nutrient-dense foods—SuperFoods—give the greatest number of nutrients for the least number of calories and the lowest cost. When 637 foods were analyzed using a nutrient-to-price ratio, it was fresh produce—one of the biggest categories of SuperFoods—that was the biggest nutritional bargain (based on daily values for 16 nutrients.)[10] It's good to know that the foods that are keeping your body healthy are also doing their bit for your pocketbook.

you'll be drinking it frequently. Make sure you have enough to tuck a few teabags into your purse or briefcase or to store at your workplace. Take them with you when you travel. You can get a cup of hot water most anywhere, and it's great to have a lovely cup of tea to sip.

- **Canned tomatoes.** Do you like to cook with canned tomatoes? We have some terrific recipes using them that you'll enjoy so pick up a couple of cans. Look for diced or whole tomatoes that are low in sodium. Read the labels carefully to be sure you don't buy tomatoes with added sweetener like high-fructose corn syrup.

- **Nuts.** Choose two or three types of nuts that you enjoy. Walnuts, almonds, and pistachios are three types that are delicious and very versatile. They can be in pieces or whole; it doesn't matter. Be sure to choose unsalted, dry roasted, or raw nuts. Nuts can go rancid so make sure you buy nuts from a store with a rapid turnover.

- **Breakfast cereals.** If you are choosing a SuperFoods breakfast that features a cereal, put that cereal on your list. If you're going to choose oatmeal I'd suggest in order of preference: steel-cut oatmeal, long-cooking oatmeal, instant oatmeal. Avoid any oatmeal varieties that have added fruit, flavoring, or sugar. You'll be adding your own. Do buy some 1-ounce instant oatmeal packets. They sure help when you're on the go and really help keep that portion control in check!

- **Oils.** Extra-virgin olive oil. You may also want to buy grapeseed and/or canola oil. Buy your oils in small quantities and store away from light and heat.

Use Your Bean. Beans are an important part of the SuperFoodsRx Diet and they're a fantastic cupboard staple. They're inexpensive and they can sit in the back of the pantry until you need an instant soup, dip, salad, or main course. Probably the best beans are those you cook yourself after soaking because their texture is usually best and they'll be the lowest in sodium. But, if you're short on time, canned beans are an excellent substitute. Given the power of beans to help you lose weight I think it's important to find a brand you like if you don't already have one. Here's an exercise I recommend: Find the two beans that you like best, say garbanzo and black beans. Select two or three brands of those beans in the smallest can size available. When you get them home open them all, rinse them and taste them. You will probably find one brand that you think is superior. That's your brand! This experiment will cost you just a few dollars but it's a good investment in your health if it encourages you to frequently add beans to your diet.

Yogurt. Choose plain low fat or nonfat yogurt. Look for hormone-free and organic if it's available and affordable. You'll add your own fixins'. I even have my favorite blueberry compote recipe for you on page 238 so you can create your own version of "fruit on the bottom" yogurt.

Canned pumpkin. Be sure you don't choose pumpkin pie mix, which has sugar and other ingredients in it. You want plain, canned pumpkin.

Soy milk. Scan the SuperFoods Meals to see if you'll be using soy milk. Many people find it's an excellent and healthy change from cow's milk on oatmeal or cereal. (Remember that each quart of milk, even nonfat milk, contains 12 grams of sugar.) Try a few brands—Silk, Organic Eden, Trader Joe's, Costco (organic), Soy Dream, VitaSoy are popular and tasty—until you find one you prefer. Look for a variety that's low in fat and sugar. Look for no more than 10 grams of sugar per serving; less than or equal to 7 is better. And give the unsweetened varieties a try—they are really tasty and the sugar is reduced, while the protein tends to be a little higher in an equal volume. As your taste buds acclimate to a naturally flavored diet, you will find sweetness in places you never imagined.

🌿 **Miscellaneous spices, salad dressings, and condiments.**
I've provided some recipes and suggestions for delicious salad dressings
on pages 307–312. I also like to keep on hand a selection of dried herbs
and spices as well as some no-salt seasoning blends for instant flavor
enhancement. Here are some seasonings you can find in your local grocery store that I use frequently:

- Italian Seasoning (salt free)—The Spice Hunter
- Herbes de Provence (salt free)—The Spice Hunter
- Citrus Herb (salt free)—Spice Islands
- Mrs. Dash®—Garlic and Herb
- Red Pepper (ground cayenne)—The Spice Hunter

SuperFoodsRx Fresh Choices

🌿 **Vegetable snacks.** For your prep week you're going to choose one or two
SuperFoods vegetable snacks that you enjoy. Baby carrots are a great choice.
Bell pepper slices are terrific. Cherry tomatoes are the ultimate "poppables."

🌿 **Fruit snacks.** Oranges are your SuperFoods fruit of choice for the Prep
Week as well as the SlimDown. If you prefer you could substitute sidekicks including tangerines, kumquats or white or pink grapefruit. Apples
are another excellent, readily available, and tasty choice. Choose one or
two of these items.

🌿 **Fresh vegetables.** Your prime fresh vegetables this week are going to
be spinach, broccoli, tomatoes, and their sidekicks (see page 3). Choose
those you like for your Prep Week and be sure that you've listed those
that you may need for the SuperFoods Meal choices that you've made.

🌿 **Blueberries,** fresh or frozen. If you're lucky enough to have fresh blueberries available in your market or blueberry sidekicks such as strawberries, purple grapes, raspberries, or cherries then you should stock up on
these treats. You'll be enjoying them for breakfast and in various recipes.
Remember that frozen berries—be sure they have no added sugar—are
excellent substitutes for fresh.

🗸 **Turkey and/or its sidekick, skinless chicken breast.** Depending on what appeals to you in the SlimDown menus, you can choose fresh or frozen skinless breasts, nitrate-free and nitrite-free deli slices, cutlets, or lean ground meat. Applegate Farms sells a very nice variety of tasty turkey slices and Honeysuckle White brand has a fat-free sliced turkey available at deli counters.

🗸 **Salmon and its sidekicks** are top choices but unless you're relying on frozen fish, you'll be buying it the day or the day before you prepare it. Canned salmon, on the other hand, can always be available in your pantry. Most canned salmon is wild. Look for low or no-sodium-added varieties. Vital Choice brand offers a good selection.

Your SuperFoodsRx Shopping List

- Plastic storage bags
- Plastic or glass containers with lids
- Beans
- Canned tomatoes
- Canned pumpkin
- Blueberries and their sidekicks
- Oatmeal
- Tea—green and/or black
- Nuts
- Extra virgin olive oil
- Yogurt
- Soy milk
- Baby carrots
- Bell pepper
- Oranges
- Spinach
- Broccoli
- Cherry and larger tomatoes and their sidekicks
- Turkey or chicken, skinless breast meat
- Salmon
- Spices
- Garlic
- Fresh herbs
- Salad dressings
- Ingredients for the 3 SuperFoodsRx meals you chose on page 108.

Setting Up Your SuperFoods

You're back from the market and your kitchen table is cluttered with bags. Here are some kitchen setup tips.

- Nuts should be stored in a cool spot. If you have a large quantity, it's best to store them in the freezer in a heavy plastic bag. Smaller amounts can go into a small plastic storage container to keep in the fridge.

- Remember those snacks—the oranges, apples, bell peppers, baby carrots, and cherry tomatoes? You aren't going to just shove them into the crisper! You're going to prep the foods (wash them, slice the peppers, quarter the oranges) and put them in clear storage containers *at eye level* in the fridge. Need a snack? You're all set!

- Fresh vegetables go into the crisper. The exception to the crisper rule is tomatoes, which should be stored on the countertop to retain flavor and texture. Don't wash your vegetables until you're ready to use them because excess moisture on them can cause mold.

- Frozen foods of course go into the freezer.

- Turkey or chicken breast, if fresh, go in the coldest part of the fridge if you're going to eat them in a day or two; if not, store them in the freezer.

- The canned foods—pumpkin, tomato, beans, and such—go into the pantry. I usually mark the date purchased on the top of cans with a permanent marker so I can use the older purchases first.

Fresh Versus Frozen. These days frozen fruits and vegetables can often be as tasty and nutritious as fresh. And of course they're often far more convenient. If you're craving a vegetable that's out of season or not readily available in your area, don't hesitate to buy a frozen version. Just be very careful that you're not buying frozen fruits or veggies with added ingredients like sodium or high-fructose corn syrup. Manufacturers have caught on that we're looking for convenience and they've found lots of enticing ways to package fruits and vegetables—sometimes even with health claims on the packages. But read the labels! You'll often find long list of added ingredients and these "convenience" foods are to be avoided. Stick to simple, unadorned frozen options. They're the best for your health and your taste buds.

Some of my clients like to decorate the fridge with notes, photos, and tips that keep them going when the going gets tough. Here are a few examples that they've shared with me:

- Notes with reminders like: Do you really want to eat that? Don't forget to put that in your food diary! Are you really hungry?

- Photos: of themselves looking trim, fit, and happy or of a reward to look forward to when a certain goal is reached.

One client told me she had a photo of her children with a little text box that said "You're doing great, Mom!" A glance at the photo made her smile and reminded her of the importance of her food goals, making it easier for her to stick to them.

Step 3: Your SuperFoodsRx Kitchen SlimDown

"It's hard work to change the way you eat and put activity into your life. There's no magic pill or remedy. But it's amazing how fast you feel the benefits, rewards, and peace of mind from this diet. I'm doing it one day at a time and I'm not letting anything or anyone distract me. I'm doing it for me."
—Lynn M., wife and stay-at-home mom

Focusing on eating the SuperFoods is going to be your expressway to effective long-term weight loss. But if you want to get in the fast lane, make your kitchen work for you. You've probably been living with cues to overeat and impediments to limit food intake that have made it ever more difficult for you to lose weight. Research shows that we are generally unaware of how many decisions we make about eating in the course of an average day and second, we are unaware of the influence our environment—our kitchens—have on these decisions.[11] All the distractions to a healthy eating plan take a measurable toll on your ability to make good choices and achieve success.

Here are some tips on how to make your kitchen your SlimDown friend. It's really important that you make your environment as positive as possible to help you reach your goals.

Consider downsizing your dinnerware. How big are your dinner plates? Many people have huge, Frisbee-sized plates that are invitations to overindulge. In one interesting study at Cornell researchers asked nutrition professors, grad students, and department staff members to serve themselves to ice cream. Some of these folks got large bowls and others small bowls; some large spoons and others small spoons. The large-bowl contingent served themselves 31 percent more than those who got the smaller bowl. And the

Cues to Overeat[12]

They can vary depending on the person, setting, or circumstance, but here are a few of the more common cues to tune into:

- **Variety**—Too much variety can actually create impulses to overeat. Multiple types of food, flavors, and textures in the food can create interest, but also an impulse to overeat in some instances. And how about those buffets we've all been to. Have you ever said, "I'll just try a little bit of everything"? What happens when there are 20 little bits versus 7 versus 4 to try?

- **Alcohol**—When there is a variety of foods to choose from, consuming alcohol appears to increase choices for higher fat and calorie foods. This is once reason aside from calories that alcohol can become such a diet trap.

- **Social settings**—Be aware that eating with family and friends can influence or inspire overeating if you're not careful and committed to your own goals. Eating with others tends also to extend the duration of meal and provide a more pleasurable eating environment versus eating alone.

- **Distraction**—Television, eating while at the computer, doing multiple things at once with food being one of them are major triggers for overeating.

- **Emotion**—Many individuals overeat in response to emotions like stress, anxiety/nervousness, depression, and boredom.

- **Situational cues**—In addition to those already listed above, some people find there are specific personal situations where they are inclined to overeat. It's important and very helpful to think about and identify them so you can take charge when they are present.

when they used a larger scoop plus a large bowl the people served themselves a whopping 57 percent more ice cream than the small bowl plus small spooners. Most interestingly, the large-bowl folks—and remember, these study participants were nutrition professionals—didn't think they had served themselves more than the small bowl people.[13] The implications of this are clear: If you use a large plate, you'll fill a large plate and you'll eat most everything on your plate. Consider it a law of consumption. So the goal is to use smaller plates. But let's be realistic about this. Some folks recommend that you use an appetizer-sized plate, which is surely counterproductive: It's just too small and you'll either go back for seconds or pile it so high that it's actually awkward to eat from it. I recommend you simply downsize to a 9- or 10-inch dinner plate from the common 12- or 13-inch plates. Your healthy portions will fit comfortably on the plate and you won't feel deprived. Put your SlimDown-sized plates in the front of the cabinet where you can readily grab them. What about that huge tub you refer to as your cereal bowl? Many people get in the habit of eating a massive amount of "healthy" cereal because their bowl is so big! Take those huge bowls and stack them up on high shelves. Find some bowls that are pretty and smaller—bowls that will make an appropriate serving of cereal or yogurt look comfortable.

Time for Some Measure Magic. This will take you back to your elementary school science days. It's a fun and truly valuable exercise and I strongly recommend that you do it during the Prep & Practice Week because it's an important step in retraining your eye (and ultimately your stomach) to appreciate appropriate serving sizes. If you can't actually see it in front of you, it's just theory. Take a bowl—it can be a giant tub if you're accustomed to using that—and put your typical amount of morning cereal in it. Go ahead: Pour it in. Now take a measuring cup and see how much you've poured. Check the label to see what a serving size is according to the package and now put that amount in the bowl. Most people are shocked to realize that they've been doubling and tripling their serving sizes. Do the same thing with pasta. You can do it with uncooked elbow macaroni if you don't have any cooked pasta around. Pour the amount of macaroni you'd typically eat for dinner into a bowl. Measure. Now, check to see what the serving size should actually be. Read about portion control starting on page 33 and you'll learn more amazing facts about why losing weight may have been so difficult for you in the past.

Arrange your SlimDown bowls in easy reach in your cupboard

- Make your fridge your friend. Keep those clear containers with snack veggies in a place of prominence. Keep some fresh fruit right up front. Check your crispers regularly so they don't become science experiments. Keep your water—whether it's seltzer, a pitcher of cool water, or serving size bottles of water—in easy reach.

- Fruit bowl as art. Consider making a glass bowl or pretty basket a feature of your countertop. Fill it with fresh fruits like oranges, lemons, and apples that don't need refrigeration. It will be a pleasing visual reminder of your goals and an encouragement to enjoy fruit daily.

If you work in an office it will be well worth the effort to SlimDown your workplace. The good news is that more and more people are eager to upgrade the food options and temptations at school and work. I recently spoke with a teacher who told me that her elementary school was making a concerted effort to improve the children's food choices at lunch and at snacktime. It quickly became apparent that it was important for the teachers to serve as examples to their students so no more cookies and candies in the teachers' lounge! Everyone is benefiting from the new standards. If your workplace is filled with food traps, you can at least rid your own area of these temptations and substitute healthy choices. Get rid of that bag of M&MS in your bottom desk drawer and substitute individual serving-size bags (or one individual serving bag if more is too tempting) of nuts and dried fruit for snacking. Make sure you have an ample supply of green and black tea on hand. Keep some baby carrots and pepper slices in the office fridge. If you can, you might even find a SuperFoods buddy at work who will take a walk with you at lunch and distract you when the coffee cart is tempting.

Look Ahead to Your SlimDown

Here's your last task before you begin your SuperFoods SlimDown next week:

Using the chart on pages 118–119, fill out your meal selections for next week. Make sure you have all the SuperFoods on hand to take you through a week. Plan your shopping so that you know you'll be able to buy any fresh foods—salmon, for example—when you'll need them.

Weekly Plan

	MONDAY	TUESDAY	WEDNESDAY
Date			
Breakfast			
SuperNutrient Booster	SuperNutrient Booster	SuperNutrient Booster	SuperNutrient Booster
Lunch	*With Without*	*With Without*	*With Without*
	Soup & Salad		
Snack			
Dinner	*With Without*	*With Without*	*With Without*
Special Notes	Soup & Salad Monday		Veggie Wednesday
Comments... **Exercise** 　**Activity:** 　**Duration:** 　**Steps:** **How are you feeling?**			

THURSDAY	FRIDAY	SATURDAY	SUNDAY
SuperNutrient Booster	SuperNutrient Booster	SuperNutrient Booster	SuperNutrient Booster
With *Without*	*With* *Without*	*With* *Without*	*With* *Without*
With *Without*	*With* *Without*	*With* *Without*	*With* *Without*
	Don't forget—lunch and dinner are ALWAYS interchangeable.		Prepare for the Week Ahead.

Sample Shopping List

Jot down your own personalized shopping list on a sheet of paper now. Here's a sample:

	MENU	SHOPPING LIST
Breakfast	Yogurt with berries	Nonfat plain yogurt Fresh or frozen blueberries or strawberries
	Oatmeal	Long-cook oats or 1-ounce instant packets
	Cereal	Two good choices are Kashi® GOLEAN® or Nature's Path® Optimum Power®
Lunch	Asian Broccoli Salad with Asian Inspired Red Pepper Sesame Dressing Side of Quinoa	**Salad:** • Broccoli (head) • Carrots • 15-ounce can hearts of palm • Medium red bell pepper • 10-ounce can mandarin oranges • Toasted soy nuts (or sliced almonds) **Dressing:** • Rice wine vinegar • Low-sodium soy sauce or Bragg's Liquid Aminos • Sesame Oil • Grapeseed Oil • Ground red pepper (cayenne) • Scallions (bunch) **Side:** • Quinoa (or brown rice can be alternative)
Dinner	Ginger Grilled Turkey Tenderloin with Medium SuperFoodsRx Salad	**Entrée:** • ½ pound turkey breast tenderloin (skinless, boneless) • Rice wine vinegar • Low-sodium soy sauce or Bragg's Liquid Aminos • Ginger (fresh) • Red pepper flakes • Peanut oil or other nut or seed oil (sesame or olive oil) **Salad:** • Bag of spinach or romaine • Baby carrots • Cucumber • Raisins (bulk or mini ½-ounce boxes) • Salad dressing (SuperFoods approved or home-made—can use same dressing from lunch!)

Step 4: Practice! What Do I Eat This Week?

Congratulations! You've taken the first, exciting step to a new you. You're better prepared than you've ever been to meet the challenge of a healthy lifestyle. It feels good, doesn't it? Your kitchen is now a new, healthy, welcoming place. You've done the prep; now it's time to practice.

What, exactly, does "practice" mean? Life is practice. You're making countless decisions every day about numerous issues that involve everything from what you should wear, how you spend time with friends and family, and how you can best accomplish your daily obligations. If you did the same thing, ate the same thing, wore the same thing every day, life would be much simpler. And, of course, far more boring. But making the right decisions that will lead you to your goal isn't always easy. It takes practice. That's why this first week of our new eating plan incorporates some practice as well as prep. You're going to practice your new eating skills.

Your eating this week will follow the basic SuperFoodsRx philosophy: It's more about what you should *include* than what you should *avoid*. This week the emphasis will be on introducing some of the SuperFoods into your regular rotation while you try and make SuperFoods in general the backbone of your diet. You learned about portion sizes in chapter 2 and it's important to review that. (Most clients are astounded by what they learn about portions!) You're not going to worry too much about particular recipes this week (except the three SuperFoods recipes that you've chosen for the week) or about calories or menu plans. You're just going to focus on *upgrading* your choices: getting more of the great foods that pay big dividends and removing foods that don't help (and may even hurt) you.

All SuperFoods, All the Time!

SuperFoods are the backbone of this eating plan. They're delicious, readily available and have proven their worth as among the most nutritious foods on the planet. They're going to be the foods you focus on this week on the Prep, next week on the SlimDown and, I hope, for the rest of your life. Once you begin to eat them regularly, you'll become a SuperFoods convert. And remember that each of the SuperFoods has "sidekicks," which are foods with a similar nutrient profile. One of the delights of eating SuperFoods is that if you don't like one, you probably will like one of its sidekicks. If you're not crazy about pumpkin, or want to take a break from it, grab some carrots or a sweet potato.

Prep & Practice Week Foods to Avoid

Here is a handy list of the foods that you're going to avoid on the SuperFoodsRx Diet. Try to start eliminating them from your diet on the Prep & Practice Week:

- White bread (any bread other than whole grain)
- Cookies
- Cakes & pastries
- Doughnuts
- Candy
- Ice cream
- Soft drinks
- Salty snacks like pretzels, chips, popcorn
- White rice
- All fried foods
- All fast foods

Step 5: Hydrate!

Did you know that increasing the amount of water you drink can be one of the easiest ways to help lose weight? Beginning immediately you're going to reform your fluid intake. It's easy to do and you'll see immediate benefits. Remember the SuperFoods Glow we talked about in the Introduction? Here's where it's going to begin. During the Prep & Practice Week you're going to begin to drink six glasses of water daily. That's at least 48 ounces. You're going to start first thing in the morning and continue, consciously, through-out the day to sip water. You're also going to increase your green and black tea consumption. You can have it iced or hot, with or without lemon. I'd like you to avoid added sweeteners but if you need to wean yourself from sweet drinks you can use just a bit of sugar or honey to start.

Why do fluids matter so much? Over the years our pattern of fluid con-sumption has shifted. Today, too many of us are drinking fluids that are high in calories like sodas and juices. Indeed, research has shown that adults today are drinking about 20 ounces more caloric beverages a day[14]. In fact, caloric beverages now make up 21 percent[15] of our total calorie intake and sodas and fruit drinks alone account for 43 percent[16] of our total added sugars in the diet (18 of those 42 teaspoons of sugar we eat daily!). That adds up to a tre-mendous number of calories in a year. And unfortunately most of us don't count those calories. Moreover, because liquids are less filling than solid foods, those high-cal drinks aren't even satisfying. By skipping the mocha frappuccinos and substituting a glass of water or club soda with lemon or lime, you'll reach your weight-loss goals a lot faster. One study found that dieters who replaced virtually all sweetened drinks with water lost an average of 5 pounds more in a year than those who did not. Moreover, those who drank more than four cups of water a day lost an additional 2 pounds com-pared to dieters who did not drink that much.[17]

Not only will you eliminate all the calories of other drinks when you sub-stitute water, you may also improve your health, your mind and your metab-olism. As little as 2 to 3 percent dehydration during aerobic exercise has been shown to increase cardiovascular strain and impair normal heart function-ing, impair cognitive performance including short-term memory and concen-tration, as well as alter metabolism.[18] Though not all research supports the idea that water can actually *increase* metabolism, one study did show a tempo-rary increase in metabolism by as much as 30 percent for a temporary time (approximately 30–40 minutes) after 16 ounces of water were consumed lead-ing to an additional 24 calories burned.[19] While this finding may have more to do more with overall hydration status, water has been shown to affect and alter metabolism. If what the researchers showed applied to you, the scientists estimated that this could mean if you drank about seven cups (51 ounces) of

We don't want to pick on any particular coffee emporium but do you have any idea how many calories are in some of those blended coffee drinks? The Caffè Vanilla Frappuccino® drink at one popular chain packs a staggering caloric wallop: 320 calories plus 10 grams of fat (6 of them saturated fat). That's for the smallest size!

water a day you could theoretically burn an extra 48 daily calories—equivalent of 17,400 calories, or about 5 pounds over the course of a year. I suggest you check on your current daily water consumption. If you're not getting at least four cups a day, you could benefit from eliminating any sweetened beverages and upping your intake, aiming for six-plus daily cups of water.

Step 6: Your Prep & Practice Food Diary

Your Prep Week is the best time to begin your Food Diary, which you read about in the previous chapter, the SlimDown. Your Prep Week SuperFoodsRx food diary is just practice. Don't be hard on yourself; just be honest. The point of beginning your diary in your Prep & Practice Week is threefold: it will help you find a format that works for you; it will get you in the habit of recording your food choices; and finally, and perhaps most significantly, it will give you an overview of your food choice patterns. You'll be able to learn the answers to some very important questions and these answers will help you personalize your SuperFoodsRx Diet. For example:

- Do you eat when stressed?
- Do you "graze" all day?
- Do you overeat while watching TV?
- Do you nibble when bored?
- Are you "starving"' for a snack at 4:00 p.m.?

It's amazing how many of us are oblivious to our own diet downfalls. If you don't recognize that your conviction—some call it willpower—does a vanishing act at 10:00 p.m. or you're desperate for a sweet every afternoon or you can't cook without "tasting" a meal's worth of calories, you can't prepare for it.

Your food diary should be honest. You need to look squarely at what you're eating so you can deal with both the good and the not so good. You can't change your behavior if you're not sure what your behavior is. You diary will be an amazingly effective tool that will help you see patterns in your eating habits. It really will change they way you view your daily diet. You will no longer be a "mindless" eater. Even when you get to the point where you don't record daily you'll still retain a consciousness that what you're eating *counts.* This sense of the value of your choices will give the stamina you need to live your new healthy lifestyle.

PostScript to Prep and Practice Week

Congratulations! You've laid a terrific foundation for your new SuperFoodsRx lifestyle. You now feel empowered and eager to begin your SlimDown. You have one more bit of housekeeping to take care of first:

- Check the meal listings starting on page 89 for your SlimDown and make your selections.

- Make a shopping list of the foods you'll need for your personal Slim-Down and make sure you have them on hand so that your first week on your new SuperFoodsRx lifestyle will be a resounding success.

Chapter 5

The SuperFoodsRx Diet FlexPlan

Welcome to your FlexPlan—your strategic guide to healthy everyday eating and continued weight loss in the real world. You can expect to see steady and continued weight loss on the FlexPlan. Most dieters continue to lose 1 to 3 pounds a week on the FlexPlan.

....

The SuperFoodsRx Diet FlexPlan is not a quick hello and good-bye. Unlike most diets that abandon you after a period of time or after you reached a certain weight, the FlexPlan will be your eating style forever. And that's a good thing! First of all, you already know the drill. If you've completed at least 2 weeks on the SlimDown and maybe more, you know the basic tenets of the FlexPlan. The only real change, as you cycle into this second phase of The SuperFoodsRx Diet, is that you can now slot extra food choices into your weekly meal plan and still enjoy continued success. This could be a dessert or perhaps wine with dinner or perhaps cheese and crackers at a friend's house or just an extra snack in the afternoon. Or maybe you've got a cocktail party scheduled and you want to try one of the pigs in a blanket. The Flex-Plan is all about adding those foods you love to a diet that's already working for you. The FlexPlan will give you strategies to incorporate these extras into your life without finding yourself on the slippery slope to a diet disaster. So the FlexPlan will support you while you continue to lose weight eating healthy foods and enjoying an occasional "extra."

Your rate of weight loss on this phase of the diet will depend on you and your choices as there's a certain amount of flexibility built in. One SuperFoodsRx dieter, a 51-year-old middle school librarian, lost a total of 30 pounds and 4 inches from her waist after 10 weeks on the diet. Another woman, a 43-year-old mom, has enjoyed slower results. She lost just over 26 pounds after 16 weeks on the diet but by then she was within 9 pounds of her goal (she has since hit her goal and is maintaining!). She commented that even though her weight loss had slowed toward the goal, the important thing is that she's stuck to the diet through various major family events and life transitions. For her, the flexibility of the FlexPlan allows her to continue dieting and moving forward even though she had not been as stringent as she'd expected to be.

Here's why the FlexPlan is going to be the eating plan you can succeed with indefinitely. Most diets are notoriously temporary. You go on them, lose weight and then go off them. Once you're "off" a diet, you tend to revert to whatever your old eating habits were and too often these very habits are what allowed you to gain excess weight in the first place. This process is terribly discouraging and demoralizing. But don't worry: that's not going to happen this time. You're going to continue enjoying all the wonderful health benefits of the SuperFoods while you continue to lose weight and inches. You'll still lose steadily, although not as quickly as you did on the SlimDown but you will be able to enjoy special occasions, travel—any change in your routine that used to derail your best eating intentions.

Some people cycle regularly back and forth in 2-week sessions between the SlimDown and the FlexPlan until they reach their final goal. Others stay on the SlimDown until they meet their interim goal (see page 42). Still others create their own personal SuperFoodsRx Diet schedule. That's the beauty of this plan: You make it work for you—for your lifestyle and your tastes.

Managing Moderation

We all know we should eat in moderation. But that word seems to mean different things to different people. The FlexPlan will show you how to live happily with a level of moderation that's right for you. You've worked hard on the SlimDown and have no doubt made progress but the hard part is learning how to continue to eat healthfully once you're on a less restrictive plan. It's interesting how many of us who struggle with weight can live with restrictions for a while to achieve a goal but find it far more challenging to manage choices when the restrictions are lifted. When it comes to dieting, many of us tend to be all-or-nothing types. It's been my routine experience working with dieters that they are very willing to closely follow a well-designed eating plan for a period of time but the hard part comes from worrying about what to do when the time comes to go "off" the plan. That's what the SuperFoodsRx Diet is about. Giving you the tools and strategies to be flexible and successful with your weight goals for life. You're never "off" this plan, nor will you want to be!

> The FlexPlan in a tiny nutshell—perhaps a pistachio shell—is simply integrating the strategic elements of the SlimDown with specific planned added options of *your choice*.

Here's one way to look at it: You used to live in the black-and-white world of "dieting." You had your "on the diet" restrictive days and your "not on the diet" free-for-all days. There was no in between. Those days are over. Welcome to the world of vibrant, rich color blending one day to the next. The SlimDown is all the colors of the rainbow—blueberries, red peppers, orange carrots, green leafies—and the FlexPlan is all those colors *plus* . . . your choice! A luscious mug of chocolaty steaming cocoa? A bowl of juicy red watermelon? Perhaps a forkful or two of luscious raspberry pie shared with friends at a restaurant? They're all part of your FlexPlan if you so choose. You're painting your own picture of the "fit you" and you're adding the finishing touches.

So let's get started on the FlexPlan.

The FlexPlan encourages you to add five choices—Flexes—in the course of a week to your SuperFoods SlimDown meals and snacks. You can fit your Flexes in anywhere in the week as long as you space them so that you don't have more than two in any one day. Why are they spaced like this? Because people tell me that when they have the option to add five additional foods to their plan over a 7-day period it feels absolutely luxurious. It makes it easy to stick with the plan because it's satisfying, both physically and emotionally, to have the freedom to include personal favorites in a planned way. The common response from

SuperFoodsRx dieters is that these additions seem generous, and some people have even commented that they are shocked that they can make these choices and still comply with a weight-loss plan.

So many people have told me that they've lived with frustration, trying to make healthy choices but struggling in the absence of clear guidelines on which "variations" from a healthy plan are appropriate and which are too much. What's the solution? In the past it was dieting or non-dieting—that all-or-nothing approach. But now on the SuperFoodsRx FlexPlan, while you could say you are *limiting* yourself to five Flexes a week, a better way to think of it is that you are also *allowing* yourself five Flexes in the week—no guilt, all pleasure—and this will help you stay on track overall with the guidelines of the eating plan. It also reduces the likelihood that you'll experience any increase in cravings since if you want something, you can *have* it—with a plan of action. Of course, your Flexes should be healthy and nutritious, relying heavily on the SuperFoods and their sidekicks, but in fact you can choose any food you'd like, as long as your selection is less than 150 calories. This is the only time in the SuperFoodsRx Diet that you need to pay any attention to calories and, if you stick with the list of suggested Flexes, you'll *never* have to count a calorie.

So first we'll look at the FlexPlan Guidelines, which are really virtually identical to the SlimDown Guidelines though now you can be more inventive if you desire, so long as you follow the portion control and SuperFoods categories 1, 2, 3, *plus* the addition of your personal Flex choices scattered as you like throughout your week:

You should feel right at home with these general guidelines. That's the beauty of the diet that becomes your lifestyle: You've practiced it and it's just what you *do*—comfortably and easily. The only difference now is the addition of the FlexPlan Options, so let's take a look at how they work.

Here is how the FlexPlan differs from the SlimDown:

FlexPlan Options

There are three options in your FlexPlan:

- The FlexPlan Flexes
- The FlexPlan "2 for 1" Options
- The FlexPlan Exercise Options

Each of these options gives you an opportunity to choose additional foods and beverages—called *Flexes*—beyond the basic structure of your diet. They've been chosen because they're generally healthy foods and they're in portion sizes that fall within caloric guidelines that will support continued weight loss and healthy weight management over the long run.

- **The FlexPlan Flexes** You can choose any five Flexes to add any time in your week but preferably they should be planned so that you have no more than two in one day and no more than two in one meal. Why? Because you don't want to make the mistake of adding too much in one day and then finding yourself in an all-or-nothing frame of mind tomorrow. You'll feel wonderfully self-indulgent *and* successful adding 1 or 2 Flexes in a given day, I guarantee it. So, for example, you might choose as your 5 Flexes to have ½ cup of fruit sorbet for dessert, a biscotti with your tea, an extra ¾ cup of pasta, an energy bar, and a glass of wine. But these would be spaced throughout your week. As much as possible, you would plan ahead where to incorporate these when you make up your Weekly Menu Plan, but of course you could deviate from your plan on a whim as long as you stayed within the portion guidelines and the general recommendations. You could grab a glass of wine one evening or a Super-Foods Blueberry Oatmeal muffin one morning—two Flexes from the list—or you could decide to simply share a spoonful or two of a chocolate mousse dessert while dining with friends. For a complete list of these FlexPlan Flexes, see page 135.

- **The FlexPlan "2 for 1" Options** is a list of foods that you can choose to include in your weekly plan, the same as the regular Flexes, but at double the rate. It's like bargain shopping: Every 2 items from the "2 for 1"

What is a **Flex**? A Flex is your choice for adding something to your overall healthy and nutritious SuperFoodsRx diet plan. It is in addition to your well-planned portion controlled meals. A Flex is individual and is what you want and enjoy in your life. You choose 5 Flexes every week on the FlexPlan—which can be from the Flexes lists themselves and/or a combination of the Flexes, the "2 for 1s," and the Exercise options.

lists counts as 1 of your 5 Flexes for the week. You can have 2 items together or simply add them individually however you want! Each "2 for 1" counts on it's own as $\frac{1}{2}$ a Flex. So one of your "2 for 1" Options could include an extra slice of bread to make your half a turkey sandwich into a whole sandwich complete with two slices of bread (of course the amount of turkey will remain the same). Or perhaps you'd prefer two Lindt® mini chocolate squares and a nonfat cappuccino to enjoy together ($\frac{1}{2} + \frac{1}{2} = 1$ of your 5 Flexes). See how simple it is? If you selected *only* from the "2 for 1" Options in a given week, you would have a total of 10 extra food selections to add to your menu plan. As you can see, the whole point of the FlexPlan is to be able to choose those foods *you* enjoy within certain guidelines. Most people mix and match, choosing selections from both the "2 for 1" and the regular Flexes. You might include one of your Flexes one day at a meal, another Flex during the week alongside a planned snack, and yet another of the five Flexes just because you feel like it at any time you choose. Just remember that planning and keeping track are important elements in success with flexibility. There's no one monitoring you but you! See page 141 for a complete list of the FlexPlan "2 for 1" Options.

FlexPlan Exercise Options includes exercise equivalents for various food choices so that you can "burn off" some foods if you'd like. Again, you have to stay within general guidelines: This isn't an opportunity to eat *anything* and make up for it with exercise. Rather it's a great opportunity to see how you can occasionally balance your activity levels with some extra food. To take advantage of the Exercise Options you must have already met your overall exercise goals. So in order to include one or two maximum extra Flexes in your Weekly Menu Plan, you would

No "Cheating" and No Guilt. These are two notions I'd like you to banish from your mind. There is no "cheating" and no "guilt" on the SuperFoodsRx Diet. The primary and guiding focus is healthy SuperFoods and their sidekicks but any food that's eaten in an appropriate amount—which is just a little if it's a bit of dark chocolate and a generous bowl if it's a luscious green salad—is fine. What if you're at a party or special occasion and you overdo it with, say, cake or chicken wings? Well, you just dust yourself off and get back on the plan. Maybe you'll be motivated to get in some extra walking. Or maybe, if you're on the FlexPlan, you'll forgo one or two of your options. But it's really nothing to make a major issue of. Sometimes we overdo it when exercising, sometimes when eating, sometimes when dancing at a wedding. The sun will still come up the next day and the SuperFoods will be there. Adjust your Weekly Menu Plan and move on.

have to add exercise over and above your basic daily and weekly goals of 45 to 60 minutes on five or more days weekly. You can use this strategy to add 1 or 2 maximum additional Flexes to your week for a grand total of 6–7 weekly. The food choices that you can select from if you want to use the Exercise Option are those in the basic Flexes although you could also choose from the "2 for 1" lists if you prefer. For a complete list of the FlexPlan Exercise Options, see page 154.

Plan, Plan, Plan

The promise of this phase of the SuperFoodsRx Diet is flexibility. That's the "Flex" part. But the crucial element is the "Plan" part. You've no doubt done well on the SlimDown because it's carefully calibrated to promote rapid weight loss. Your belt is probably looser and you're enjoying the positive feeling of control and accomplishment. Congratulations! Let's remember now, as you phase into the FlexPlan, that a big part of what helped you succeed on the SlimDown was *planning.* You looked ahead to your week and slotted in meals

> Using the FlexPlan changes everything. I don't see my extras as 'cheats' anymore, but 'choices'.—D. S., 42-year-young business-woman

and snacks and exercise. Planning is a critical component of success in weight control. So while you're going to be able to choose and enjoy additional foods on the FlexPlan, you'll still want to stick with the habits and practices you worked on in the SlimDown, including planning your week ahead and choosing meals, snacks, and Flexes.

You have already found a day that works best for you to plan your week ahead and fill out your menu plan. Most people find that Saturday or Sunday mornings are good choices. Make a point of finding some quiet time and sitting down with your Weekly Menu plan. Think about your upcoming week and the obligations you'll face that could affect your meals. Slot in as many meals as you practically can from the SuperFoodsRx Meals Lists (pages 188–215). Think about your Flexes and where you might like to enjoy them. Consider your options. In the beginning, keep it simple and specific just like you did at the beginning of the Slim-Down when you were practicing meals from your choices and limiting the variety in your weekly plan. Keep it simple so you can practice and internalize your choices. Many clients have told me that they find it easier to say "no" to some foods when they've already planned something else to enjoy later in the day or week. The cookie from the conference table at work is less tempting if you've already planned to have a sorbet with the kids at the ice cream shop after work or a glass of wine with dinner. It's not about deprivation; it's about your personal choice.

What about spontaneity? Well, of course, once you become comfortable living in the FlexPlan mode, you can make spur-of-the-moment choices. Life is filled with unplanned delights and you will be able to enjoy them. But it's still an important practice to sit down each week and lay out your food choices as best you can. The simple practice of doing this will remind you of your goals and restore your focus,

> There truly is no reason why a person should not continually follow the SuperFoods Flex-Plan. My advice for others is to always have the SuperFoods and the plan readily available. If not, you are setting yourself up to choose the wrong foods. The FlexPlan has allowed options that if not on the diet program I would have felt guilty of eating. Knowing I have these options has allowed me to make the SuperFoodsRx program a lifestyle not just a diet.
> —Brenda C., active wife of 40 years

Each Flex choice tops out at approximately 150 calories. If you'd prefer to choose something that isn't on the lists I've included here, you can do that. Just aim to stay within the general SuperFoodsRx Diet in terms of real, whole, quality foods and keep the calorie level of your choices in the neighborhood of 120–150 calories.

helping you to maintain the progress you've already made. It will soon become second nature to you.

Keep Your Fingers off Your Triggers

Most of us seem to have foods that we find virtually impossible to walk away from. Maybe it's that bowl of peanuts at a cocktail party or the chips a friend puts out while you watch a game. Or maybe it's that coffee ice cream lurking in the back of the freezer. If certain foods are an absolute challenge for you, I advise you to simply cross them off your Flex list. There are still so many things you can choose to enjoy, every day if you like. It's just not worth the risk. The SuperFoodsRx Diet is all about a whole new lifestyle and a genuine honesty with yourself. So go to the Flex list and eliminate those one or two foods that you just know will be too difficult for you to enjoy in a healthy amount—for now. Making priorities about what you choose to eat is empowering. You can always revisit this decision in the weeks or months to come.

The FlexPlan Flexes

Guidelines for your Flexes:

- FlexPlan options are listed by general category (snacks, drinks, and so on) for easy reference to quickly locate items you are interested in.

- Each item in a general category below counts as 1 Flex. You choose 5 for your week. You can choose the same Flex more than once among your 5 selections for the week.

- Not more than 2 at one meal; not more than 2 in one day (or equivalent using the "2 for 1" list on page 141)

- Plan, count, and record! Make a conscious choice.
- Enjoy!

Snacks

- 1 snack from SuperFoodsRx snack list (page 214)
- 1 energy bar (look for 120–150 calorie options) such as:
  - Kashi® TLC bar (sold 6 to a box)
  - Cascadian Farms® organic energy bar (various flavors)
  - Luna® Z-Bar Organic for Kids or similar
  - See energy bar guidelines on page 339
- One 4–6-ounce yogurt (150 calories max, no high-fructose corn syrup or artificial sweeteners such as sucralose or aspartame)
- Nuts (one of the following):
  - 18–20 almonds
  - 10–11 walnut halves
  - 23 peanuts
  - 14 pecans
  - 25 cashews
  - 140 pine nuts (about 1½ tablespoons)
  - 42 pistachios
  - 8 macadamias
  - 16 hazelnuts
  - 5 Brazil nuts
- 1½ tablespoons nut butter (peanut butter, almond butter, etc.)

Drinks

- Hot drinks
  - 1 nonfat milk or soy double latte, 12 ounce
  - 1 cappuccino with low-fat milk or low-fat soy

- Hot cocoa—2 teaspoons dark chocolate cocoa mix made with 6 ounces nonfat milk or low-fat/nonfat soy milk
- Fruit juice and Smoothies
  - ½ breakfast smoothie option (page 224)—make ½ recipe
  - 8 ounces fresh orange juice or other 100% fruit juice (try to choose SuperFoods-based juices like blueberry, pomegranate, unfiltered apple)
- Alcohol drinks
  - 1 glass wine (5 ounces)
  - 4 ounces sake (rice wine)
  - One 12-ounce beer
  - 1½ ounces liquor (with water—flat or sparkling—or on the rocks)

Soups

- 1 cup SuperFoods Soup Base Option 1, 7, 10 (recipes page 284)
- ¾ cup Four-Bean Chile (recipe page 293)

Extra Sides—Fruits and Veggies

- 1 serving Sweet Potato & Asparagus with Orange Glaze (2 cups)—recipe page 247
- 1 serving (1 cup) All Season Fruit Salad (recipe page 236)
- 1 serving Almond Green Beans (recipe page 242)
- 1 serving Modern Ambrosia for One (recipe page 241)
- ½ cup Confetti Salad (recipe page 249)
- Dried Fruit
  - ¼ cup raisins
  - ¼ cup dried blueberries
  - ¼ cup dried cranberries, tart cherries, or dried plums (prunes)
  - 6–8 dried apricots

Protein Add-Ons

- Additional 3 ounces turkey, salmon, poultry, or other lean animal protein (deck of cards!)
- Additional 5–6 ounces tofu
- $\frac{1}{2}$ cup edamame (boiled soybeans)—just the beans, out of the pod
- $\frac{2}{3}$ cup edamame (boiled soybeans)—measured in the pod
- $\frac{1}{2}$–$\frac{2}{3}$ cup cup plain, cooked beans—black, lentils, etc.
- $\frac{1}{2}$ cup SuperFoodsRx Cooked Lentils (recipe page 219)
- One 4–6 ounce yogurt (150 calories max, no corn syrup or artificial sweeteners)
- See also bean-based **Spreads and Dips** in the "2 for 1s" on page 141.

Grains . . . and other crunchy snacks

- 3–4 cups air-popped or 94%+ fat-free microwave popcorn
- $\frac{3}{4}$ cup whole wheat pasta (cooked)
- 1 serving (tennis ball portion—$\frac{1}{3}$–$\frac{1}{2}$ cup) grains additional in your day
- $\frac{2}{3}$ cup brown rice
- One 6" corn on the cob
- 1 medium (tennis ball portion) sweet potato (remember it's not really a grain, but we treat it like one)
- $\frac{1}{3}$ cup wheat germ
- 1–1$\frac{1}{2}$ ounce oatmeal ($\frac{1}{3}$–$\frac{1}{2}$ cup dry)
- $\frac{1}{4}$ cup steel-cut oats
- 1 Thomas'® bagel—regular size (multigrain, cinnamon raisin)
- 2 mini bagels (about 2" diameter, approximately $\frac{3}{4}$ ounce-size)
- 12–15 baked tortilla chips
- Soy crisps such as:
  - Genisoy® brand—1 ounce is approximately 17 chips
  - Glenny's® brand—3-ounce bag

🌿 1 SuperFoodsRx Blueberry Muffin with Walnuts (recipe page 318)

🌿 1 SuperFoodsRx Pumpkin Walnut Muffin (recipe page 320)

Nuts, Seeds, Cheese and Oil

🌿 Nuts (one of the following):

- 18–20 almonds
- 10–11 walnut halves
- 23 peanuts
- 14 pecans
- 25 cashews
- 140 pine nuts ($1\frac{1}{2}$ tablespoons)
- 42 pistachios
- 8 macadamias
- 16 hazelnuts
- 5 Brazil nuts

🌿 $\frac{1}{8}$ cup (3 tablespoons) sunflower seeds (salt free or reduced salt)

🌿 $\frac{1}{4}$ cup soy nuts (unsalted)

🌿 $1\frac{1}{2}$ tablespoons nut butter (peanut butter, almond butter, and such)

🌿 $1–1\frac{1}{2}$ ounces cheese

🌿 2 tablespoons low-fat cream cheese

🌿 1 tablespoon olive oil

Breakfast

🌿 $\frac{1}{2}$ SuperFoodsRx breakfast—$\frac{1}{2}$ of any SuperFoods breakfast option; $\frac{1}{2}$ recipe—e.g. $\frac{1}{2}$ bowl of cereal, with berries, etc.

🌿 $\frac{1}{2}$ breakfast smoothie option (recipe page 224)— make $\frac{1}{2}$ recipe

🌿 Additional 1 ounce ($\frac{1}{3}$ cup dry) oatmeal to regular breakfast

🌿 3 tablespoons SuperFoodsRx Granola (recipe page 222)

Sweets

- 1 SuperFoodsRx Blueberry Muffin with Walnuts (recipe page 318)

- 1 SuperFoodsRx Pumpkin Walnut Muffin (recipe page 320)

- 2 SuperFoodsRx Dark Chocolate Chip Cookies (recipe page 313)

- 1 Oatmeal Cinnamon Bar (recipe page 314)

- 2 Pumpkin Dessert Crepes with Yogurt Sauce (recipe page 315)

- 1 dessert serving Blueberry Compote Crumble (recipe page 318)

- $\frac{1}{2}$ cup "fruit first" sorbet (fruit must be the first ingredient on the label)

- $\frac{1}{2}$ cup nonfat, frozen yogurt (natural, no HFCS) with $\frac{1}{4}$ cup blueberries

- 1 commercial biscotti

- 1 average cookie (2$\frac{1}{2}$"– 3" diameter)

- 2 whole grain (natural) fig bars such as:
  - Barbara's Bakery® Whole Wheat Fig Bars
  - Whole Foods 365® Every Day Value™ Organic Fig Bars

- 1 ounce 70% or higher dark chocolate
  - Tip: Buy 1-ounce bars so you don't run into personal portion challenges! One ounce is $\frac{1}{4}$"x3$\frac{1}{2}$"x1$\frac{1}{2}$"—Scharffen Berger® makes a 1-ounce bar and 4–5 small Lindt® Excellence Minis (1"x1"x$\frac{1}{8}$") = 1 ounce

- 1$\frac{1}{2}$–2 tablespoons dark chocolate chips—mixed into your homemade trail mix (nuts and dried fruit) baggies for the week (see SuperFoodsRx Snack list, page 214) OR melted and used for dipping with some fresh strawberries!

- 2–3 regular forkfuls (modest really) of a restaurant dessert—aim for something with real fruit in it.
  - Tip to remember: First bite is taste, second bite is for flavor, and the third is for pleasure and savoring and then you're done. This is a good option when you can share a dessert. Don't make this more than 1 out of 5 of your weekly FlexPlan options

The FlexPlan "2 for 1" Choices:

Guidelines:

- Each counts as ½ of a Flex. Two of the choices listed below equal one of your five weekly Flexes.
- Not more than 4 at one meal; not more than 4 in one day
- Plan, count, and record! Though they may be a "bargain," they still have calories and do count toward your overall weekly intake and long-term success. Make a conscious choice.
- Enjoy!

Snacks

- Nuts (one of the following):
  - 8 almonds
  - 5 walnut halves
  - 11 peanuts
  - 7 pecans
  - 12 cashews
  - 70 pine nuts (approx. 2 teaspoons)
  - 21 pistachios
  - 4 macadamias
  - 8 hazelnuts
  - 2 Brazil nuts
- Dried Fruits:
  - 2 tablespoons raisins, cranberries, or blueberries
  - 2–3 dried apricots

Drinks

- Hot drinks
  - Nonfat cappuccino (8–12 ounces)

- ✐ Cold drinks
  - Juice Sparkle: 4 ounces 100% juice + 4 ounces sparkling water
  - Gentle juice: 4 ounces 100% juice + 4 ounces water
  - SuperFoodsRx Fruit Tea: 4 ounces 100% blueberry, pomegranate, or unfiltered apple juice mixed with 4 ounces green tea—served warm, room temperature or over ice
  - ¾ cup vanilla Silk® Soymilk
  - ¾–1 cup nonfat soy milk
  - ½ cup 100% fruit juice
- ✐ Alcohol drinks
  - Wine spritzer—2–3 ounces wine + sparkling water

Soups

- ✐ 1 cup simple SuperFoodsRx Soup Base (recipe page 284)
- ✐ ¾ cup Sweet Potato Soup (recipe page 289)
- ✐ ¾ cup SuperFoodsRx Soup Base Options 2, 4, 5, 6, 8, 11 (recipes pages 285–288)

Veggie Extras

- ✐ 1 cup Broccoli and Cauliflower Salad (recipe page 243)
- ✐ 1 serving Roasted Broccoli (recipe page 244)
- ✐ 2 Slow Baked Tomatoes (recipe page 245)
- ✐ 2 servings (whole recipe) Steamed Carrots with Dill (recipe page 246)
- ✐ 3 tablespoons avocado
- ✐ 8–10 olives
- ✐ 1 cup pumpkin

Fruit Extras

- ✐ Fruit: (one of the following):
  - 2 cups watermelon

- ½ grapefruit
- 1 large kiwi
- ½ large orange or 1 small
- 1 cup raspberries, strawberries or blackberries
- ¾ cup blueberries
- 1–2 tangerines
- 2 plums
- ½ banana (4"–5")
- 12–15 cherries
- 1 small apple
- Other: approximately ½–1 cup of any fruit

- Baked Apple (recipe page 237)
- Cold Fruit Soup (recipe page 292)
- ¼ cup Fresh Blueberry Compote (recipe page 238)
- ¾ cup natural applesauce (no sugar added)
- Dried Fruits:
  - 2 tablespoons raisins, cranberries, or blueberries
  - 2–3 dried apricots

Protein Add Ons

- ½ cup nonfat cottage cheese (low sodium)
- 1 egg
- 4 egg whites
- See also bean-based Spreads and Dips on page 145

Grains . . . and other crunchy snacks

- 1 (80-calorie) slice of whole grain bread (e.g. to make your half sandwich a whole sandwich)
  - Tip: Stick to 80-calorie (not 100) whole grain bread if you use this option.

- 🌿 Crackers (one of the following):
  - 2 whole grain rice cakes
  - 3 Wasa® crackers
  - 3 Ak-Mak® crackers
  - 2 rye crispbreads
  - 4 low-sodium Triscuits®
  - 9 Hain® Wheatettes
- 🌿 One 3" corn on the cob
- 🌿 ½ cup corn
- 🌿 1 medium (tennis ball) or ½ cup sweet potato or other potato
- 🌿 1 whole grain (75–80 calorie variety) toaster waffle
- 🌿 One 6" corn tortilla
- 🌿 1 whole wheat, low-carb (6"–8") tortilla
- 🌿 8 Homemade Tortilla Chips (recipe page 251)
- 🌿 7–8 baked tortilla chips (commercial varieties)

Nuts, Seeds, Cheese and Oils

- 🌿 Nuts (one of the following):
  - 8 almonds
  - 5 walnut halves
  - 11 peanuts
  - 7 pecans
  - 12 cashews
  - 70 pine nuts (2 teaspoons)
  - 21 pistachios
  - 4 macadamias
  - 8 hazelnuts
  - 2 Brazil nuts
- 🌿 2 tablespoons ground flaxseed (added to smoothies, soups, salads, muffins, oatmeal, etc.)

- 1 ounce goat cheese, feta cheese
- 3½ tablespoons shredded parmesan
- 2 Laughing Cow® light wedges
- 1 Laughing Cow® Mini Babybel cheese
- 1 ounce string cheese or other natural snack cheese
- ⅛ cup part-skim ricotta cheese

Spreads/Dips

- ⅓ cup Creamy Spinach Dip (recipe page 297)
- ⅓ cup Black Bean & Mango Salsa (recipe page 296)
- ½ cup Smoked Salmon Spread (recipe page 298)
- ¼ cup Yogurt Banana Strawberry Spread (recipe page 298)
- ⅓ cup Garlic Lovers Dip (recipe page 299)
- ⅓ cup Great Northern Bean Dip (recipe page 300)
- ⅓ cup Hummus (recipe page 301)
- ¼ cup "Refried" Beans (recipe page 302)
- ½ cup Roasted Pepper Puree (recipe page 303)
- ⅓ cup Salsa Bean Dip (recipe page 304)
- ¾ cup Year Round Salsa (recipe page 305)
- ¼ cup "Brocco-mole" (recipe page 300)

Sweets

- 1 SuperFoodsRx Dark Chocolate Chip Cookie (recipe page 313)
- 1 Pumpkin Dessert Crepe with Yogurt Sauce (recipe page 315)
- 3 tablespoons Spicy Pumpkin Butter (recipe page 239)
- ¼ cup Fresh Blueberry Compote (recipe page 238)
- 1 tablespoon dark chocolate syrup—for berry or banana dipping, add to plain yogurt or a SuperFoodsRx smoothie (add to ½ cup nonfat yogurt and count 1½ Flex options)

- 1 tablespoon dark chocolate chips
- 1½ tablespoons maple syrup
- 1 tablespoon honey
- 2 Lindt® Excellence 70% or 85% cocoa mini squares (1"×1" sold in a 20-count bag)
- 2–3 tablespoons all fruit preserves

Let's Get Strong! FlexPlan Exercise

You've already started your exercise program in the SlimDown when you began to walk (or continued with whatever exercise you already enjoy). Now it's time to add a bit more movement to your day so you can enjoy the fullest benefits of exercise on your weight-loss program.

There's no getting around it: Exercise is the linchpin that holds your whole SuperFoodsRx healthy lifestyle together. It will boost your optimism, build your muscles as well as your confidence, and, of course, it burns calories. Exercise makes every day better. Some people are discouraged when they're urged to exercise. They envision a toned, muscular body in spandex, sweating through a marathon. Some people find this type of exercise exhilarating, but working at that duration and intensity is not at all a requirement of the SuperFoodsRx lifestyle. If you can walk around the block—or work up to it—you can succeed at the SuperFoodsRx exercise plan. You've already started walking in the first phase of the diet—the SlimDown. But now I'll explain why exercise is so important to your SuperFoodsRx healthy lifestyle and I'll provide some strategies to help you move to the next step on your own exercise program.

Perhaps the single most important thing to know about how exercise helps you lose weight is the fact that exercise builds muscle and muscle burns more calories than fat. That's right. It takes one to three calories a day to sustain a pound of fat but 40 to 120 calories a day to keep a pound of muscles going. Given this, it's obvious that the more muscle you have on your body, versus fat, the more calories you'll burn even while you're sitting at the computer working or laying down sleeping.

On the flip side, it's sobering to know that sedentary people can lose 23 to 35 percent of muscle mass over the course of their adult lives.[1] This loss not only may contribute to becoming overweight but can also cause a loss of strength and balance as well as an overall physical decline.

Consider these facts about exercise and weight, which will inspire you to lace up your sneakers:

- According to researchers, women 40–66 years of age who accumulate 10,000 or more steps a day have a significantly lower percent body fat, waist, and hip circumference, waist-to-hip ratio, and body mass index compared to inactive women.[2]

- Individuals who successfully lose weight exercise enough to burn an average of 2,600–2,800 calories per week.[3] This may seem like a lot, but let's break it down:

  - 2,800 calories a week equals 400 calories a day equals . . .

  - an average 4 miles per day . . . or close to

  - 10,000 steps per day . . . or better yet—

  - an average over the course of a week of 70,000 steps—no matter how you get there—more some days, less other days

- and the most common activity, reported by 75 percent of those who successfully lose weight and keep it off, is walking.[4]

Here are some of the benefits of exercise that have been demonstrated by research:

- Higher energy levels. Once you get through the initial adjustment from adding more exercise into your life, you'll likely find that your energy levels pick up so you can be more productive and enjoy more of what life offers.

I fit in extras by watching quantity and quality. I may have dessert, but small portion to taste or take bites of something where before I ate it all. Also, I go for better choices with the Flex-Plan . . . And my progress hasn't really slowed either, not even with a few of the challenges we've had like moving and getting our children off to college and entered into new schools. I just decided to step up and be accountable with the FlexPlan and I maintain my motivation, my progress and weight loss.
– Dana M., 51-year-old husband and father

- *Better performance.* Your daily activities like lifting, bending, reaching, and climbing stairs will all become easier. Your strength, stamina, balance, and coordination will all improve.
- *Clearer mind.* Exercise can help boost your brainpower—allowing for better concentration, attention, and cognitive functioning.
- *Improved mood.* Exercise has been shown to help boost moods while also helping to decrease mild-to-moderate anxiety and depression.
- *Better self-esteem.* Exercise not only improves your energy but also boosts self-confidence.
- *Sleep.* Physical activity can help improve the quality of your sleep, so you awaken more rested, restored, and energized for the day ahead.

If you haven't been exercising at all up to now, this might seem like a lot of activity. But if you weigh the importance of regular daily exercise to your short-term as well as long-term health and also to your weight loss goals, you'll appreciate that it's time well spent. Most SuperFoodRx dieters find that they soon become so accustomed to the good feelings and good results they get from their daily exercise that they make time for it no matter what else is happening in their lives.

Now, after you complete at least 2 weeks of the SlimDown, it's time to work to boost your walking time. Your new exercise goal on the FlexPlan is 45 to 60 minutes of daily aerobic exercise (simply increase your walking if you're doing the SlimDown 30 minutes) 5 or more days weekly. Of course, if

Compelling recent research has revealed that exercise can actually help boost brain health. We've seen some evidence in the past that those who exercise do better on memory tests, but now evidence gathered with the use of MRIs shows that exercise can actually stimulate the growth of new cells in the area of the brain associated with memory and what researchers refer to as cognitive aging. And through stimulating these new cells to form in the brain, exercise may even help *restore* some memory that has been lost as a result of stroke![5]

So those steps you're taking every day to help lose weight may also be giving your brain a lifesaving workout, too.[6]

you're participating in some other exercise, simply make sure that you're getting this amount of time in aerobic activity at least 5 days a week. Don't forget to record your progress in your food diary.

Strength Training

Strength training will amplify all the healthy positives you're already enjoying now that you've completed at least 2 weeks of the SlimDown. You're already walking, or actively participating in another cardiovascular exercise program of your choice, and you're no doubt seeing the difference that exercise makes in your life. You're also going to be boosting your exercise program on the FlexPlan in duration as mentioned above and also by adding strength training to your schedule. No exercise regimen is complete without a strength-training routine. Perhaps you're already doing some strength training because you've read about all the recent research demonstrating its significant benefits for your bones, your muscles, your metabolism, and your overall health. If not, now's the time to start.

Strength training is for everyone, no matter your age, weight or fitness level. It can easily be done at home in 20-minute sessions that will pay major long-term dividends to your overall health. One benefit for women in particular: One study demonstrated that strength training can actually increase metabolism not only during the exercise session itself but for up to 2 hours *after* strength training ended—resulting in an additional 100 extra calories burned![7] And I've already mentioned how lean muscle tissue burns more calories than fat. A regular program of strength training can reduce your body fat, increase your lean muscle mass, and help you to burn calories more efficiently. But perhaps the most significant benefits of strength training are the long-term bonuses: Strength training can ensure your future independence and overall ability to enjoy life. Strength training today can mean a future filled with activities and pleasures that are sometimes denied to those who lose strength, motion, and functional abilities.

Here are some of the powerful benefits you'll enjoy as strength training will help you:

- Maintain and increase your muscle mass as well as your overall strength. Most people don't realize that they begin to lose muscle mass around age 30 if they aren't actively engaging the muscles on a regular basis. By the time they reach their late thirties or early forties, most people are losing muscle mass at a rate of about a quarter pound a year. Most people also think that muscle weakness is an inevitable result of age while in fact it is in large part a result of disuse.

- Create and maintain stronger bones. By stressing your bones, strength training increases bone density and reduces the risk of osteoporosis. If you already have osteoporosis or osteopenia, strength training can lessen its severity and, in some cases, reverse it. Research shows that strength training (along with your nutrient-dense SuperFoodsRx Diet) can also help minimize any bone loss that is sometimes experienced as the result of weight loss.

- Control your body fat. As you lose muscle, your body burns calories less efficiently, which can result in weight gain or slowed weight loss. The more toned your muscles, the easier it is to control your weight.

- Reduce your risk of injury. Building muscle protects your joints from injury and facilitates recovery from falls. It also helps you maintain flexibility and balance as you age.

- Boost your stamina. As you grow stronger, you won't fatigue as easily. This will be especially noticeable with your general daily activities like carrying groceries or walking up stairs.

The great news about strength training is that research shows you don't have to put in as much time as we used to believe. In fact, today it's generally accepted that doing 1 effective set of approximately 12 repetitions of an exercise—or to muscle fatigue—is sufficient to experience the real benefits of strength training.[8]

- Improve your sense of well-being. Strength training can boost your self-confidence, improve your body image and reduce the risk of depression.

- Get a better night's sleep. People who strength train regularly are less likely to struggle with insomnia.

- Reduce the signs and symptoms of a variety of diseases and health conditions including arthritis, back pain, heart disease, depression, diabetes, osteoporosis, and obesity.

How to Get Started

Space limitations prevent me from presenting a full strength-training program for you here. You really need visuals—photos or a video or an actual trainer—to fully understand and customize the simple techniques you will incorporate in your strength-training program. But it's easy to find resources to help you get started. There are excellent sources of information online and in video and book format in your library and at your local bookstore. Three good online resources include:

- The Centers for Disease Control and Prevention Web site offers a detailed strength-training program developed by experts from Tufts University and the CDC. Explore: http://www.cdc.gov/nccdphp/dnpa/physical/growing_stronger/. While this program was originally designed for older people, it could be used by anyone who's beginning a strength-training program. It provides animated photos of exercises and detailed guidelines on how to proceed.

- The American College of Sports Medicine provides a free brochure called "Selecting and Effectively Using Free Weights." You can download it from: http://www.acsm.org/Content/ContentFolders/Publications/

Brochures/FreeWeightsbrochure.pdf or you can write for it by sending a self-addressed, stamped, business-size envelope to: ACSM National Center, P.O. Box 1440, Indianapolis, IN 46206-1440.

🖋 Miriam Nelson, PhD, Director of the Center for Physical Activity and Nutrition and Associate Professor of Nutrition at the Friedman School of Nutrition Science and Policy at Tufts University, is an authority on strength training and nutrition in the aging population. She has several books and a Web site with well-designed and effective strength-training exercises for fitness, strong bones, back strength, and weight management. Her Web site: http://www.strongwomen.com, provides specific exercises and more information.

Here are a few points about your strength-training program:

🖋 Get your doctor's okay to begin a strength-training program, particularly if you're over 40 years of age or if you've been inactive.

🖋 Consider a few sessions with a personal trainer to be sure that you are exercising correctly and efficiently. Physical therapists, athletic trainers, and certified exercise/fitness specialists have been specifically trained in strength-training techniques and can help you design appropriate routines to fit your needs. Look for certification by the American College of Sports Medicine (ACSM) or American Council on Exercise (ACE).

🖋 Establish clear and concise goals for each exercise and an overall goal for your total strength-training program. Tailor these goals and the total plan to your individual and changing fitness needs and abilities.

🖋 Make sure to include all of your major muscles in your strength-training regimen—abdominals, legs, chest, back, shoulders, and arms. Pay attention to strengthen the opposing muscles in a mindful, balanced way—for example, the front of the leg with the back of the leg.

🖋 Remember to aim for 10–12 reps of each exercise. This number should feel like the maximum before fatiguing each muscle group, and is effective for strengthening and toning. One set is sufficient for each muscle group.

- Try not to fling, jerk, or rock the hand weights up and down. Raise and lower with control—slowly. In this way, you will be more effective at and working the muscles specifically and safely.

- Do not hold your breath during strength-training exercises. Exhaling during the release phase and inhale as you begin the movement. Breathing freely throughout the exercises can help with relaxation and prevent blood pressure irregularities.

- Make sure to give yourself one full day in between working out the same muscle group. Rest 48 hours between strength-training sessions. You can alter upper body one day, lower body the next day—but rest 48 hours between sessions on a given area.

- In order to build new muscle, three or more times per week of strength training is recommended.

- Always wear shoes with good treads and support.

- Use stable equipment—chairs, doors, walls, or exercise equipment. Check it out before using it with your body for exercises.

- Learn the difference between muscle fatigue and muscle strain or pain.

- Have fun!

Flexibility: A Few Words on Stretching

You've no doubt seen a cat or dog stretching upon rising from sleep. They know instinctively what we sometimes have to learn: Stretching your body prepares it for motion, helps to minimize or avoid injury, and increases your range of motion. And after you've exercised, stretching helps prevent muscle cramping and also reduces soreness. Stretching also, quite simply feels good. Here are some tips on stretching:

- Try to fully stretch your body at least three times a week.

- Do a few simple stretches every morning and every evening.

- Stretch regularly—at home or the office—especially after you've been immobile for a period of time.

Here are some simple stretches:

- Ankle twists: Try slowly writing the letters of the alphabet with each foot.

- Wrist stretch: Make full wide circles in both directions with your wrist.

- Calf stretches: Holding a wall or other stable support and using a 1-inch or larger book on the floor, rest your toes on the book and lean gently forward with your legs straight.

- Hamstrings: Do straight-leg toe touches while standing, sitting on the bed or floor or bending over in a chair.

- Quads: Hold onto a stable desk or table and put a sturdy chair behind you. Place the top of your foot on the chair seat and hold that position. Alternatively, you can use a towel to wrap your foot and pull your heel toward your buttocks and hold it briefly in position.

- Abdomen: Lay on the floor on your back and point your toes while extending arms over your head.

- Lower back: Sit in a chair, feet flat on floor and knees bent at a 90-degree angle. Lean forward, bringing your chest toward your lap and letting your arms dangle to the floor.

- Shoulders: Roll your shoulders forward five times and then backward five times in a smooth motion, bringing your shoulders up toward your ears and then back down toward your belly button.

The FlexPlan Exercise Options

Here's where you can use a bit of extra exercise to balance a little more food in your diet. This gives you yet more flexibility as you follow the FlexPlan. Here are the FlexPlan exercise option guidelines:

- The Exercise Options can be employed only if you've already met your weekly basic daily and weekly goals of 45 to 60 minutes on 5 or more days weekly.

- Don't use the Exercise Option more than twice a week. (For a maximum of 2 additional Flexes.)

- Plan, count, and record! Make a conscious choice.

- Remember, sometimes you can choose to simply count those extra calories burned in additional activity as a leap toward your weight-loss goal.

- The exercises listed below are based on the time it takes a person weighing 150 pounds to burn approximately 150 calories doing that activity. If you weigh more, you'd be burning more calories; less, fewer calories. Nonetheless, I recommend you stick with these general guidelines for simplicity's sake.

Earn 1 additional Flex[9] (no more than twice weekly) for:

39 minutes of walking (3 mph; approximately 4 calories/min)

16 minutes of jogging/running (5 mph; 9.5 cal./min)

13 minutes of running (6 mph; 11.5 cal./min)

21 minutes of biking (10–12 mph, slow, light effort; 8 cal./min)

18 minutes of swimming (laps, slow, light to moderate effort)

20 minutes of elliptical (moderate)

16 minutes of elliptical (vigorous)

26 minutes of dancing (approximately 6 cal./min)

15 minutes of jump roping (10 cal./min)

37 minutes of golf with cart

28 minutes of golf, no cart, carrying own clubs

51 minutes of Hatha style yoga (3 cal. /min)

16 minutes of tennis, singles

42 minutes of strength training (moderate)

30 minutes of gardening

30 minutes of raking leaves

23 minutes of mowing lawn

42 minutes of general housecleaning

36 minutes of active housecleaning—vacuuming, mopping, scrubbing

Think Twice About the Following:

You have lots of latitude on your FlexPlan: Really, nothing eaten in appropriate portions is off limits unless you decide it is. But there are some choices that can take a bigger toll than you might think so let's take at look at them.

Alcohol

While alcohol is not included on the SlimDown, it can be a part of the FlexPlan as long as you recognize certain considerations. For one thing, alcohol is not considered a nutrient-dense food (even though it offers some nutritional benefits like the antioxidants in red wine). It therefore is not a featured player in the SuperFoodsRx Diet. If you do choose to have alcohol on the FlexPlan, you should try to limit yourself to no more than one drink on any given day. This recommendation is based on good research, on behavioral factors, and on good sound reasoning for long-term weight and waist management. My general rule is that one drink can fit just fine but the second is really just extra calories. Moreover, if alcohol is going to interfere with your good food choices, then it really should be avoided. Pay particular attention to fancy cocktails. Some are as high as a dessert in calories—or in some cases even close to your total meal calories! *If* you choose to have an alcoholic beverage, make your decision in advance—and don't forget to count it among your FlexPlan options. Keep it simple—a glass of wine or a 12-ounce bottle of beer will keep the calories in check. If you are looking for a cocktail, try one with sparkling water/club soda and a "splash" of cranberry juice or other 100 percent juice if available along with a couple wedges of lime. Stick to one drink, preferably with the meal.

Specialty Coffee Drinks

The nonfat latte or soy cappuccino is fine once in a while, but watch out for sugary coffee and tea beverages, whipped and blended coffee "shakes" with whipped cream and even chai tea lattes, which are often poured from a box containing chai tea and sugar already blended into a sweet syrup. Instead try a plain tea, a small nonfat latte or make your own chai tea latte by steeping 2 chai tea bags in water, adding nonfat or low-fat milk or soy and even a packet or two of sugar in the raw—the 16–32 calories from sugar and 20–40 calories from the milk will ring in as half a Flex (a "2 for 1") and a far better choice than the high-calorie specialty coffee drinks.

Energy Bars and Granola Bars

Energy sounds great, right? Well, on a label, "energy" simply means "calories." So when you're shopping for a calorie bar, make sure you choose one with the right ingredients and take a careful look at the calories. Some have over 200 calories or more. Search for bars that have 150 or less calories. Then check the ingredients. Avoid those with artificial flavorings, artificial sweeteners, high-fructose corn syrup or trans fats. Try to find bars with less than 15 grams of sugar (even lower is better—some like Kashi® TLC bars have only 6 grams) and at least 2 grams of fiber. Finally, look for a bar that includes SuperFoods like oats, nuts, berries, ground flax, or other natural ingredients. Finally, limit your use of these bars to an occasional choice, say, when traveling, and not part of your daily routine. They're handy and convenient but so are little snack bags you can make up in a flash with mixed walnuts and dried blueberries in just the right portions for you.

Doughy Things

Pastries, muffins, croissants, bagels . . . consider carefully before choosing one of these. For one thing, they would each count as 2–3 Flexes. A bakery muffin (even if it has blueberries) can run as high as 650–800 calories with over 7 teaspoons of oil (the unhealthy kind) and over 10 teaspoons of sugar. They sure feel "grab and go" convenient at times, but they're not going to add much to your SuperNutrient intake. If you must choose this type of food, do try for something with whole grains and minimal fat and sugar, eat a half or even better, a third and top it with a tablespoon of peanut or almond butter instead of butter or cream cheese.

Mayonnaise . . . the Healthy Eater's Mayo-nightmare

When we think of the SuperFoods, it's easy to imagine all the SuperNutrients being absorbed into our bodies when we eat them. But certain other foods challenge this vision. Mayonnaise is a common food that performs a specific function—it imparts moisture, binds foods like tuna, and adds some flavor—but it really serves the food more than our bodies. Mayonnaise contains nearly 12 grams of fat and more than 100 calories in a single tablespoon. So look for a better binder and "food-moisturizer" that tastes good without the negatives of mayonnaise. Try yogurt. You can use thick nonfat Greek yogurt or make your own Yogurt Cheese (recipe on page 217). You can flavor it with herbs and seasonings, add some mustard or chopped onion and not only do you get a great binder and versatile spread for your sandwich, but you get great SuperFoods nutrients as well. Bean spreads—like hummus or black beans—and red pepper spread are other great alternatives to mayonnaise.

Salad Dressing

Salad dressing can make a salad go from 0 to 60—or in this case from 50 to 150 (calories) with merely a drizzle. Look for low-calorie dressings—40–60 calories per 2 tablespoons—but avoid ingredients like color dyes, trans fats, corn syrup, sodium and MSG. Dilute dressings—even lower calorie varieties—to make the most of the "flavor spread" to your lettuce leaves and when at home, measure the dressing and then toss the salad. Also consider using a spray bottle for thinner dressings. In a restaurant, use fruit wedges like oranges, limes, or lemons or use balsamic vinegar or a salsa to add flavor to your salad.

Flavored Sugar Drinks, Sports Drinks, Sweetened Tea

Don't fall into the trap of drinking your calories because clever advertising convinces you that you need to replenish your electrolytes. You won't get instantly smarter from "smart" water or faster from sports drinks or healthier from teas that have lots of artificial sweeteners or corn syrup. If you want to sweeten a beverage, use a teaspoon of honey or add $\frac{1}{2}$ inch of 100 percent juice to your water or fresh brewed tea. If you count it as a half a Flex (2 for 1), you can combine 4 ounces of any 100 percent SuperFoods juice to your water or tea. And unless you're out there exercising for more than 60 minutes doing cardiovascular, aerobic exercise on a regular basis, you generally don't need a sports drink. Instead, flavor sparkling water with fruit slices or squeeze a lemon or orange into it. If you are on the FlexPlan, you can make a Juice Sparkle by adding the sparkling water in the glass first and topping off with up to 4 ounces of 100 percent juice. You can also make a Green Tea and Citrus Soda, by putting half and half green tea and sparkling water and topping off $\frac{1}{2}$–$\frac{3}{4}$ inches of the glass with juice from a hand-squeezed orange or lemon.

Crackers and Baked Chips

These can be great FlexPlan choices but check the package carefully. Aim for whole grains, make sure they are baked and not fried, and watch out for sodium and other artificial ingredients or preservatives. For a snack, your portion is 50–70 calories worth of the crackers or chips (along with whatever, if anything, you will eat it with—your recommended Flex serving amount of

A Word About Smoothies. Smoothies are a great way to get fruit and yogurt—terrific SuperFoods—into your diet. While they're not included on the SlimDown except as a breakfast meal option, they're a good choice for the FlexPlan. But keep in mind that a typical smoothie from a commercial smoothie shop is 16 ounces and up. A 16-ounce smoothie would count as approximately two Flexes due to their high calorie count. A better choice would be to make your own smoothie using one of the recipes on pages 224 and 327 which would count as one Flex. If you do buy a commercial smoothie, exercise your healthy choice and stick to an 8-ounce portion. Ask them to serve you only this much, share a 16-ounce serving with a friend or you may have to sometimes discard the excess. Reaching your goal is worth it.

cheese, bean dip, salsa, hummus, peanut butter, etc.) Your FlexPlan portion should usually be about half of the "serving size" typically listed on the box or bag. Remember that air-popped and 94 percent-plus, fat-free microwave popcorn are also great crunchy alternatives to the baked chips.

"Diet" or Low Fat Foods

With the exception of dairy products, in which the fat is "skimmed" off (especially the saturated fat, which is unhealthy to consume in quantity), diet and low-fat foods are notorious for getting the chronic dieter in trouble. They typically contain large amounts of sugars, often in the form of corn syrup and, as mentioned previously, research has shown that when people eat "diet" foods they tend to consume greater amounts and more calories than if they

Do Frozen Meals Fit?

Sometimes a SuperFoodsRx dieter will ask me a version of the following: "I'm so busy during the week, sometimes I've relied on frozen meals in the past. Are there any frozen meals that are okay on my SuperFoodsRx Diet?"

The answer is "Yes, but. . ." First, as you know already, fresh, whole foods are the best and a bit of planning can help make home-made SuperFoods, especially soups, an easy and quick meal during a busy week. But if you're really pressed and a frozen meal is where you're headed, use this approach.

First check out the 15-Minute SuperFast SuperFoods Recipes (page 328) just to be sure you really can't *throw something together* that's quick and fresh and easy. Then, for

an occasional back-up plan, here are the guidelines for choosing a SuperFoodsRx–approved frozen meal.

- Make sure there are two or more SuperFoods in the meal
- Look for ones with around 300 calories or less
- Aim for less than 450 milligrams sodium (600 as an absolute maximum)
- And the secret SuperFoodsRx solution? Have something *fresh* alongside your frozen meal so you can feel great about your compromise. Examples: an apple, a small salad, a cup of berries, celery and peanut butter, veggie crudités, or a selection from column D in your menus on page 208.

were eating the real thing. In fact some researchers have suggested that people eat as many as 50 percent more calories when the food is labeled as "diet." People often think that "low fat" foods are roughly 40 to 50 percent lower in fat and calories, when in fact they are usually only 15 to 30 percent lower. My best advice: Eat real food and watch your portions!

FlexPlan Guidelines*:

The Food:

- Breakfast is mandatory, the simplest, easiest long-term approach is to stick with one of the breakfast options provided (page 188).

- Carbohydrates in the form of grain and fruit or just fruit at breakfast.

- Grain carbohydrates at lunch or dinner, *but not both*. You'll refer to these as **with** and **without** (grains, that is). But *now* a FlexPlan option that is a grain could technically be added to your **without** meal with advance planning.* Call it your "**without** meal plus FlexPlan grain" to stay on track mentally.

- SuperNutrient Booster every day at mid-morning (or you can vary the time if you insert a FlexPlan option mid-morning instead and as long as you still plan and include your SuperNutrient Booster daily*).

- Afternoon snack every day with a SuperFood or sidekick on most days.

- Eat from your SuperFoodsRx Meal Lists or follow *carefully* the SuperFoodsRx Meal Template (page 178).*

- SuperFoods salad or soup or both every day.

"The FlexPlan is working for me. And it's nice to be able to add a few things in each week. For example, when my parents were in town for a visit, we ate out quite often. I made healthy choices at the restaurants and kept on track. It's lovely to be able to enjoy a sorbet with fresh berries on a hot summer day. I think I enjoyed it more knowing it fit my SuperFoods diet. I lost a steady $3\frac{1}{2}$ pounds a week on the SlimDown but I'm still losing about $1\frac{1}{2}$ pounds a week on the FlexPlan. I'm down nearly 30 pounds after 10 weeks."
—Carol C., wife and mother of four grown children—four sons and a daughter

*Designates guidelines unique to SuperFoodsRx FlexPlan

- 🌿 Monday is Soup & Salad Day.
- 🌿 Wednesday is Veggie Day.
- 🌿 5 SuperFoodsRx FlexPlan Options added at your discretion to weekly menus.*
- 🌿 No food after dinner.
- 🌿 Beverages: Water and Tea.
  - Alcohol is a FlexPlan option and must be planned.*
  - Caloric beverages—100% juice is a FlexPlan option and must be planned.*
  - Up to 1 cup coffee daily (try to shift to tea).
  - Low-fat or nonfat milk or soymilk is okay as a snack or as part of a meal.
  - Green or black tea—1 or more brewed cups daily.
  - 6 + cups water daily—*throughout* your day.

The Behaviors:

- 🌿 Plan your week in advance, selecting from the SuperFoodsRx Meal Lists and highlighting any meals that may be eaten in a restaurant or require a review of the criteria for constructing a SuperFoodsRx meal (page 179).
  - 3 meals, 1 SuperNutrient Booster, 1 snack daily.

If you're a male, very active or have 20 or more pounds to lose here are some extra guidelines for you:

- Add one snack from the list (page 214) daily, either with your morning SuperNutrient Booster or at another time in the afternoon. Space the snack at least 2 hours apart from another snack or meal. So for example, you might have a snack at 3:30, another snack at 5:30, and dinner at 7:30 or 8.

- Add one tennis ball of additional fruit—a SuperFoods fruit or any other choice as long as you're meeting your other SuperFoods Rx Diet goals. This can be added to a meal or stand alone.

- Breakfast variety: minimum 2 different breakfasts weekly.
- Lunch variety: minimum 2–3 different lunches weekly.
- Dinner variety: minimum 3–4 different dinners weekly.
- Lunches and dinners are *interchangeable*.
- Choose your 5 weekly FlexPlan options *
- Will you choose from the original FlexPlan categories?*
- Will you choose a "2 for 1"?*
- Will you choose a FlexPlan exercise option?*

- Daily recording in your Food Diary.
- Do not skip meals or snacks. Eat to boost your metabolism.
- Stop eating within 2, preferably 3 hours of bedtime.
- Monday & Friday weight checks.
- Monday waist measure check.
- Exercise 45 to 60 minutes daily, at least 5 days a week.*
- Do your strength-training program and flexibility exercises.*
- Sleep—aim for a minimum of 7 hours nightly.

Your Weekly FlexPlan Menu Plan

You're probably surprised at how easy the FlexPlan is. It really is a simple, real-life guide to eating. And I know it can be your foolproof system of enjoying a whole new, healthy way to eat and maintain your healthy weight for the rest of your life. Here's your sample FlexPlan Weekly Menu for you to fill out. It will help you track your five Flexes on a weekly basis. It will be your outline for lifelong SuperFoods health. Happy eating!

*Designates guidelines unique to SuperFoodsRx FlexPlan

Weekly Plan/Food Diary for FlexPlan

	MONDAY	TUESDAY	WEDNESDAY
Date			
Breakfast			
SuperNutrient Booster	SuperNutrient Booster	SuperNutrient Booster	SuperNutrient Booster
Lunch	*With Without*	*With Without*	*With Without*
Snack			
Dinner	*With Without*	*With Without*	*With Without*
Special Notes	Soup & Salad Monday		Veggie Wednesday

Comments...
 	
Exercise
  Activity:
  Duration:
  Steps:
 	
How are you feeling?			

FlexPlan
  5 per week
  Remember
  2 max on any
  one day
	FlexPlan 1:
	
	FlexPlan 2:
		FlexPlan 1:
		
		FlexPlan 2:
			FlexPlan 1:
			
			FlexPlan 2:

THURSDAY	FRIDAY	SATURDAY	SUNDAY
SuperNutrient Booster	SuperNutrient Booster	SuperNutrient Booster	SuperNutrient Booster
With *Without*	*With* *Without*	*With* *Without*	*With* *Without*
With *Without*	*With* *Without*	*With* *Without*	*With* *Without*
	Lunch and dinner are ALWAYS interchangeable.		Prepare for the Week Ahead.
FlexPlan 1: FlexPlan 2:	FlexPlan 1: FlexPlan 2:	FlexPlan 1: FlexPlan 2:	FlexPlan 1: FlexPlan 2:

Chapter 6

The SuperFoodsRx LifePlan

This is where you pull all the pieces together. The SuperFoodsRx lifestyle is about more than food; it's about all the aspects of your life than affect your health, sometimes in surprising and significant ways. LifePlan is your blueprint for a healthy future.

....

It's important to know that, despite the almost exclusive interest paid to it, losing weight isn't solely about what you eat. While eating SuperFoods in healthy portions will help you make tremendous strides toward reaching your weight loss goals, you'll achieve your best success if you also pay attention to other factors in your daily life. You already know that exercise is important and you'll want to view that as a critical part of your overall LifePlan. But you shouldn't neglect the important roles stress management and sleep play in keeping your body in balance and primed to shed pounds, and I'll cover those two topics here. I'll also give you some suggestions on how to build a terrific SuperFoodsRx meal anywhere, as well as tips on eating while traveling, dining out, and enjoying parties and social gatherings. These will all ultimately provide you with the keys to long-term SuperFoodsRx Diet success in your LifePlan.

....

My effort of course has been to guide you to healthy, permanent weight and waist loss. Perhaps in the past you've come to the point in a diet where the topic is "maintenance," or how to keep the weight off. But there is a better way to think about this topic. Real maintenance is not about keeping *down*, it's actually about keeping *up*. So let's shift the focus to *genuine* maintenance—

keeping up. You keep up the lifestyle and you'll keep down the weight. People who are most successful at maintaining their weight loss are those who generally focus not only on their weight but rather on "keeping up" the positive eating and lifestyle habits that have helped them reach their goals. LifePlan is your guide to keeping up.

Honor your body. Nourish your body. Inside and out.
That's the goal of the SuperFoodsRx Diet:

- Nourishment on the inside from the SuperFoods and the power of the SuperNutrients, which promote optimum health, weight, endurance, and strength.

- Nourishment from the outside with the LifePlan: exercising, reducing stress, getting sufficient sleep, embracing friends and family, and thus building confidence, self-esteem, and personal power.

There's often someone out there who'll tell you how totally *simple* it is: You eat less—or eat different—and you lose weight. Done. Well, of course, those who've struggled with their weight know there's nothing simple about it. A common issue surrounding weight loss is anxiety about what happens later. Sometimes this anxiety begins the very day you begin the plan. You "bite the bullet" for a period of time and you see results but inside there is a doubtful voice that says, "you know that this can't last." You'll have to go back to "normal" at some point. Then what? Will you regain the weight? Will you "fall off the wagon?" Will you have to feel deprived forever? How do you choose between the thrilling benefits of how you look and feel after losing some excess weight versus your desire to give in to the moment with food choices that may not be in your best long-term interest? These are very stressful concerns, even if they're only bubbling below the surface.

Here's the simple naked truth: Maintenance takes work. Once you've achieved your goal weight, you can't go back to your old habits. Fortunately, with the SuperFoodsRx Diet you won't feel any inclination to. Why? Because after all of your practice with the foods and strategies of this plan, when you "fall back" it will be right back to the tried and true SuperFoods meals and behaviors that are now part of your life. Those old habits will be a distant memory. You'll wonder *was that even me?* New habits will be formed, reinforcements will be in place, and your daily strategies and built-in reminders will anchor your weeks. It won't be difficult to make a daily commitment to your goals and to foster an attitude that recognizes, "this is me today, and I like it. I'm going to do what it takes to be the size I want to be, have the energy I want to enjoy, and the freedom and power to honor my body and live healthfully."

Remember that your SuperFoodsRx lifestyle honors your body today—*and* in the future. Here's where the crucial benefit of this concept comes into play: This is a *lifetime* plan that's all about choice—your choice—to eat well and live well. And, as we've seen and you yourself have proven, this has nothing to do with willpower; it's about learning how to work *with* your body both to lose weight and to learn behaviors that reinforce your good choices and amplify their benefits.

So let's take a look at the LifePlan and how your lifestyle choices are going to deepen your commitment to your SuperFoodsRx healthy life. Here are the topics we'll explore in the LifePlan:

- Keys to Long-Term Success on the SuperFoodsRx Diet
- Stress and Your Diet
- Sleep and Your Diet
- SuperFoodsRx Eating in the Real World
- Help: I'm on a Plateau and I Can't Get Off!

Keys to Long-Term Success on the SuperFoodsRx Diet

Here are the keys to living the SuperFoodsRx lifestyle every day. I've discussed some at length previously; others I'll discuss in more detail here.

- **Eat SuperFoods.** Not only will the SuperFoods cut your risk of long-term disease, but many of them—the foods and the nutrients they provide—will help balance your metabolism and directly or indirectly promote long-term weight loss. Eat them every day—remember the 1, 2, 3 Categories—and you will succeed.

- **Use the SlimDown.** This is your "express" to healthy weight and waist loss. Use it in 2-week cycles until you reach your interim weight goal, or for longer periods if you like until you reach your final goal.

- **Use the FlexPlan.** This is your basic weekly diet. It gives you lots of options to include planned and spontaneous extras in your menu. Use it in 2-week cycles, alternating with your SlimDown if you choose. And then use it *forever*, after you reach your interim or final goal.

- **Don't Skip Meals or Snacks.** Keep your metabolism revved up and your energy on an even keel.

- **Think Category 3 SuperFoods if You're Hungry.** The Category 3 SuperFoods will fill you up and help you reach your goals. Follow the steps to managing hunger in the SlimDown on page 87, *if* hunger strikes.

- **Always Use Portion Control.** Remember your deck of cards and tennis ball. They will remind you to eat for the size you want to be.

- **Learn How To Diet SuperFoodsRx-Style, Anywhere, Anytime.** See page 178 for your general guidelines to building a SuperFoodsRx diet-friendly meal that's "not on the list"—*anywhere, anytime.*

- **Eat Slowly.** Remember, it takes up to 20 minutes for your brain to register that food's "on board" and you're being satisfied. In one study when women took more time to eat, they consumed on average 70 fewer calories than women who ate more quickly.[1] Think about that! This can add up to a lot of calories daily and weekly.

- **Monitor Your Body.** Check and record your weight and waist measurements twice a week—Mondays and Fridays—to help keep you on track. It's impossible to "get lost" when you're checking your map regularly.[2]

- **Monitor Behaviors.** Your food diary will ensure you maintain your weight-loss goals. It's a great asset. Once you're on the FlexPlan, you can work out a recording schedule that works for you—4 days a week? Every other day? As long as you record you'll be rewarded. Some folks who have achieved their weight-loss goal record three or four days every other week. Whatever works for you is fine, but make sure you're recording at least every other week. That way you won't let months roll by again where you weren't paying attention. Record your daily exercise as well, right alongside your food diary or as an independent log.

Exercise. We have taken a look at some of the empowering and extraordinary benefits of exercise. Now, it's simply crucial to acknowledge that exercise—regular daily and weekly exercise—must be a part of your SuperFoodsRx lifestyle. Wear a pedometer. (See page 78.) Record your steps. Work up to at least 60 total minutes of exercise and activity daily for the long run. Research has shown that 60 to 90 minutes is what it takes. If this still seems overwhelming, remember that you should just start where you're able now and work up to this goal little by little, every day, over time. Remember, too, that you can break your exercise into smaller bits and it will still count.

Manage Stress. Stress management is as important to a healthy lifestyle as exercise and choosing the right foods. And it plays a significant role in your ability to maintain a healthy weight. I'll give you some tips below on how to approach this important issue.

Sleep. We'll take a closer look at sleep below. For now, the most important thing you need to know is that adequate sleep actually *favors* healthy weight loss while lack of sleep can make your efforts to lose weight ever more challenging. Get seven to eight hours every night. You really do need it.

Believe in Yourself. Eat for and live the life of the person you are and aspire to be. Visualize your success, make choices that favor your personal goals, and know you can get there. Maintain a positive attitude and positive outlook and practice positive self-talk. Everyone has ups and downs, tough days and easy days. But each small step in the right direction gets you closer to your goal. One day, one step, one minute, one blueberry at a time.

Reflect, Recap, Refocus. Many of us hurtle from day to day, checking things off our to-do lists and never looking back. While this may feel efficient, it's an approach that doesn't really help when it comes to weight loss. Your long-term success is a lifetime goal. Keep your eyes on the prize, but reflect on how far you've come. Develop the habit of reflecting on your day, and, perhaps—at least at the outset—writing down three successful things you did—*three small successes*, I like to call them. If you like, it should be easy enough to jot them down in your food diary. Look back on the healthy choices you've made for your life and refocus on where you want to be tomorrow, in 1 week, 1 year, and 5 years. Visualize a decade ahead, too. See yourself living healthfully, actively, successfully maintaining your SuperFoodsRx lifestyle.

Stress and Your Diet

Stress has become such a familiar part of our daily vocabulary—raise your hand if you're stressed out—that it's easy for us to ignore its effects. But stress is a real and a serious threat to your overall health as well as your efforts to lose weight.

To better understand some of the consequences of stress, let's take a look at what happens when your body copes with a threat. Your body is constantly trying to maintain a state of internal stability, called homeostasis. You sweat to cool yourself on a hot day and shiver to stay warm when it's very cold. If thunder cracks, you jump. If your child is about to fall you instinctively reach out to grab him. When your body feels stressed, it struggles to compensate for the real or perceived threat that's created the stress. This response can involve a complex series of biochemical changes that struggle to bring you back to your pre-stressed state. For example, when you're stressed your body releases various hormones and chemicals including adrenaline, cortisol, and others that shift your body into a flight-or-fight response. These hormones increase your metabolism, your heart rate, respiration, blood pressure, and muscle tension. If these bodily changes are channeled into a physical activity—fighting a lion or running a marathon—the stress can be resolved. If, however, the stress is a chronic and unresolved part of your life, like a difficult boss or an unhappy relationship, or even an inevitably backed-up daily commute, the effects on your body are ongoing and dangerous.

Long-term, unresolved stress of the kind that many of us endure daily makes us vulnerable to hypertension, coronary heart disease, osteoporosis, and other disorders. Most significant to those of you working hard to lose weight, unresolved stress also has been linked to developing insulin resistance (a risk factor for diabetes) as well as developing the "belly fat" associated with inflammation. Excess cortisol may also contribute to leptin resistance. Leptin is a hormone that is recognized as a "turn off signal" to hunger. Though the complex mechanisms of hormonal interactions are not yet fully understood, it is generally accepted that leptin has a strong potential to suppress appetite. Leptin resistance makes appetite control a continuing challenge. Chronically elevated cortisol in conjunction with adrenaline can also encourage your body to hold on to fat,[3] and lead to elevated insulin levels or insulin resistance thereby favoring fat storage, particularly around the abdomen. These complex interactions throw yet other obstacles before you as you try to reduce fat and inches in, on and around your body. High cortisol levels stimulated by stressful situations can also play a contributing role in bone loss over time.

So how do you deal with stress? You de-stress whenever possible! I know it seems easier said than done but if you teach yourself to adopt some simple stress-reducing strategies, you really can reduce the physical effects of stress.

In essence you need to become stress resistant *and* stress resilient. It's like rolling with some of the punches while learning to dodge others before they're even thrown. An effective three-prong approach to managing stress and keeping cortisol levels in check include: first, following the SuperFoodsRx Diet, which is rich in foods that will reduce the effects of inflammation and internal stress on the body; second, getting regular adequate exercise, which will help dissipate unfavorable chemical responses created by stress while simultaneously releasing favorable "feel good" chemicals; and third, incorporating some specific stress-reduction techniques and practices into your daily life.

Just as you will customize your FlexPlan options in your SuperFoodsRx Diet, you need to customize your stress-management practices to fit your lifestyle. Meditation and journaling and other activities can be great solutions for some individuals but not the right fit for others. Choose a method or two that suits you and practice it regularly to help reduce chronic stress. You'll find that these techniques will ultimately reduce your body's physiological response to stress and will also become pleasurable interludes in your daily routine.

....

Here are a few activities that can be part of your stress-management routine:

- Relaxation techniques: meditation, mindful walking, power naps
- Mind-body techniques: visualization, guided imagery, qi gong (traditional Chinese breathing exercises)
- Hobbies: journaling, scrapbooking, playing or listening to music, reading, learning a language, etc.
- Exercise: tai chi, yoga, walking, and all forms of exercise
- Using your mantra: posting and saying your SuperFoods mantra of "honor your body" and establishing a very personal mantra about your health and your goals
- Complementary health care: massage, acupuncture, biofeedback, counseling

While day-to-day behaviors and practices should be part of your Super-FoodsRx weight-loss program and lifestyle overall, sometimes you just need a quick fix to defuse a momentary or acute stress. Knowing what to do in a

Research has shown that relaxation techniques can have a direct impact on the body's immune system. Mind-body techniques including meditation have been associated with higher levels of infection-fighting antibodies, improved wound healing, lower blood pressure, reduced anxiety and nausea, and promoting a healthy immune system.[4]

pinch can bring you back to center. Try to pick one or two of these activities that appeal to you and use them whenever you find yourself at wit's end.

Quick Activities for Relieving Temporary Stress and Anxiety

- Get up and walk. Walk around the block, up and down the hall if you're at the office, or up and down a flight of stairs.

- Drink a glass of cool water or a cup of tea.

- Breathe deeply. Close your eyes and take 10 deep breaths: first 5 in and out of your nose; second 5 in through your nose and out through your mouth.

- If you're alone, throw your arms up into the air and exclaim from deep inside with lots of breath, "Aarggh." Repeat four or five times.

- Standing up straight with feet shoulder-width apart, starting with your hands, clench all your muscles tight (hands to arms to shoulders to neck to jaw then clenching stomach to legs to feet) and hold for a count of 3. Release, bending forward into a shrug until you are completely limp. Repeat.

- Force a laugh of exasperation (Ha, ha, ha, ha, ha! Ha, ha, ha, ha, ha!) so that you sound like a sinister character in a movie.

- Close your eyes for a full minute, picture the ocean with waves crashing, and imagine pieces of the stress being cracked as each wave breaks hard against the sand. Let the pieces float away.

- Call a friend.

- Try one of your own favorite stress-reducing activities—e.g. listening to music, reading, etc.—for 5 to 10 minutes.

There, don't you feel better?

Sip your stress away, with tea. In one study in London, men who drank 4 cups of tea daily over the course of 6 weeks showed lower cortisol levels after performing tasks designed to be stressful compared to drinking a placebo beverage. The tea drinkers also reported increased feelings of relaxation after stressful tasks compared with the fake-tea placebo.[5] While you're at it, make it green tea. Ahhh, what a relaxing Super-Food.

Sleep and Your Diet

Chronic stress and reduced or impaired sleep often walk stressfully and drowsily hand in hand. Sleep deprivation can create stress and stress can interrupt sleep patterns, which can in turn generate more stress. And that's not all: Both chronic stress *and* sleep deprivation each play an independent role in our struggles with overweight and obesity.

Most people who are struggling to lose weight never stop to consider the effect that sleep could be having on their efforts. In fact, I've even heard from clients who ask if getting *less* sleep might be helpful as they'd burn more calories if they were awake more hours. While this could seem logical at first blush, research has demonstrated that the exact opposite is true: A good night's sleep—a restful 7 hours for most people—actually favors a healthy weight and body mass index while inadequate sleep can make losing weight ever more difficult while simultaneously having other negative health consequences. We've long known that sleep seems to refresh the brain but we now know that sleep, or the lack thereof, affects a host of bodily systems including our metabolism, our hormones, and our immune function. The interplay of these effects can actually promote weight gain. Just as significant for individuals working to control their weight, inadequate sleep can also negatively affect decision-making about food choices and exercise. Consider these facts:

- Research has shown that approximately 7 hours of quality sleep are necessary for good health and weight control.[6] Researchers also suspect that chronic sleep loss may accelerate the onset and increase the severity of symptoms and conditions related to aging including memory loss, diabetes, high blood pressure, and obesity.[7] Conversely, too much sleep has been associated with increased mortality, heart disease, and other health concerns like depression.

- One large scale study following more than 68,000 women for 16 years showed that those who slept *less than* 7 hours on average per night put on *more weight* during middle age than women who slept 7 hours.[8] In addition, over the course of the study those women who slept only 5 hours a night were nearly one-third more likely to gain significant weight (33 pounds or more).

🌿 Another study found that adults who slept 4 hours or less per night were 73 percent more likely to be obese than those who slept between 7 and 9 hours each night.[9] And those who got between 5 and 6 hours of sleep had a 50 percent and 23 percent higher risk of serious overweight or obesity, respectively, than those who were getting their full night's rest.

🌿 Individuals reporting less than 7 hours were also more likely to be obese and have higher than average body mass indexes.[10]

🌿 Sleep deprivation

- Can impair insulin sensitivity (a diabetes risk factor) and carbohydrate tolerance, and therefore potentially increase the risk for diabetes[11]

- Is associated with increased levels of ghrelin (the "turn on" switch for appetite) and decreased levels of leptin (the "turn off" switch for appetite), thus increasing both hunger and appetite[12]

- Can increase cortisol—the stress hormone associated with promoting obesity[13]

🌿 Less than 4 hours of quality sleep nightly and chronic sleep loss overall have been shown to have a harmful effect on carbohydrate metabolism.[14]

An occasional night of disrupted sleep can be overcome from a metabolic standpoint. But constant, chronic lack of sleep can ultimately result in a disrupted metabolism that encourages more fat storage and especially fat storage in those areas of the body that increase disease risk. Chronic sleep deprivation can also promote metabolic disorders related to blood sugar/insulin regulation. This is not to mention the hormonal shifts in perceived hunger and appetite that can promote behaviors that may ultimately encourage more eating along with reduced efforts to exercise due to general fatigue.

Is there hope? Absolutely! The human body is a finely tuned machine. If you can arrange your life such that you can plan on getting at least 7 hours of restful sleep most nights, you'll be taking one more step to promote weight loss.

Tips for Better Sleep

Here are some suggestions that will help you get a restful night's sleep:

- Create a wind-down ritual to prepare yourself for bed. Try herbal tea, dimmed lights, quiet reading, or a warm bath.

- Your sleep environment really matters. Make sure your bedroom space has good window coverings for darkness, is uncluttered and well ventilated.

- No TV near bedtime and preferably no TV in the bedroom.

- No work in bed or bedroom. The bedroom should be reserved only for sleeping, resting, and sex.

- Avoid eating within 3 hours of bedtime.

- If you take a calcium supplement, take at least part of your dose in the evening as calcium is a mineral that can help with sleep.

- Alcohol can affect sleep. You may fall asleep faster after drinking, but your sleep may be less restful. Limit or eliminate alcohol.

- Caffeine is a nervous system stimulant and affects your production of the sleep hormone melatonin. If you're sensitive to the effects of caffeine, time your intake so it won't interfere with sleep. For some people this means no caffeine after 3:00 p.m., for others it's noon.

- Scents can help you sleep. Lavender has been shown to be particularly effective.

- Cooler room temperature can help promote sleep.

- *Hang your worries at the door* before entering the bedroom—they'll be there to pick up in the morning (and amazingly there are usually fewer to pick up the next day after a good night's sleep). Visualize this and practice. When you cross the threshold, you are entering a "stress-free" zone. Your worries and stressors may not go away altogether but at least ban them from the bedroom.

- Practice a stress-management technique that can also help with sleep: guided imagery, meditation, and breathing exercises can be effective choices.

- Invest in a quality alarm with a backup battery. You'd be surprised at how many people wake up frequently in a near panic, worrying that they've overslept or slept through their alarm.

- Try using a sleep mask and make sure you have a good comfortable pillow and mattress.

- Sound machines with soothing sounds can also be helpful. Some people like the sound of the ocean, others the sounds of nature, and others prefer "white noise." Find what appeals to you.

SuperFoodsRx Eating in the Real World

It's one thing to eat at home, following your SuperFoodsRx menus and recipes. But there will be many times when you will be eating out—at friends' homes, in restaurants—and also many occasions like parties and holidays that require certain tactics to enable you to stick to your healthy lifestyle. We'll provide LifePlan tips for each of those situations.

Building a SuperFoodsRx–friendly meal— anywhere, anytime

Let's begin with a general rule that will be true for dining in restaurants, during travel and at parties. Besides following the overall guidelines of whichever phase—SlimDown or FlexPlan—you're following, along with your daily and weekly goals and your portion-control guidelines, here is how you can adapt the SuperFoodsRx Diet to any situation:

- Breakfast—Choose and stick with a SuperFoodsRx breakfast option. Review the various choices and follow portion guidelines using your deck of cards and tennis ball as your visual reminders. Most SuperFoodsRx dieters find this very simple.

- Lunch/Dinner—Choose Either/Or (**with** grains or **without** grains at one or other—lunch OR dinner, but not both), then proceed:

  - **With** grains (lunch or dinner): 1 tennis ball carbohydrates, 1 deck of cards protein, 2 tennis balls vegetables/fruit

    Aim in general for <u>one</u> Category 1 SuperFood; <u>one</u> Category 2 Super-Food and <u>two</u> Category 3 SuperFoods.

  - **Without** grains (lunch or dinner): 1 deck of cards protein, 2 tennis balls vegetables; 1 tennis ball fruit

    Aim in general for 1 Category 2 SuperFood and 2–3 Category 3 SuperFoods.

The Social Whirl

Let's face it, if eating were just about nutrition and providing fuel to your body, it wouldn't be so hard to stick to a plan, right? But eating is so much more. It's social, it's business, it's holidays and special occasions, it's convenience, it's vacation, it's spiritual, and of course it's your sustenance, too. Because of all these varied issues that both enhance and complicate the practice of eating, you can at times feel at risk of diet derailment. When restaurant portions are huge, party fare is high-calorie, and you're constantly surrounded by temptations to abandon your efforts, you can sometimes feel like you must make a choice between being lean and healthy or having a social life. You're not alone with this dilemma: socializing has been estimated to be one of the top reasons people eventually fail on a diet. But take heart: With a little effort you can prevail and beat the odds. Here are some strategies you can adopt as your own to help keep you on track in various social and travel situations.

> **Deck of Cards** = 3 oz. cooked/prepared
>
> **Tennis ball** = $1/2$–$2/3$ cup

Restaurant Tips

Americans eat out on average four times weekly. According to a report recently published by a nonprofit group called the Keystone Center, we spend almost half of our food budgets on foods eaten outside the home and these foods provide more than one-third of our daily calorie intake.[16] While you'll probably find it harder to stick to your SuperFoodsRx Diet if you eat out frequently, there's certainly no harm in enjoying an occasional restaurant experience. The trick is in knowing how to navigate your way to a healthy meal. The two keys to successful restaurant dining are SuperFoods and Portion Control.

- Ask if the restaurant offers a special "heart healthy" or "low-fat" menu and, if so, apply your portion control expertise to make the amount right for you.

- Order first unless you're the host, so you're less tempted to say "I'll have what she's/he's having." You'd be surprised how you can set the course of action for the table by ordering a fresh-brewed iced tea or sparkling water with orange instead of wine. You'll gain confidence and feel proud of sticking with your goals—and you might even find others at the table saying, "I'll have what she's/he's having" since many of us really want to be healthy but just need a little inspiration.

- Consider asking the waiter to package half of your portion in the kitchen for you to bring home. Consider splitting an entrée with someone at the table and ordering separate appetizers.

- Try ordering a "custom" meal: Ask the waiter what fish or turkey or chicken is fresh or particularly recommended that day. Order it simply prepared—preferably grilled—accompanied by a selection of fresh seasonal vegetables. When you create your own meal you are less likely to be overwhelmed by menu choices and more likely to make your waiter's job easier. Endlessly "editing" a restaurant menu becomes tedious for those with you and those who work at the restaurant.

- Choose a zero-calorie beverage like water or seltzer with lemon or orange or a splash of 100-percent juice.

- Remember the SuperFoods 1, 2, 3 Categories. Start by determining what Category 3 foods you will choose and work backward from there. Inserting lower calorie foods in your meal, especially those Category 3 Super-Foods, can help boost nutrition and satisfy you while cutting overall calories. Small salads, healthy portions of one or more vegetables, or a non-cream, vegetable-, broth- or tomato-based soup are great options. Do a quick mental check on how the day is stacking up in terms of your daily goals.

- Grilled, lean fish or poultry are the best choices and they're SuperFoods. Just be sure to remove the skin from chicken or fish before eating.

- Is this a *with* or *without* grains meal? If it's a *with* grains meal—stick with one type of grain. Whole grain bread or pasta or corn tortilla or brown rice. Choose one, visualize that tennis ball serving on your plate, and you'll be fine.

- If you're ordering a side salad along with a meal, hold the cheese and croutons. If the side salad is part of your meal (for example, along with a soup or shrimp cocktail, or to accompany a piece of grilled salmon or grilled chicken breast), it can include some cheese but no more than 2 tablespoons. Otherwise, the cheese should be counted as a FlexPlan option. Order low-fat or nonfat salad dressing and dilute it, or even try salsa as a dressing substitute. Use balsamic vinegar and 1 teaspoon (measure at the table—take control!) of extra virgin olive oil. Use some wedges of lemon, lime, or orange to spread flavor and moisture.

- Request that all vegetables be steamed or very lightly sautéed

- Ask if you can substitute healthier items for less healthy side dishes: sweet potato instead of fries, fresh sliced fruit instead of hash browns, brown rice instead of white rice or bread, a side of vegetables instead of coleslaw.

- Assume that every main dish constitutes two or three servings or meals. Ask for an extra plate and serve yourself "family style" onto that plate. Then either get rid of the extra food or leave it in the middle of the table for others to share if they like. This is an especially great strategy for lifelong members of the *Clean Plate Club*.

- Request all dressings and condiments *on the side* so you'll have control.

- Avoid alcohol. If you're on the SlimDown, remind yourself of your goal: no drinkable calories—alcohol or otherwise. And if you're following the FlexPlan, know your choices. Choose in advance and stick to the program and you'll succeed and feel great. Whatever you do, avoid the "mega cocktails." Super grande margaritas and large daiquiris and piña coladas can run 400 or more calories.

- Berries are a great dessert choice. Forgo any cream or sauce.

Party Tips

Parties and special events can be challenging. Gatherings of family and friends are often centered on eating and many traditional party foods are not especially healthy. For many people, social situations are the most challenging hurdles for those trying to stick to a healthy eating plan. What to do? Here are some tips to help you manage special occasions:

- Make a short list of what you've accomplished thus far toward your weight-loss goals and the four or five reasons you want to continue your success. Write down your short list. The act of doing so confirms that these goals are important to you.

- Stick with your SuperFoodsRx Diet. If you're on the FlexPlan, plan ahead on what options you might choose to include at the party.

- Don't go to a party starving. Eat a SuperFoodsRx snack before you go and drink a tall glass of water about a half hour before the party.

- It's not a party without SuperFoods! Most parties these days include a vegetable platter. You can always offer to bring one for everyone to enjoy.

- Adjust your daily and weekly menu. If you have one or two parties scheduled in a week, consider them when you create your weekly menu. You might want to plan some lighter meals and skip some FlexPlan Options on non-party days. If you're going to an evening party, have a lighter lunch that day. Perhaps party day might be a good choice for a Soup & Salad day.

- Keep your hands full. Keep a drink—sparkling water with lemon or lime—in one hand and some veggie treats in the other.

- Limit alcohol. If you're on the FlexPlan, decide in advance what, if any, alcohol you'll drink. Enjoy that drink and then shift to sparkling or flat water or tea.

- Visit with people, not food. Don't linger at the food table. Make a point of catching up with friends and/or meeting new people.

- Practice saying "no thank you" before you even leave for the party. This sounds funny, but it's truly helpful.

- Party with a buddy. If you have a SuperFoodsRx Diet buddy who'll be at the party, check in with one another for support.

- A party does not count as exercise! Don't use it as an excuse to skip a workout. Skipping exercise can sometimes do more damage to your progress than a few extra nibbles at a party.

- Keep on monitoring. Even if you feel you've made some poor choices, don't avoid recording your weight and waist on Monday and Friday as usual. It's those skipped measurements that can lead to backsliding.

- Have fun. If you overeat on an occasion, let it go. Start off again on the right foot immediately and get back to moderation. Lighten up—in mind and body—and enjoy the success you've achieved.

Travel Tips

Travel can mean changes in your eating schedule and challenges that differ from your routine ones. But a little focus, attention, and planning will help you stick to your SuperFoodsRx Diet no matter where you are. Here are some tips and strategies:

- If you're flying and a meal is provided on the flight, consider ordering a special meal. Low-fat/low-cholesterol and vegetarian options are often healthier and more nutritious than the standard fare.

- Whether you're traveling by train, plane, or car, consider packing your own meals. A healthy peanut butter and all-fruit preserve sandwich on whole wheat bread or a hummus and veggie wrap on a whole wheat tortilla, along with a piece of fruit, is an excellent, healthy meal.

- Don't forget to pack snacks. Resealable plastic bags with trail mixes, whole grain crackers, veggies like carrot sticks and cherry tomatoes are great, metabolism-boosting snacks. See the SuperFoodsRx Snacks (page 214) for a full list of possibilities.

- Drink plenty of water, especially when flying. Flying dehydrates you and extra healthy fluids are important. Avoid sodas and alcohol.

- Choose healthy options from an airport deli. Try a lean turkey sandwich loaded with veggies or a vegetarian sandwich. Other choices include: low-fat yogurt, grilled chicken breast sandwich on whole grain bread, vegetable wraps, and fresh fruit. Remember: Skip the mayo!

- Take advantage of travel to walk, walk, walk. Use layover time in airports for a brisk walk around the terminal. Skip the moving sidewalks. If you're in a new city, walking is the best way to explore. If you're on a car trip, stop regularly to stretch your legs and log some steps on your pedometer.

- Avoid mini bars at hotels. They're expensive and tend to feature high-calorie, low-nutrient-density foods. Request a room without a mini bar or ask that the mini bar be emptied before you arrive so you can fill it with bottled water, veggies, or fruit snacks.

- Remember your Veggie Day. It will help keep you mindful of your SuperFoodsRx lifestyle. If you're traveling abroad or domestically, you'll often find interesting vegetarian choices that will make your Veggie Day a memorable pleasure. Remember though that 'vegetarian' doesn't *always* mean healthy so use your SuperFoodsRx Diet as your guide to the best choices.

Are you a stress eater? One study showed that nearly three-fourths of survey respondents reported increased snacking when under stress. The shift was more toward snack foods and away from fruits, vegetables, and protein sources like meat and fish. Dieters also more frequently reported stress overeating than non-dieters.[17] The lesson? Have healthy SuperFoods readily available and work on keeping stress at bay—every day!

- Pick your splurges. Decide in advance when you want to try a special dessert or interesting menu entrée. If you plan it, there's no reason to feel guilty later. Use your FlexPlan Options and get some extra walking in to compensate for any extra choices.

- Don't deprive yourself of regional specialties, but try to enjoy them in small amounts. Remember that the biggest pleasure is in that first delicious bite.

- Always pack your sneakers and your pedometer. Make any trip an active one by choosing hotels with fitness centers and walk, walk, walk wherever you find yourself. If you're on a business trip, make a point to schedule time for exercise. There's always a spare hour in the morning, the evening, or even at lunchtime. Conduct your meetings in motion when you can: Walk and talk. Walk while you use your cell phone. Walk at the end of the day to wind down and refresh.

- Resistance bands and water-filled hand weights are two exercise aids that travel well and will keep you on target with your strength-training exercises.

Help! I'm on a Plateau and I Can't Get Off!

Those last few pounds always seem so hard . . . this is the point when many people can feel discouraged. But don't lose heart! There are some real reasons your weight loss may have slowed down. For one thing, as you approach your goal, fewer calories are needed to feed a lighter you. For every pound you've lost, you require about 8 calories less to maintain your current weight. This doesn't seem like too much but if you've lost 20 pounds that adds up to 160 calories or one FlexPlan Option equivalent. Remember, the FlexPlan is designed to help you to continue to lose weight but if you get too "flexible," adding an extra option or two, or ignoring portion control you'll find the needle on your scale stuck. Here are some strategies to get you off that plateau:

- Recognize peaks and valleys. The path to long-term healthy weight loss doesn't always run smooth. You may be losing inches while the scale doesn't budge. Muscle weighs more than fat and so you could be increasing muscle mass—a good thing—while you weight doesn't change.

- Record your intake. Your food diary is one of the best techniques for getting off a plateau. Your food diary eliminates mindless eating. The sandwich crusts from your toddler's plate, the handful of nuts at a party . . . . You'll think twice when you know you're logging it all.

- Review your portion control. Some people relax about portions as they approach their goals. This can stall weight loss. Pay attention to the amounts you eat—eat for the weight you want to be—and you'll see progress.

- Keep it simple. The exciting SuperFoodsRx menus and options may have you overcompensating with your shopping to ensure you have all the ingredients necessary. Make sure to sit down and plan your weeks in two week cycles with plenty of, but not too much, variety (see page 90 for a reminder). Too much food in the house can sometimes lead to too much food in the mouth.

- Boost your exercise. Getting in a half hour or 45 minutes daily? Terrific. Now add 10 or 15 minutes to that. Sometimes just a bit of extra movement will turn the tide.

- Keep your focus. It's sometimes harder to stick with your new eating habits as time moves on, simply because we all crave change and freedom. Here's a suggestion that can help: Break out! Try a new SuperFoodsRx recipe. Try some SuperFoods that you've never tasted. Treat yourself to a beautiful prepared bowl of cut-up fruit at the supermarket. Try a new brand of yogurt or green tea. Keep it interesting and fun.

Reflect. You're better off than you were a month ago, right? Sometimes we forget how much we've accomplished. Take some credit for what you've already achieved. You've already taken steps to honor your body and keep in mind that the scale isn't the best or only measure of your achievement.

I hope that you've found these LifePlan discussions helpful. I know, and successful SuperFoodsRx dieters tell me, that it's far, far easier to reach a weight-loss goal when you transform your notion of "diet" from "eating less" to "living well." The Life-Plan will help you achieve this in your own life.

We invite you to visit **www.superfoodsrx.com** for more information and updates on the SuperFoodsRx Diet.

> "A person has to realize that she is losing weight for herself and not for anyone else. Others will reap the benefits, but ultimately I realized I'm doing it for me."
> —Shelly, 42-year-old medical coder and mother of two

Chapter 7

SuperFoodsRx Menus, Meals, and Recipes

Ease, flavor, and interchangeability were our guidelines in creating a delicious selection of SuperFoodsRx dining options. We have organized the meal options and recipes ahead so you can quickly find what *you* like to eat and to easily reference in order to plan, shop, prepare, and stay committed to your SuperFoodsRx Diet. We've even provided a list of 15-Minute SuperFast recipes along with ways to make "trades" in particular instances when you want to even *spice it up* further after a bit of practice.

Breakfast Selections

Guidelines:

- Choose 2–3 breakfasts for every 2-week cycle from the options below.
- Pencil them into your weekly food plan.
- Include the simple ingredients on your shopping list.
- Eat breakfast every day and ENJOY!

Meal "Types." *Most of us have a breakfast "style"—maybe you're a yogurt person or a cereal gal. Maybe eggs are your thing or your morning toast. Whatever your breakfast style, you'll find enough variety here to fit your SuperFoods SuperNutrient needs!*

- Oatmeal
- Yogurt and Cottage Cheese
- Cereal and Milk
- Muffin Plus
- Eggs
- Toast Plus
- Smoothies

Oatmeal

Remember: You can substitute the sidekicks.

Oatmeal with Blueberries and Almonds (no milk)

1 ounce dry (1 packet or ⅓ cup) oats (make with water)

¾ cup blueberries (fresh or frozen)

1 tablespoon slivered almonds

¼ teaspoon cinnamon

2 teaspoons honey

Oatmeal with Blueberries, Ground Flaxseed, and Milk/Soy Milk

1 ounce dry (1 packet or ⅓ cup) oats (make with nonfat milk or soy milk)

¾ cup nonfat milk

¾ cup blueberries (fresh or frozen)

¼ teaspoon cinnamon

1 tablespoon ground flaxseed

You can substitute 1½ tablespoons chopped walnuts or sliced almonds for ground flaxseed.

Oatmeal Swirl

Swirl in ¼ cup Fresh Blueberry Compote* or Spicy Pumpkin Butter* or dice and add a Baked Apple* to 1 ounce dry (1 packet or ⅓ cup) oats (make with water) and 2 tablespoons chopped or sliced nuts (or ground flaxseed).

Yogurt and Cottage Cheese

Yogurt, Strawberry, and Chopped Walnut Breakfast Parfait

Layer:

¾ cup plain nonfat yogurt

½ medium banana, sliced (3½")

1 cup sliced strawberries, fresh or thawed frozen (or ½ cup blueberries)

2 tablespoon chopped walnuts (or sidekick)

1 teaspoon honey

*Indicates a SuperFoodsRx Diet recipe available starting on page 217

Fruit on the Bottom Yogurt

1 cup nonfat or low-fat plain yogurt

¼ cup Fresh Blueberry Compote* or 3 tablespoons Spicy Pumpkin Butter*

Add one of the following: 2 tablespoons slivered almonds OR ¾ cup whole grain cereal or have a hardboiled egg on the side

Baked Apple*

with 1 cup nonfat or low-fat plain yogurt (or ¾ cup no-salt added nonfat cottage cheese) and 2 tablespoons ground flaxseed or chopped/slivered nuts

SuperFoodsRx Granola* ⅛ cup

1 cup plain nonfat yogurt (or ¾ cup 1% fat (or nonfat) cottage cheese–no salt added; All Season Fruit Salad* 1 serving

SuperFoodsRx Blueberry Muffin with Walnuts* and Yogurt (or Cottage Cheese)—see opposite page

SuperFoodsRx Pumpkin Walnut Muffin* and Yogurt (or Cottage Cheese)—see opposite page

Also see options under Muffins Plus on page 191 and Smoothies on page 193.

Cereal and Milk

Kashi® GOLEAN® or Nutritious Living® Hi-Lo™

1 cup cereal

¾ cup nonfat or low-fat milk or soy milk

¾ cup blueberries (or sidekick)

Indicates a SuperFoodsRx Diet recipe available starting on page 217

Nature's Path® Optimum Power Flax-Soy-Blueberry or Cascadian Farm® Great Measure or Cascadian Farm® Raisin Bran or Barbara's® Multigrain Shredded Spoonfuls

¾ cup cereal

¾ cup nonfat milk or soy milk

1 cup raspberries (or sidekick)

Cheerios® or Post® Shredded Wheat or Cascadian Farm® Organic Clifford Crunch

1 cup cereal

¾ cup plain nonfat or low-fat soy milk or nonfat milk

¾ cup blueberries (or sidekick)

1 tablespoon sliced almonds

Substitute berries with an orange on the side for any cereal breakfast.

Muffin Plus

SuperFoodsRx Blueberry Muffin with Walnuts* and Yogurt (or Cottage Cheese)

1 cup plain nonfat yogurt (or ¾ cup 1% fat (or nonfat) cottage cheese–no salt added

1 tablespoon ground flaxseed, or 1 teaspoon sliced almonds or chopped walnuts

SuperFoodsRx Pumpkin Walnut Muffin* and Yogurt (or Cottage Cheese)

1 cup plain nonfat yogurt (or ¾ cup 1% fat (or nonfat) cottage cheese–no salt added

1 tablespoon ground flaxseed, or 1 teaspoon sliced almonds or chopped walnuts

You can also choose a natural, whole grain muffin with berries that is 150 calories maximum.

Eggs

Egg Frittata with Cherry Tomatoes, Spinach, and Cheese*

1 slice of whole grain toast (80–100 calories/slice)

1 tablespoon all-fruit preserves (low sugar/no sugar added)

"Eggsellent" Spinach, Mushroom & Onion Scramble*

1 slice of whole grain toast (80–100 calories/slice)

1 tablespoon all fruit preserves (low sugar/no sugar added)

½ cup blueberries

Cheddar Cheese, Egg, and Tomato Toast

1 slice whole grain bread, lightly toasted (80–100 calories/slice)

Layer and toast:

1 whole egg (poached or scrambled)

2 tablespoons grated sharp cheddar (= ½ ounce)

1 medium tomato, sliced

Enjoy with: an apple, orange, or ¾ cup berries.

Toast Plus

Cheddar Cheese, Avocado and Tomato Toast

1 slice whole grain bread, lightly toasted (80–100 calories/slice)

Layer and toast:

2 tablespoons avocado, mashed

2 tablespoons grated sharp cheddar (= ½ ounce)

1 medium tomato sliced

Enjoy with an apple, orange, or ¾ cup berries.

*Indicates a SuperFoodsRx Diet recipe available starting on page 217

Almond Butter and Banana Toast

> 1 slice whole grain bread, lightly toasted (80–100 calories/slice)
>
> 1½ tablespoons almond or peanut butter
>
> ½ medium banana (approx. 3½ inches)
>
> *Assemble on fresh or toasted bread. Cut banana into "coin" and enjoy open-faced or as a half sandwich.*

Cheddar Cheese, Egg, and Tomato Toast (see Eggs on previous page)

Smoothies

Fruit Delight Breakfast Smoothie*

SuperFoodsRx Pumpkin Smoothie*

Lunch and Dinner Selections

Sandwiches, Pitas, Wraps, Tacos, Pizza
  Guidelines
  Options

Soups and Salads: Mix-and-Match
  Guidelines
  Options

Entrée Salads (Cold Entrée) and Hot Entrée Meals
  Guidelines
  Entrée Salads (Cold Entrées)
  Hot Entrées

SuperFoodsRx Diet Exchange Tables for Sides and Grains
  Non-Grain *Trades* for Recommended Sides and Accompaniments in the
  SuperFoodsRx Meal Options
  Change the Grain

Introducing the SuperFoodsRx Lunch and Dinner Meal Selections

A whole new way to diet deliciously, optimize your health, and live in the real world.

You want versatility. You want to lose weight *and* enjoy your meals. Well here you are! Lots and lots of SuperFoodsRx dieters' (not to mention their unknowing families', friends', and colleagues') taste buds, stomachs, and appetites have been deliciously satisfied with the many selections here. Why? Because the menus and recipes consist of easy, scrumptious, satisfying, and practical, everyday SuperFoods recipes and sides designed for your good health and ready for you to insert your own personality.

And as the newest member of the SuperFoodsRx Diet experience toward weight loss and improved health, you will include these selections into your weekly plan. After you practice with the menus for several weeks, you can also choose to customize the sides you select by referring to the handy *trades* charts starting on page 207. Be sure to mark your favorites: You'll want to prepare them again and again!

Guidelines:

🌿 Remember to choose your lunch and dinner meals—one **with** grains and the other **without**. You decide. Will it be lunch **with** and dinner **without**? Or will you reverse that? Decide when you're planning your weekly menus and making your shopping list. It's easy—7 **with grains** meals and 7 **without**.

- Remember Monday is Soup & Salad day at one of your meals. Select your meal from the *Mix-and-Match* meal options.

- Wednesday is your Veggie Day: Select one **with grain** and one **without grain** meal as usual, just choose from the options with the 🌿 symbol.

- Keep it simple. You can have the same meal twice (cook once, eat twice) or stick to familiar items for a while until you have them mastered. There are dozens of possible meal options here, not to mention all the various *trades* you can make for your sides. Include the trades with the already more than 100 specifically designed options of soups, salads, sandwiches, hot and cold entrées and you have variety to last you through every phase of your weight-loss journey and for lots of healthy years to come!

- Stick to the sides (or permitted "trades" starting on page 207) suggested for each entrée.

- Each *complete meal* as recommended is *interchangeable* on your daily plan with another meal option and equal in SuperNutrient balance and great nutrition for your optimal weight and health.

Sandwiches, Pitas, Wraps, Tacos, Pizza

Guidelines:

- When you feel like a sandwich, pita, wrap, taco, or pizza option, choose from these!

- Each of these options should be counted as your **with grain** meal for lunch or dinner for the day.

- *Easy* is great for being successful in eating well with a busy life. Each of these meals is interchangeable with any other item including any **with grain** meal in the diet—hot or cold!

- Plan these into your weekly food plan as **with grains**.

- Include the simple ingredients on your shopping list.

Options:

1. **SuperFoodsRx Turkey Spinach Pita***
   Ginger Orange Dressing*
   2 stalks of celery (7–8 inches) with 1 tablespoon almond butter

2. **Salmon Taco with Mango & Avocado***
   $\frac{1}{2}$ cup plain yogurt, $\frac{1}{2}$ cup berries, and 1 teaspoon honey

3. **Grown-Up PB and Strawberry Sandwich***
   $\frac{1}{2}$ cup low fat (or nonfat) milk or 15 baby carrots

4. **Bean and Veggie Burrito***
   $\frac{3}{4}$ cup red grapes (approximately 20) or **Corn Salsa***

5. **Pear, Feta, and Pecan Stuffed Pita***
   $\frac{3}{4}$ cup blueberries

6. **Cold Vegetable Tortillas (Green, Red, or Orange)***
   Garlic Lover's spread*
   10–12 almonds or $1\frac{1}{2}$ tablespoons grated cheese in the wrap
   1 cup watermelon balls or $\frac{1}{2}$ cup blueberries

7. **Fresh and Light Tacos***
   1 cup red grapes (25)

8. **Thanksgiving Open-Faced Sandwich***
   Medium SuperFoodsRx side salad* or **All Season Fruit Salad***

9. **Roasted Vegetable Pita***
   Modern Ambrosia*

10. **Greek Salad Roll Ups***
    Tuscan Bean Soup*
    Alternate to soup: $\frac{1}{3}$ cup black beans and whole apple.

11. **Tofu "Eggless" Salad* Sandwich**
    2 sliced whole grain bread, 1 sliced tomato, romaine lettuce
    All Season Fruit Salad* or **Modern Ambrosia***

12. **Poached Salmon in Spinach Tortilla Wrap***

    Great Northern Bean Dip*

    20 carrot and celery sticks

    Alternate to veggies and dip: All Season Fruit Salad*

13. **Hummus and Roasted Pepper Sandwich***

    Four Bean Chile (1 cup)*

    Alternate to soup: Medium SuperFoodsRx side salad* and whole orange.

14. **Thin Crust Turkey Pizza on Corn Tortillas***

    Small SuperFoodsRx side salad*

Eating SuperFoods on the Fly—Find a Subway® Sandwich Store

SUBWAY® 6" Veggie Delite

One 6" Veggie Delite Sub sandwich (order whole grain bread and ask for extra vegetables)

1 medium apple

1 tablespoon almonds (8–9)

Alternate for apple: ½ banana (4–5"), ¾ cup blueberries or 15 grapes (big handful)

Any variety of nut (1 tablespoon) can be substituted for almonds

Subway® 6" Veggie Max

One 6-inch Veggie Max Sub sandwich (order whole grain bread and ask for extra vegetables)

2 medium stalks (7–8") celery

Alternate for celery—5–6 baby carrots (a handful)

Indicates a SuperFoodsRx Diet recipe available starting on page 217

Soups & Salads
Mix-and-Match

Guidelines:

- Include a soup or salad (or both) every day as part of your SuperFoodsRx lifestyle

- Expand your definition of salads to include any combination of vegetables, combinations of fruits, or even simple preparations of your Category 3 SuperFoods and sidekicks, along with the newer additions of apples, onions, kiwis, pomegranate, and dried SuperFruits.

- Remember your *Soup and Salad Monday* for a lunch or dinner meal, and include Soup and Salad *Mix and Match* meals anytime during your week.

- Plan your soups and salads into your weekly food plan as **with grains** or **without grains** appropriately.

- Include the ingredients on your shopping list.

- Prepare a soup or two in advance and store in single servings to enjoy during the week.

- Soup and Salad combinations make for a SuperNutrient dense and delicious meal anytime. Great for your SuperFoodsRx Diet, great for your long-term health!

You will find a variety of versatile soups and salads to choose from. My clients regularly tell me they enjoy eating soups and salads but like to customize their choices. They describe the challenge of deciding how to coordinate the ingredients they have on hand, their personal tastes, and their intentions to stay on track with their weight and health goals.

Here's your solution! See the *Mix-and-Match* Soup and Salad options on opposite page. Select any one of the simple salads and any soup from the same group and *voilà*—a perfectly balanced, supernutritious, SuperFoodsRx Diet meal!

You will find additional entrée salads and meals with salad accompaniments starting on page 204 and recipes on pages 230–235.

Soup & Salad Meals
Mix-and-Match

Group 1

SOUPS (SELECT ONE)		SALAD/FRUIT/VEGETABLE PAIRING (SELECT ONE)
Turkey Meatball Soup* ⊰ Turkey Sausage and Tortellini Soup˟ (1½ cups)	**Enjoy with:**	Small SuperFoodsRx Just Veggies side salad* Grilled Fruit Kabobs* (3) Broccoli and Cauliflower Salad* ⊰ Corn Salsa* ¾ cup blueberries Large Orange

Group 2

SOUPS (SELECT ONE)		SALAD/FRUIT/VEGETABLE PAIRING (SELECT ONE)
Turkey Pumpkin Chili with Roasted Pumpkin Seeds* (1 cup) SuperFoodsRx Soup Option #10 Turkey Chili* (2 cup)	**Enjoy with:**	Medium SuperFoodsRx side salad* Modern Ambrosia* Crunchy Coleslaw* All Season Fruit Salad* No Cook Vegetable Kabobs*

⊰*Denotes Grain meals*
*Indicates a SuperFoodsRx Diet recipe available starting on page 217.

Group 3

SOUPS (SELECT ONE)		SALAD/FRUIT/VEGETABLE PAIRING (SELECT ONE)
SuperFoodsRx Soup Option #1 Garbanzo Vegetable* (2 cups)		Stuffed Tomato with Curried Tuna Salad* (or alternates) Half orange (wedges)
SuperFoodsRx Soup Option #2 Lentil Vegetable* (2 cups)		Broccoli and White Bean Salad with Crushed Red Pepper*
⇥ SuperFoodsRx Soup Option # 4 Italian Vegetable* (2 cups)		Medium SuperFoodsRx side salad*
⇥ SuperFoodsRx Soup Option #5 Seafood Gumbo* (2 cups)	Enjoy with:	1 heaping tablespoon nuts Crunchy Coleslaw*
⇥ SuperFoodsRx Soup Option #7 Tortellini Vegetable* (2½ cups)		Small apple Small SuperFoodsRx side salad*
⇥ SuperFoodsRx Soup Option #8 Mexican Chowder* (2 cups)		1 cup red grapes (25) ⇥ ½ cup Confetti Salad* (Note: ½ serving)
SuperFoodsRx Soup Option #9 Turkey Vegetable* (1½ cups)		20 baby carrots or ¾ cup berries
Four-Bean Chili* (1¼ cups)		

⇥Denotes Grain meals
*Indicates a SuperFoodsRx Diet recipe available starting on page 217.

SUPERFOODSRx MENUS, MEALS, AND RECIPES

Group 4

SOUPS (SELECT ONE)		SALAD/FRUIT/VEGETABLE PAIRING (SELECT ONE)
SuperFoodsRx Soup Option #6 Asian Vegetable* (2 cups) Tuscan Bean Soup* (1¼ cup) ⊰⊱ SuperFoodsRx Soup Option #7 Tortellini Vegetable* SuperFoodsRx Soup Option #11 Edamame Vegetable* (2 cups) SuperFoodsRx Soup Option #12 Tofu Vegetable* (2 cups)	**Enjoy with:**	⊰⊱ Confetti Salad* (1 cup) Asian Inspired Broccoli Salad* No Cook Vegetables Kabobs* ½ cup plain nonfat yogurt, ½ cup sliced berries, and 1 teaspoon honey Medium SuperFoodsRx side salad* 2 stalks celery with 1 tablespoon peanut butter Spicy Tofu Salad* Chicken Salad with Thyme, Walnuts & Grapes*

Group 5

SOUPS (SELECT ONE)		SALAD/FRUIT/VEGETABLE PAIRING (SELECT ONE)
⊰⊱ Turkey Sausage and Tortellini Soup* (¾ cup) (Note: ½ serving) SuperFoodsRx Soup Option #10 Turkey Chili* (1 cup) SuperFoodsRx Soup Option #12 Tofu Vegetable* (1½ cups)	**Enjoy with:**	Large SuperFoodsRx side salad* ½ cup berries or 1 cup watermelon balls Broccoli and White Bean Salad with Crushed Red Pepper* Sliced apple

Group 6

SOUPS (SELECT ONE)		SALAD/FRUIT/VEGETABLE PAIRING (SELECT ONE)
⇥ Sweet Potato Soup* (1½ cups) Four Bean Chili* (½ cup) (Note: ½ serving) SuperFoodsRx Soup Option #3 Spicy Vegetable* (2 cups)	**Enjoy with:**	Marvelous Mediterranean Salad* ⇥ Confetti Salad* Apple or ¾ blueberries

Group 7

SOUPS (SELECT ONE)		SALAD/FRUIT/VEGETABLE PAIRING (SELECT ONE)
Tuscan Bean Soup* (½ cup) Cold Fruit Soup* (1 cup) SuperFoodsRx SoupBase* (1 cup)	**Enjoy with:**	Marvelous Mediterranean Salad* Layered Turkey (or Chicken) Entrée Salad*

Entrée Salads (Cold Entrée) and Hot Entrée Meals

Guidelines:

🌿 Remember to choose your meals—one **with** grains and the other **without.** You decide.

🌿 Wednesday is your Veggie Day: Select one **with** and one **without grain** meal as usual, just choose from the options with the ⇥ symbol.

⇥ Denotes Grain meals
*Indicates a SuperFoodsRx Diet recipe available starting on page 217.

- Keep it simple. You can have the same meal twice (cook once, eat twice). Become comfortable with a few great recipes and increase your repertoire little by little over time.

- Variety minimum two to three different lunches and three to four different dinners for each 2-week cycle.

- Stick to the sides (or permitted "trades" on page 207) suggested for each entrée.

- Each complete meal is interchangeable on your daily plan with another and equal in SuperNutrient balance and great nutrition for your optimal weight and health.

- Several of these recipes can be made in advance and are very quick and easy.

- Plan your meals into your weekly food plan as *with grains* or *without grains* appropriately.

- Include the simple ingredients on your shopping list.

Entrée Salads (Cold Entrée) Meals

ENTRÉE SALAD (COLD ENTRÉE) MEAL OPTIONS	TO MAKE YOUR MEAL A *WITH GRAIN*, ENJOY THE FOLLOWING:	TO MAKE YOUR MEAL A *WITHOUT GRAIN*, ENJOY THE FOLLOWING:
1. **Marvelous Mediterranean Salad***	• Small whole wheat pita or slice of whole grain bread	• ½ cup plain yogurt, ½ cup berries, and 1 teaspoon honey or 1 cup red grapes (25)
2. **Layered Turkey (or Chicken) Entrée Salad***	• 2–3 whole grain crackers	• ¾ cup blueberries or an apple
3. **Spicy Tofu Salad***	• **Grilled Corn on the Cob*** • **Almond Green Beans***	• **Almond Green Beans*** 1 cup red grapes (25)
4. **Stuffed Tomato with Curried Tuna Salad*** (or alternates)	• ½ cup quinoa or brown rice • **All Season Fruit Salad***	• 2 stalks of celery (7–8 inches) with 1 tablespoon peanut butter • **All Season Fruit Salad***
5. **Chicken Salad with Thyme, Walnuts, & Grapes***	• 2 cups spinach • 3–4 whole grain crackers, • ¾ cup berries or **Baked Apple***	• 2 cups spinach • 15–20 baby carrots • Sliced whole apple or **Baked Apple***
6. **Asian Broccoli Salad***	• ⅓–½ cup cooked quinoa ½ cup berries or small orange	• ½ cup Great Northern beans • ½ cup berries or small orange
7. **SuperFoodsRx Entrée Salad***	• Small whole wheat pita or slice of whole grain bread • ½ cup plain yogurt, ½ cup berries, and 1 teaspoon honey	• ½ cup black beans • ½ cup plain yogurt, ½ cup berries, and 1 teaspoon honey

*Indicates a SuperFoodsRx Diet recipe available starting on page 217

Hot Entrée Meals

HOT ENTRÉE MEAL OPTIONS	TO MAKE YOUR MEAL A *WITH GRAIN*, ENJOY THE FOLLOWING:	TO MAKE YOUR MEAL A *WITHOUT GRAIN*, ENJOY THE FOLLOWING:
1. Stuffed Turkey Breast Sicilian Style*	• ½ cup whole wheat couscous	• Small SuperFoodsRx side salad*
2. Grilled Vegetable Kabobs with Shrimp or Tofu*	• ½ cup whole grain pasta or 1 small whole wheat pita	• Grilled Fruit Kabobs* • ¼ cup yogurt and 1 teaspoon honey for dipping or 2 tablespoons Yogurt Banana Strawberry Spread*
3. Pan Roasted Stuffed Turkey Breast With White Bean Sauce*	• ⅓–½ cup baked sweet potato • ½ cup blueberries	• Honey Ginger Carrots* • ½ cup sliced strawberries
4. Peanut Glazed Shrimp*	• ½ cup brown rice • 1 cup steamed broccoli	• 1 cup steamed broccoli • All Season Fruit Salad*
5. Orange Flaxseed (or Sesame) Salmon*	• Confetti Salad* • 2 cups steamed spinach	• Medium SuperFoodsRx side salad* or ½ cup Cooked Lentils* • 1 cup broccoli
6. Papillote (Turkey/Chicken) with Veggies*	• ½ cup cooked quinoa	• ½ cup black beans or Cooked Lentils* or SuperFoodsRx Spicy Vegetable Soup*
7. Tofu Stir Fry*	• ½ cup whole wheat couscous • 20 grapes (¾ cup)	• ½ cup black beans or Cooked Lentils* • ½ cup blueberries
8. Ginger Grilled Turkey Tenderloin*	• Citrus Apricot Couscous* • 1 cup steamed baby bok choy (2 small, halved) • 1 cup mixed berries and 2 tablespoon yogurt cheese or 1 cup grapes (approx. 25)	• Almond Green Beans* • 1 cup mixed berries and 2 tablespoon yogurt cheese or 1 cup grapes (approx. 25)

HOT ENTRÉE MEAL OPTIONS	TO MAKE YOUR MEAL A *WITH GRAIN*, ENJOY THE FOLLOWING:	TO MAKE YOUR MEAL A *WITHOUT GRAIN*, ENJOY THE FOLLOWING:
9. Broiled Salmon with Lemon Herb* (or other variations)	• **Sweet Potato & Asparagus with Orange Glaze*** • $\frac{1}{2}$ cup nonfat plain yogurt with 2 tablespoons **Fresh Blueberry Compote***	• **Crunchy Coleslaw*** • $\frac{1}{3}$ cup white beans or **Cooked Lentils***
10. Grilled Salmon with Yogurt Dill Drizzle*	• **Grilled Corn on the Cob*** • **Small SuperFoodsRx Side Salad*** • **Grilled Fruit Kabobs*** or whole orange	• $\frac{1}{3}$ cup black pinto beans (or other bean) • **Small SuperFoodsRx Side Salad*** • **Grilled Fruit Kabobs*** or whole orange
11. Great Northern Shrimp Salad*	• **Steamed Carrots with Dill*** • Slice of whole grain toast	• **Steamed Carrots with Dill*** • 1 cup cherries or grapes (approx. 25 of either)
12. Lemon Roasted Turkey*	• **Broccoli and Cauliflower Salad*** • 1 medium **Baked Sweet Potato*** or $\frac{1}{2}$ cup brown rice	• **Broccoli and Cauliflower Salad*** • **All Season Fruit Salad*** or 1 tablespoon (8) almonds and 2 tablespoons raisins
13. Chicken Croquettes*	• (Burgers) Whole grain dinner roll, sliced tomato, onion, lettuce • **Small SuperFoodsRx side salad*** or **Broccoli and Cauliflower Salad***	• $\frac{1}{3}$ cup black beans (or other) • **Small SuperFoodsRx side salad*** or **Broccoli and Cauliflower Salad***
14. Asian Stuffed Salmon Fillet*	• **Slow Baked Tomatoes*** • Small whole wheat pita or $\frac{1}{2}$ cup brown rice	• **Crunchy Coleslaw*** • $\frac{1}{2}$ orange (slices) or 8–10 sliced strawberries

*Indicates a SuperFoodsRx Diet recipe available starting on page 217

HOT ENTRÉE MEAL OPTIONS	TO MAKE YOUR MEAL A *WITH GRAIN*, ENJOY THE FOLLOWING:	TO MAKE YOUR MEAL A *WITHOUT GRAIN*, ENJOY THE FOLLOWING:
15. Poached Salmon*	• **Modern Ambrosia*** • **Baked Sweet Potato*** or $1/3$ cup brown rice	• **Modern Ambrosia*** • $1/2$ **cup Cooked Lentils*** or $1/2$ cup **Four Bean Chili***
16. Lentil Meatballs or Burgers*	• Whole grain dinner roll for burger sliced tomato, onion, lettuce • **Small SuperFoodsRx side salad*** or **Broccoli and Cauliflower Salad*** *(see also Turkey Meatballs and Pasta Meal for alternative **with grain** pairing)*	• **Small SuperFoodsRx side salad*** or **Broccoli and Cauli-flower Salad*** • **All Season Fruit Salad***
17. Turkey Meatloaf with Tomato Gravy*	• **Sweet Potato Soup*** • 3 tablespoons **Toasted Pumpkin Seeds or Pine Nuts*** • **Roasted Broccoli***	• **Roasted Broccoli*** • **Modern Ambrosia***
18. Turkey (of Tofu) Meatballs*	• $1/2$ cup tomato sauce (no salt added) • $1/2$ cup cooked whole grain pasta • **Small SuperFoodsRx side salad***	• **No Cook Vegetable Kabobs*** • Sliced Orange

Non-Grain **Trades** for Recommended Sides and Accompaniments in the SuperFoodsRx Meal Options

Are you out of a certain ingredient but want to make a particular entrée recipe? Or do just simply feel like having something different than is recommended in one of the menu selections? No problem! Find the recommended side in the chart below and substitute something else *from the same column* and you have your own customized meal!

E.g.—Interchange one side from column C for another in column C, or one side from column D or another in column D, etc.

🍃 Be sure to follow the measurements as recommended and only for items in the table.

🍃 These *trades* are non-grain sides that you may find in a **with grain** or **without grain** meal but should not be substituted <u>for</u> a grain.

A	B	C	D	E
¼–⅓ cup plain yogurt (2-3 tablespoons yogurt cheese)	½ cup plain yogurt	¾ cup plain yogurt + 1 teaspoon honey	½ cup plain nonfat yogurt, ½ cup berries, and 1 teaspoon honey	¾ cup plain nonfat yogurt, ½ cup berries, and 1 teaspoon honey
1 teaspoon olive oil	½ cup low fat or nonfat milk	½ cup nonfat or low fat cottage cheese	2 stalks (7–8") celery + 1 tablespoon peanut (or nut) butter	**SuperFoodsRx Soup Option #12 Tofu Vegetable*** (1½ cup)
1 cup baby bok choy	**Steamed Carrots with Dill***	**SuperFoodsRx SoupBase*** (1 cup)	**SuperFoodsRx Soup Option #3 Spicy Vegetable*** (2 cups)	1 cup **SuperFoodsRx Soup Option #10 Turkey Chili*** (*Note:* ½ serving)
2 cups steamed spinach with ½ teaspoon olive oil	**Honey Ginger Carrots***	**Tuscan Bean Soup*** (½ cup)	½ cup **Four-Bean Chili*** (*Note:* ½ serving)	**No Cook Vegetable Kabobs*** (2)

Indicates a SuperFoodsRx Diet recipe available starting on page 217

A	B	C	D	E
2 cups broccoli	**Slow Baked Tomatoes***	**Cold Fruit Soup***	**Almond Green Beans***	**Slow Baked Tomatoes*** *(Note: whole recipe is 2 tomatoes)*
1 cup broccoli with ½ teaspoon olive oil	**Roasted Broccoli***	**Broccoli and Cauliflower Salad***	½ cup **Cooked Lentils***	**SuperFoodsRx medium side salad***
15–20 baby carrots	**No Cook Vegetable Kabob*** *(Note: 1 kabob or ½ serving)*	**SuperFoodsRx small side salad***	1 cup assorted vegetables with 1 serving **SuperFoodsRx Spread/Dips***	**Steamed Carrots with Dill*** *(Note: whole recipe is 2 servings)*
3 table-spoons beans (kidney, black, garbanzo, etc.)	¼ cup black beans (garbanzos, pintos, kidneys, etc.)	¼ cup **"Refried" Beans***	½ cup black beans (gar-banzos, pintos, kidneys, etc.)	**Crunchy Coleslaw***
¼ cup mango	¼ cup **Cooked Lentils*** *(Note: ½ serving)*	⅓ cup black beans other	½ cup **Broccoli & White Bean with Crushed Red Pepper Salad*** *(Note: ½ serving)*	**Modern Ambrosia***
2 table-spoons **Fresh Blueberry Compote***	½ cup blueberries	¾ cup blue-berries	¼ cup **Fresh Blueberry Compote***	**All Season Fruit Salad***

A	B	C	D	E
2 table-spoons **Yogurt Banana Strawberry Spread***	**Super-FoodsRx Spreads*** with beans and **Roasted Pepper Dip***	**Fresh Blueberry Compote*** (2 table-spoons) with ½ cup nonfat plain yogurt)	2 table-spoons **Spicy Pumpkin Butter*** with ¾ cup nonfat plain yogurt	
3 table-spoons **Spicy Pumpkin Butter***	**Grilled Fruit Kabobs*** (2)	**Baked Apple***	¼ cup **Spicy Pumpkin Butter***	
¼ cup grapes (10)	½ cup grapes (15)	¾ cup red grapes (20)	1 cup red grapes (25–30)	
½ orange (wedges)	Orange (3")	Large navel orange (4–5")	2 tablespoons chopped walnuts (nuts)	
½ large apple (sliced)	Medium Apple (to 3")	Large apple		
8–10 strawberries	15 strawberries	Large pear		
1 (½ oz) mini box raisins or 1 tablespoon dried fruit	1½ cups watermelon balls (about 15)	Dried fruit (2 tablespoons)		
1½ table-spoons grated cheese	2 table-spoons grated cheese	3 tablespoons grated cheese		
Year Round Salsa* (½ cup)	2 table-spoons soy nuts (⅛ cup)	3 tablespoons soy nuts		

A	B	C	D	E
Water-melon & Jalapeño Salsa* (½ cup)	**Toasted Nuts and Seeds***	1½ to 2 tablespoons nuts • Walnuts 5–7 halves • Almonds 89 • Peanuts⁺ 14 • Peanut Butter⁺ 1 tablespoon • Pecans 6–7 halves • Cashews 8 • Pine Nuts 2 tablespoons • Pistachios 20 • Macadamias 4–5		
Roasted Pepper Spread* (¼ cup)	3 table-spoons roasted pumpkin seeds			

+Peanuts are not a tree nut, but are included in the SuperFoods nuts for their SuperNutrient properties.
*Indicates a SuperFoodsRx Diet recipe available starting on page 217

Change the Grain

Including your whole grains on a daily basis is important to your energy, your diet and weight, and your long-term health. You may decide to have a healthy grain at breakfast when you make your selections from the breakfast menus, you might also choose one as part of your afternoon snack, and you'll have healthy whole grains at either lunch *or* dinner in your **with grains** meal for the day.

Here are some measurement equivalents and some substitutions you can make in the menus and recipes while staying within the guidelines of the SuperFoodsRx diet to help you reach your goals.

Remember:

- 🌿 1 serving or 1 tennis ball of grains (and potatoes).
- 🌿 1 serving is about ½–⅔ cup cooked grains with a couple exceptions listed below.
- 🌿 1 serving is about 80–100 calories.

You can exchange 1 serving of a whole grain for another from this list of equivalents (simple grains and SuperFoodsRx recipes):

- ⊰ ⅓ cup (1 ounce) dry oats
- ⊰ 1 slice whole grain bread
- ⊰ ½ cup cooked brown rice
- ⊰ ½–¾ cup whole wheat pasta (and other varieties)
- ⊰ ⅓–½ cup cooked quinoa (6 tablespoons dry)
- ⊰ ½–⅔ cup cooked kasha (buckwheat)
- ⊰ ½ cup (1 ounce) cooked barley
- ⊰ ½ cup cooked whole wheat couscous
- ⊰ ½–⅔ cup yellow corn (fresh, frozen or canned—no salt)
- ⊰ 1 small whole wheat pita
- ⊰ 2, 6–7" corn tortillas
- ⊰ 1, 6–7" whole wheat tortilla
- ⊰ 3 cups air-popped popcorn
- ⊰ ¼ cup whole grain flour

- ⇥ **Grilled Corn on the Cob*** (6–7 inches)
- ⇥ **Corn Salsa***
- ⇥ 1 medium **Baked Sweet Potato*** (2-inch diameter x 5 inches long)
- ⇥ ½ cup sweet potato
- ⇥ **Citrus Apricot Couscous***
- ⇥ **Homemade Tortilla Chips*** (8)
- ⇥ **Sweet Potato & Asparagus with Orange Glaze*** (1 grain serving plus vegetables)
- ⇥ ½ cup **Confetti Salad*** (½ serving)
- ⇥ **Sweet Potato Soup*** (1½ cups)

Snack Mix and Match

Guidelines:

- Include an afternoon snack every day as part of your SuperFoodsRx lifestyle.
- Set a time that is right for you—about 2–3 hours between meals.
- You can choose grains anytime, *whole* grains.
- Aim for a balance of some carbs, some protein, and healthy fat at most snacks.
- Make your snacks in advance—ready to grab and go!

Quick Tip:

Trying to change a *with grains* meal into a *without grains* alternative or vice versa?

Simply swap one serving of whole grains (see **Change the Grain**) for ½ cup beans or another item in Column D of the **Trades** table on page 208.

Snack combos

GRAINS, FRUITS, AND VEGGIES (SELECT ONE)		PROTEINS, NUTS, BEANS, DIPS, AND CHEESE (SELECT ONE)
• Whole grain crackers[+] • Fruit: 2 cups watermelon, $\frac{1}{2}$ grapefruit, 1 large kiwi, $\frac{1}{2}$ large orange or 1 small, 1 cup raspberries, strawberries or blackberries; $\frac{1}{2}-\frac{2}{3}$ cup blueberries, 1–2 tangerines, 2 plums, $\frac{1}{2}$ banana (4–5"); 12–15 cherries, 15 grapes, or 1 small apple (*$\frac{1}{2}$–1 cup of any fruit*) • 2 tablespoons dried fruits (raisins, cranberries, blueberries), 2–3 dried apricots • **Baked Apple*** • $\frac{1}{4}$ cup **Fresh Blueberry Compote*** • $\frac{3}{4}$ cup natural applesauce (no sugar added) • 3 tablespoons **Spicy Pumpkin Butter*** • 15–20 baby carrots • 2 cups assorted raw or blanched vegetables (especially SuperFoods) • 2 cups air-popped popcorn • Half slice of whole grain bread • $\frac{1}{8}$ cup **SuperFoodsRx Granola*** • 1, 6-inch corn tortilla • 1 whole wheat, low carb (6-8") tortilla • 8 **Homemade Tortilla Chips*** • 4 **Whole Wheat Pita Crisps*** • 7–8 baked tortilla chips • 2 whole grain rice cakes, 3 Wasa® crackers, 3 AkMak® crackers, 2 rye crispbreads, 4 low-sodium Nabisco® Triscuits® or 9 Hain® Wheatettes	Enjoy with:	• Nuts: 8 almonds, 5 walnut halves, 11 peanuts, 7 pecans, 12 cashews, 70 pine nuts (approximately 2 teaspoons), 21 pistachios, 4 macadamias, 8 hazelnuts, 2 Brazil nuts, 3 tablespoons soy nuts, 1 tablespoon peanut butter, or almond butter or other nut butter • $\frac{3}{4}$ cup nonfat yogurt or $\frac{1}{2}$ cup yogurt cheese • $\frac{1}{2}$ cup nonfat cottage cheese (low sodium) • $1\frac{1}{2}$ ounces turkey, salmon, poultry or other lean animal protein (half a deck of cards!) • 1 egg • 1 ounce goat cheese, feta cheese, light cheddar or similar • $3\frac{1}{2}$ tablespoons shredded parmesan • 2 Laughing Cow® light wedges • 1 Laughing Cow® Mini Babybel® cheese • $\frac{1}{8}$ cup (2 tablespoons) part-skim ricotta cheese • $\frac{1}{8}$ cup (2 tablespoons) or 2 slices avocado[†] • **Creamy Spinach Dip*** • **Black Bean & Mango Salsa*** • **Smoked Salmon Spread*** • **Yogurt Banana Strawberry Spread*** • **Garlic Lover's Dip*** • **Great Northern Bean Dip*** • **Hummus*** • **"Refried" Beans*** • **Roasted Pepper Puree*** • **Salsa Bean Dip*** • **"Brocco-mole"***

5-MINUTE MEAL—SUPERFAST SUPERNUTRIENTS . . . AND SUPERFILLING!

Servings: 2
    Take a 15-ounce can of Vegetarian Bean Chili (low sodium) and add a 15-ounce can of no-salt added diced tomatoes. Heat and serve with 2 tablespoons nonfat plain yogurt.

With grains: Enjoy one serving with 2–3 whole grain crackers.

Without grains: Enjoy one serving with a sliced apple.

Single Food Options and Miscellaneous Snacks

- 1 energy bar—(look for 120–150 calorie options): Kashi® TLC® bars (6 in a box); Cascadian Farms® Organic energy bars; Clif® Z-Bar® Organic for Kids or similar (see energy bar guidelines on page 339)

- Soy crisps (Genisoy®—1 ounce, approximately 17 chips or Glenny's®— 3-ounce bag)

- ½ cup nonfat plain yogurt (or ¼ cup yogurt cheese) with 1 teaspoon all-fruit preserves or honey and cinnamon

- 1 4–6 ounce yogurt (150 calories max, no corn syrup or artificial sweeteners)

- 1 SuperFoodsRx Blueberry Muffin with Walnuts (page 318)

- 1 SuperFoodsRx Pumpkin Walnut Muffin (page 320)

---

*Unless otherwise noted, enjoy 1 serving as indicated in the SuperFoodsRx recipes.
+Cracker guidelines: (1) Choose whole grain (whole is first), and (2) Look at the serving size and figure out how many crackers are equal to 50–70 calories. That is your portion.
† Avocado is treated as a healthy SuperFoodsRx fat in your snacks.

SuperFoodsRx Diet Recipes

🍃 SuperFoodsRx Diet STAPLES

🍃 BREAKFAST

🍃 COLD ENTRÉES—*without grains*

🍃 SALADS

🍃 FRUIT, FRUIT SALADS, COMPOTES

🍃 VEGETABLES AND OTHER *without grain* SIDES

🍃 SIDES *with grains*

🍃 SANDWICH, PITAS, WRAPS, TACOS, PIZZA

🍃 HOT ENTRÉES

🍃 SOUPS

🍃 SPREADS, DIPS, SALSAS

🍃 SALAD DRESSINGS and MARINADES

🍃 BAKERY ITEMS, SWEETS, DESSERTS

🍃 SUPERNUTRIENT BOOSTERS

🍃 SUPERFAST SUPERFOOD SUGGESTIONS

🕐 **SuperFast**—designates recipes that can be done in 15 minutes or less.

🌿 **Vegetarian**—are recipes that are lacto-ovo vegetarian (may include dairy and/or eggs, but do not include turkey or salmon [or sidekicks]).

🌱 **Grain**—designates recipes where grains play a prominent role in the recipe and subsequently is counted as a ***with grains*** meal when using this recipe in your diet plan.

SuperFoodsRx Diet Staples

VEGETARIAN

Yogurt Cheese

Keep yogurt cheese on hand at all times! You can also find thickened Greek-style yogurt at many grocery stores today if you prefer, but making your own is super easy and inexpensive.

Servings: Depends on amount strained

Serving Size: Depends on amount strained

Volume: ½ of amount strained (1 cup yogurt equals ½ cup cheese)

Prep Time: 2 minutes

Total Time: 4 to 8 hours depending on amount strained

Place the yogurt in a yogurt strainer or in several layers of cheesecloth or a coffee filter placed in a colander. Place the colander over a bowl to reduce the whey and make it a thicker consistency. Set in the refrigerator to drain. When ready to use, discard the whey.

Poached Chicken

Servings: 1

Serving Size: 3 ounces

Volume: 3 ounces

Prep Time: 1 minute

Cook Time: 10 minutes

Total Time: 20 minutes

4 ounces boneless skinless chicken breast

Place the chicken in a sauté pan and add enough water to completely cover the chicken. Bring to a boil and immediately reduce to simmer. Cook 8 to10 minutes. Cool the chicken in water, if time permits. Cut into bite-sized pieces and use in desired recipe.

Poached Salmon

Want an elegant dinner? Here it is!

Servings: 4	Prep Time: 15 minutes
Serving Size: 3 ounces	Cook Time: 10 minutes
Volume: 1 pound	Total Time: 25 minutes

$\frac{1}{2}$ cup chopped onions

1 (7") stalk celery, cut into $\frac{1}{2}$" slices

1 (5$\frac{1}{2}$") carrot, peeled and cut into $\frac{1}{2}$" slices

3 whole black peppercorns

1 bay leaf

1 large sprig fresh dill

2 tablespoons white wine vinegar

$\frac{1}{2}$ cup water

1 pound fresh salmon steak, 1" thick (raw weight 14–16 ounces to yield 3-ounce servings; approximately 12 ounces cooked)

In a large saucepan, bring the onions, celery, carrots, peppercorns, bay leaf, dill, vinegar, and water to a boil. In the meantime, wrap the salmon steak in a couple of layers of damp cheesecloth. When the mixture boils, reduce heat to simmer. With a large spatula, lower the salmon into the simmering broth. Cover and cook for 10 minutes or until the salmon flakes easily when pierced with a fork.

Carefully remove the steak from the broth, and discard the broth. Unwrap the salmon and remove the skin around the steak with a sharp paring knife. Cut the steak into 3-ounce portions and serve 2 portions hot. Refrigerate the remaining steak.

Cooked Lentils

Lentils are among the most ancient of all legumes. They are available very inexpensively in the dried form, but cook more quickly than other dried beans. They can be substituted cup for cup in any recipe calling for adzuki beans or split peas.

Servings: 4

Serving Size: ¼+ cup

Volume: 1¼ cups

Prep Time: 25 minutes

Cook Time: 35 minutes

Total Time: 1 hour

½ pound dried lentils (⅓ cup dry)

Place the lentils in a medium bowl and cover with cold water to a depth of 2 inches. Allow them to soak for 20 minutes, and then drain. Place the lentils in a large saucepan and add 3 cups of cold water. Bring the water to a boil, reduce the heat to low and simmer 30 to 35 minutes or until tender. Drain and allow the lentils to cool, then refrigerate or freeze them. Cooked lentils can also be used immediately as a side dish (see note).

Note: If serving as a side dish, add ¼ cup of chopped onion and 1 clove of minced garlic to the cooking water. Season with ¼ teaspoon black pepper and enjoy.

Toasted Nuts and Seeds

Toasting is like putting a megaphone to the flavors of any nuts and seeds. It also enhances crunch, so munch away!

Servings: Varies (try ½ to 1 cup
   at a time; 1 cup yields 8 tablespoons)
Serving Size: 1 to 2 tablespoons,
   depending on use
Volume: Varies

Prep Time: 1 minute
Cook Time: 35 minutes
Total Time: 6 to 8 minutes

Walnuts, almonds, pecans, hazelnuts, pine nuts, pumpkin seeds, or sunflower seeds

Preheat the oven to 400 degrees (see note below). Lay the nuts/seeds in a single layer on a baking sheet. Place the baking sheet in the oven and toast the seeds until slightly brown, 5 to 7 minutes. Smaller nuts/seeds will toast faster than larger pieces. Watch carefully through the lit oven window. Remove the nuts/seeds from the oven and place them on waxed paper to cool, or use immediately. Once completely cool, store them in an airtight container.

Note: For smaller quantities, you can toast nuts and seeds on the cook top. Place them in an ungreased small skillet over medium-high heat. Stir frequently and toast until a light brown color is achieved. Remove the nuts/seeds from the heat and store as above.

Alternative Preparation Method: Add a bit of spice to toasted nuts and seeds with a light sprinkling of cayenne pepper, cinnamon, garlic powder, onion powder, or any of your favorite snipped herbs.

Special note: Average—20 to 30 calories per tablespoon seeds; 60 calories per tablespoon nuts

Breakfast Recipes

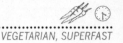

"Eggsellent" Spinach, Mushroom & Onion Scramble

Servings: 1

Serving Size: 1¼ cups

Volume: 1¼ cups

Prep Time: 5 minutes

Cook Time: 9 minutes

Total Time: 14 minutes

Olive oil spray

¼ cup sliced onions

½ cup sliced (4) mushrooms

1 egg

2 egg whites

½ teaspoon dried thyme (or 1½ teaspoons fresh)

⅛ teaspoon black pepper (3 good cranks of the pepper grinder)

½ cup spinach, chopped lightly

In a sauté pan, spray the cooking oil for 4 seconds to coat and sauté the onions and mushrooms until soft (3 to 5 minutes). In a bowl, combine the egg, egg whites, thyme and pepper. Add the chopped spinach to the pan with the onions and mushrooms and sauté for 1 minute, loosely covered, until limp. Pour the eggs over the vegetables and cook over medium heat, stirring constantly until the eggs are fully scrambled.

Tip: To make this a quick and easy daily option, cut the onions in advance and store in a designated (onions only—labeled) airtight container. Buy baby spinach, so chopping is minimal. You can even buy sliced mushrooms to make this recipe a virtual cinch.

SuperFoodsRx Granola

Low in fat and high in flavor, this simple-to-make granola can double as a breakfast cereal.

Servings: 8
Serving Size: ¼ cup
Volume: 2 cups

Prep Time: 10 minutes
Cook Time: 20 minutes
Total Time: 30 minutes

1½ cups old-fashioned oatmeal
1½ teaspoons canola oil
1½ tablespoons honey
2 tablespoons chopped walnuts
⅛ cup dried blueberries
1 teaspoon pure vanilla extract

Preheat the oven to 300 degrees. In a bowl mix together the ingredients in the order listed, thoroughly mixing after each addition. Spread the mixture on a jelly roll pan sprayed for 2 seconds with cooking spray and bake for 20 minutes, stirring the mixture every 5 minutes. Bake until the oats are a golden brown. Cool and store in an airtight container or resealable plastic bags.

Variation: Substitute sliced almonds for walnuts and dried cranberries for blueberries.

Hint: Heating the honey in the microwave oven for 8–10 seconds before adding makes it easier to incorporate when blending the ingredients.

Egg Frittata With Cherry Tomatoes, Spinach & Cheese

Servings: 1

Serving Size: 1¼ cups
Volume: 1¼ cups

Prep Time: 10 minutes

Cook Time: 20 minutes in toaster oven or
    60 seconds in microwave

Total Time: 30 minutes for toaster oven or
    11 minutes for microwave

- 1 egg
- 2 egg whites
- 1 tablespoon soy milk or nonfat/low-fat milk
- 1½ tablespoons grated cheddar or other cheese such as feta (1 rounded tablespoon)
- ⅛ teaspoon black pepper (3 good cranks of the pepper grinder)
- 4 cherry tomatoes, cut in quarters
- ½ cup fresh chopped spinach (or ¼ cup frozen, thawed, and mashed between paper towels to remove excess moisture)

In a medium bowl, whisk together the egg, egg whites and milk with a fork for 30 seconds. Mix the in cheese and pepper. Fold in the tomatoes and spinach. Grease a 1-cup oven-safe ramekin with cooking spray for 1 second. Pour the egg mixture into the ramekin. Bake 20 minutes in toaster oven at 375 degrees OR place in a microwave for 60 seconds or until done. Serve immediately with: 1 slice of whole grain toast (80–100 calories/slice) and 1 tablespoon all-fruit preserves (low sugar/no sugar added).

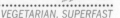

Fruit Delight Smoothie

Servings: 2
Serving Size: 1¼ cups
Volume: 2½ cups

Prep Time: 5 minutes
Total Time: 5 minutes

- ½ cup blueberries (fresh or frozen)
- ½ cup strawberries, halved
- ½ cup vanilla or plain soy milk
- ½ medium banana (approximately 3½–4")
- ½ cup nonfat plain yogurt
- 2 teaspoons honey
- 2 teaspoons ground flaxseed

Place all the ingredients in a blender and process until smooth. Adjust the consistency with water or ice, if desired. Serve immediately.

Pumpkin "Julius" Smoothie

Citrus and fruits now have to share the morning spotlight with pumpkin.

Servings: 1
Serving Size: 1½ cups
Volume: 1½ cups

Prep Time: 3 minutes
Total Time: 3 minutes

- ¾ cup soy milk
- ½ cup fresh pumpkin puree (or canned pumpkin)
- ¼ cup nonfat plain Yogurt Cheese (see recipe *page 217*)
- 2 tablespoons wheat germ or 1 tablespoon ground flaxseed
- 1½ tablespoons honey
- ½ teaspoon pumpkin pie spice
- ⅛ teaspoon ground cinnamon
- 2 ice cubes

Place all of the ingredients in a blender and puree until smooth. Adjust the thickness with more or less ice cubes or water.

Cold Entrées—*without grains*

··

Stuffed Tuna Salad Tomatoes
Basic Tuna Salad, Blueberry Walnut Tuna Salad, Curried Tuna Salad

Servings: 1

Serving Size: 1½ cups

Volume: 1½ cups

Prep Time: 5 minutes

Total Time: 5 minutes

- 1 medium beefsteak tomato
- 3 ounces canned tuna, packed in water, drained
- 2 tablespoons plain nonfat yogurt (or yogurt cheese)
  Basic, Blueberry, or Curried Salad Enhancements

Basic Salad Enhancement
- ¼ cup finely diced celery
- ⅛ teaspoon fine sea salt
- ⅛ teaspoon black pepper (3 good cranks of the pepper grinder)

Blueberry Walnut Salad Enhancement
- ¼ teaspoon lemon-pepper seasoning
- 1 tablespoon dried blueberries (about 17)
- 2 teaspoons chopped walnuts

Curried Salad Enhancement
- ¼ teaspoon curry seasoning
- 4 tablespoons diced cucumber (about 3" of cucumber)

Core the tomato and cut into quarters, leaving the bottom intact. Set it aside. In a medium bowl, mix the tuna, yogurt, and your choice of salad enhancements together. Place the tuna salad on top of the tomato.

Serving Suggestion: Place the stuffed tomato on top of ½ cup of baby spinach that has been drizzled with balsamic vinegar or fresh lemon juice.

Chicken Salad with Thyme, Walnuts & Grapes

This refreshing salad has a surprise sweetness from the grapes and orange juice along with a wonderful crunch from the walnuts. For a change, see the variation for Mango Chicken Salad.

Servings: 1

Serving Size: 2¼ cups

Volume: 2¼ cups

Prep Time: 5 minutes

Total Time: 5 minutes

3 ounces boneless skinless chicken breast, poached, cooled and diced (see recipe for Poached Chicken, *page 217*)

⅛ teaspoon fine sea salt

⅛ teaspoon black pepper (3 good cranks of the pepper grinder)

¼ cup seedless purple grapes, sliced in half (about 10 grapes)

1 tablespoon chopped walnuts

1 teaspoon fresh thyme leaves or ⅓ teaspoon dried thyme leaves

1 tablespoon orange juice

⅛–¼ cup Yogurt Cheese (see recipe *page 217*) or approx. 2–3 tablespoons plain low-fat or nonfat yogurt

2 cups baby spinach

Mix the chicken, salt, pepper, grapes, walnuts, thyme, orange juice, and yogurt. Blend well.

Serve over baby spinach.

Alternative Preparation Method: For **Chicken Salad with Mango, Soy Nuts, Cilantro, and Lime,** do not add the grapes, walnuts, and thyme. Instead substitute 2 tablespoons roasted soy nuts, ¼ cup diced mango, ½ cup roughly chopped cilantro, and 1 tablespoon fresh lime juice.

Variation—Tuna: Substitute 3 ounces of canned, drained low-sodium tuna in spring water for the 3 ounces of cooked chicken.

Spicy Tofu Salad

This easy, yet flavorful dinner can be made a day or two in advance.

Servings: 2   Prep Time: 15 minutes

Serving size: 1¼ cup   Total Time: 1 hour 15 minutes

Volume: 2½ cups

    2   tablespoons rice vinegar
 1½   tablespoons sesame oil
    1   tablespoon low-sodium soy sauce
    1   large clove garlic, minced
    1   teaspoon minced fresh ginger
  ½   teaspoon crushed red pepper
  ¾   pound very firm tofu, well drained and cut into ½" cubes*
    4   mushrooms, sliced
  ½   orange bell pepper, cut into matchsticks
    2   large lettuce leaves
    1   tablespoon minced fresh cilantro

In a jar with a tight-fitting lid, combine the vinegar, oil, soy sauce, garlic, ginger, and crushed red pepper. Cover and shake the jar vigorously to combine the ingredients. Place the tofu, mushrooms, and bell peppers in a bowl and add the marinade. Stir gently to coat the vegetables well. Refrigerate at least 1 hour and use within 3 days. To serve, place the lettuce leaves on chilled serving plates. Top the leaves evenly with tofu salad. Garnish with fresh cilantro.

*Use extra-firm light tofu when possible.

Tofu "Eggless" Salad

A healthy, adult version of old-fashioned egg salad.

Servings: 4

Serving size: ½ cup

Volume: 2 cups

Prep Time: 10 minutes

Total Time: 2 hours 10 minutes

1 (14-ounce) package firm light tofu, drained well
½ cup plain nonfat yogurt or Yogurt Cheese (see recipe *page 217*)
1 (7") stalk celery, finely chopped
1 scallion, chopped
1 teaspoon pickle relish or finely chopped dill pickles
1 teaspoon Dijon mustard
½ teaspoon garlic salt
¼ teaspoon black pepper
  Lettuce leaves

In a large mixing bowl, mash the tofu or press it in a potato masher. Add the yogurt, celery, scallions, relish, mustard, salt, and pepper, stirring to combine. Cover and refrigerate the mixture at least 2 hours to allow the flavors to meld before serving. Spread it on slices of fresh whole wheat bread and top with lettuce leaves. Cut the sandwich on the diagonal and serve immediately with Homemade Tortilla Chips (see recipe on page 251).

Alternative Serving Suggestion: Serve as a cold luncheon salad on mixed lettuce leaves with a whole wheat dinner roll on the side.

Broccoli & White Beans with Crushed Red Pepper

Servings: 2

Serving Size: 1¼ cups

Volume: 2½ cups

Prep Time: 5 minutes

Cook Time: 10 minutes

Total Time 15 minutes

- ½ cup water
- 2 cups broccoli florets
- 1 teaspoon minced garlic or 1 medium clove
- 1 cup small white beans, drained and rinsed (half of a 15-ounce can)
- ½ teaspoon extra virgin olive oil
- 1 teaspoon balsamic vinegar
- ¼ teaspoon crushed red pepper, 3 good shakes

Place the water and broccoli in sauté pan. Cover and cook the broccoli for 5 minutes. Add the minced garlic and white beans and cook until the beans are heated thoroughly. Remove the pan from the heat. Add the oil, vinegar, and crushed red pepper. Toss it well and serve.

Note: This dish is delish hot or cold.

Salads

Asian Inspired Broccoli Salad
Servings: 2

Serving Size: 1½ cups

Volume: 3 cups

Prep Time: 5 minutes

Cook Time: 3 minutes

Total Time: 10 minutes

- 2 cups broccoli florets
- ¾ cup shredded carrots
- ½ can hearts of palm, (7 ounces of a 14-ounce can), drained, rinsed, and sliced into 1" pieces
- 1 medium red bell pepper, cut into thin strips
- ½ can mandarin oranges (5 ounces of a 10-ounce can), drained
- 4 tablespoons Asian Inspired Red Pepper Sesame Dressing (see recipe *page 309*)
- ⅓ cup toasted soybeans (soy nuts)

Bring a large pot of water to a boil and add the broccoli. Cook 2 to 3 minutes or until tender. Drain and then place the broccoli in a bowl of cold water to stop the cooking process. Drain it again.

Add the carrots, hearts of palm, bell peppers, and oranges. Toss the salad gently with Asian Inspired Red Pepper Sesame Dressing. Top with toasted soy nuts.

Crunchy Coleslaw

Do not prepare ahead of time or you'll have no crunch. But since it throws together in no time at all, no problem!

Servings: 2

Serving Size: ½ cup+

Volume: 1¼ cups

Prep Time: 5 minutes

Total Time: 5 minutes

½ tablespoon low-sodium soy sauce

1 tablespoon white wine vinegar

¼ teaspoon black pepper

1 tablespoon canola oil

½ (of a 10-ounce) bag fresh coleslaw mix

1 green onion, trimmed and chopped

1½ tablespoons sunflower seeds, toasted

In a small bowl, combine the soy sauce, vinegar, and pepper. Whisk in the oil to emulsify. Set it aside. In a serving bowl, combine the coleslaw mix, green onions, noodles, and seeds. Gently toss the salad with the dressing and serve immediately.

Marvelous Mediterranean Salad

Servings: 1 entrée salad   Prep Time: 10 minutes

Serving size: 4 cups   Total Time: 10 minutes

Volume: 4 cups

2½–3 cups romaine lettuce, chopped

½ cup tomatoes, wedges or diced

¼ cup sliced red onions

¼ cup sliced or diced red bell peppers

½ cup chick peas, drained and rinsed

3 Kalamata olives, diced

2 tablespoons crumbled feta cheese

2 tablespoons Basil Garlic Vinaigrette (see recipe page 308 or Super-FoodsRx–approved dressing)

Place the chopped lettuce on a chilled dinner plate. Attractively arrange the tomatoes, onions, peppers, and chick peas over the lettuce. Sprinkle the olives and cheese over the top. Drizzle with the dressing and serve immediately.

Layered Turkey (or Chicken) Salad

Servings: 1 entrée salad

Serving Size: 3 cups

Volume: 3 cups

Prep Time: 10 minutes

Total Time: 10 minutes

 1 cup romaine lettuce or spinach leaves (or a combination)
 ½ cup diced tomatoes
 ½ cup sliced mushrooms
 ½ cup chopped broccoli florets
 3 ounces cooked turkey breast, chopped
 3 tablespoons kidney beans, drained and rinsed
 3 tablespoons shredded cheddar cheese
 2 tablespoons Rosemary Garlic Vinaigrette (see recipe page 307 or SuperFoodsRx–approved dressing)

On a chilled dinner plate, arrange the lettuce leaves, and then top with the tomatoes. Continue layering the mushrooms, broccoli, and turkey. Sprinkle the top with beans and cheese. Drizzle the vinaigrette over the salad and enjoy immediately.

Possible substitutions:

- 1 tablespoon raisins, dried blueberries or 2 apricots in place of kidney beans.
- 1 tablespoon almond slices or crushed walnuts in place of grated cheese.
- 3 ounces wild salmon or chunk light tuna in water for turkey or chicken.

SuperFoodsRx Salads

Small, Medium, Large, and Entrée

Servings: 1   Prep Time: 5 minutes
Serving Size: 1¾ to 2½ + cups   Total Time: 5 minutes
Volume: 1¾ to 2½ + cups

Small SuperFoodsRx Just Veggies side salad

Combine 1¾ to 2½ cups SuperFoods greens and assorted vegetables and 2 tablespoons SuperFoodsRx dressings (pages 307–312).

Medium SuperFoodsRx side salad:

To *Small:* Add 1 of the SuperFoods salad *add-ins* (or combination).

Large SuperFoodsRx salad:

To *Small*: Add any 3 of the SuperFoods salad *add-ins* (any combination).

SuperFoodsRx salad add-ins list:

- 1 heaping tablespoon nuts (or 2 tablespoons soy nuts)
- 3 tablespoons toasted seeds
- 1 tablespoon ground flaxseed or 2 tablespoons wheat germ
- 1 tablespoon dried fruit
- 1½ tablespoons grated cheese
- 2 hard-boiled egg whites
- 3 tablespoons beans (garbanzo, kidney, etc.)
- 8–10 sliced strawberries or ½ cup blueberries (or sidekicks)
- ½ orange (sectioned) or ¼ cup mandarin oranges
- ½ apple sliced
- ⅓ cup grapes or cherries (10)
- ⅛ avocado (2 tablespoons)

Entrée SuperFoodsRx Salad:

To Large salad, add 1 of the following:

- Deck of cards (3 ounces) turkey, chicken, salmon, tuna
- Deck of cards (5 ounces) firm tofu, cubed
- Tennis ball ($\frac{1}{3}$–$\frac{1}{2}$ cup) beans (garbanzo, black, kidney, etc.)
- Tennis ball ($\frac{1}{2}$ cup) edamame (boiled soy beans)
- $\frac{1}{2}$ cup cottage cheese
- Hard-boiled egg or 4 hard-boiled egg whites

SuperFoodsRx Salad Inspiration

Sometimes we find ourselves in a salad "rut." I have heard at times, "Oh, I'm so tired of the same old salad." Need some inspiration? Here are some wonderful salad pairings to inspire you from the SuperFoodsRx kitchen with Tammy Algood at the helm—adjust using the guidelines above as you wish! Invent your own, too, and write them down so you can refer back to them again and again.

A sampling of Small SuperFoodsRx Salad Pairings

#1—Shredded carrots, sliced mushrooms, shredded cabbage, and minced scallions over mesclun mix. Garnish with a tablespoon toasted sesame seeds.

#2—Halved cherry or teardrop tomatoes, cucumber, and watercress over spinach.

#3—Julienned orange bell pepper, whole kernel yellow corn, chopped tomatoes, and minced green onion bottoms over spinach leaves. Garnish with a sprinkling of minced fresh basil.

#4—Chopped tomatoes, diced onions, sliced beets, a handful of mung bean sprouts, and diced celery over romaine.

#5—Red and yellow cherry tomatoes, a sliced jalapeño pepper, fresh chopped cilantro and parsley, a squeeze of lime juice, and lightly toasted cumin seeds over spinach leaves.

A sampling of Medium SuperFoodsRx Salad pairings

#6—Halved red grapes (5 as $\frac{1}{2}$ *an add-in*), chopped red onions, diced celery, and snow peas over shredded hearts of romaine lettuce. Garnish with $1\frac{1}{2}$ tablespoons (*half an add-in*) of toasted sunflower seeds.

#7—Chopped onions, sliced radishes, snow peas, and green bell pepper strips over romaine. Top with a 2 slices ($\frac{1}{8}$) of fresh avocado.

#8—Chopped broccoli or cauliflower, chopped red onions, red bell pepper strips, and shredded carrots over triple hearts lettuce mix. Garnish with a tablespoon of toasted pine nuts.

#9—Drained and rinsed canned garbanzo beans (3 tablespoons), diced tomatoes, chopped scallions, chopped flat-leaf parsley, a squeeze of fresh lemon juice, and a grind of black pepper over triple hearts lettuce mix.

#10—Chopped tomatoes, chopped green onion tops, diced cucumber and minced fresh parsley over shredded hearts of romaine. Sprinkle $1\frac{1}{2}$ tablespoons of grated cheddar. Serve with lemon wedges.

#11—Minced fresh cilantro, carrot matchsticks, chopped jalapeño pepper, black beans, and a sprinkling of fresh lime juice over mesclun mix.

A sampling of Large SuperFoodsRx Salad pairings

#12—Sliced strawberries, sugar snap peas, garbanzo beans, and toasted walnuts over spinach leaves.

#13—Minced fresh chives, yellow bell pepper strips, sugar snap peas, dried blueberries, and soy nuts over romaine.

#14—Mandarin orange wedges ($\frac{1}{2}$ cup as 2 *add-ins*), red and green bell pepper strips over baby spinach. Top with sliced almonds.

Fruit, Fruit Salads, Compotes

All-Season Fruit Salad

Follow the seasons for fruit at its finest. This salad allows you to take advantage of the varying harvest and also keeps food boredom at bay!

Servings: 2

Serving Size: 1 to 1½ cups

Volume: 2 to 3 cups

Prep Time: 5 minutes

Total Time: 5 minutes

2 tablespoons Yogurt Cheese (see recipe *page 217*)

Spring:

1 cup sliced strawberries

1 cup seedless grapes

1 small kiwi, peeled and sliced

Summer:

1 cup honeydew melon, peeled, seeded, and diced

1 cup cantaloupe, peeled, seeded and diced

1½ cups seedless watermelon, diced

OR

1 cup blueberries

2 small peaches, peeled, seeded and sliced

½ teaspoon ground cinnamon

Fall:

1 apple, cored and sliced

1 cup fresh cranberries or ¼ cup pomegranate

1 pear, peeled, cored, and sliced

2 tablespoons freshly squeezed lemon juice

½ teaspoon ground cinnamon

Winter:

1 orange, peeled, seeded, and sectioned

1 mango, peeled, seeded, and sliced

1 cup fresh pineapple, peeled, cored, and cut in chunks
1 tablespoon freshly squeezed lime juice

Garnish for all salads: Place 1 heaping tablespoon of yogurt cheese on top of each fruit salad serving.

Baked Apples

Make a trip to a local orchard and you can bake the apples without any other ingredient. The natural juice from freshly harvested apples will be evident as soon as you core the fruit. Store apples in the refrigerator crisper drawer in a loosely sealed plastic bag with a tablespoon of water to keep the fruit hydrated.

Servings: 2   Prep Time: 5 minutes
Serving Size: 1 apple   Cook Time: 5 minutes
Volume: 2 fruits (tennis ball-sized)   Total Time: 10 minutes

2 small apples (such as Pink Lady, Fuji, Cameo, Empire, or Braeburn)
$\frac{1}{4}$ teaspoon ground cinnamon
1 tablespoon chopped walnuts (optional)
$\frac{1}{4}$ teaspoon pure vanilla extract

Core the apples, leaving $\frac{1}{2}$ an inch of the bottom intact. Place the apples in a baking dish that has been sprayed 2 seconds on the bottom with a cooking spray. Combine the cinnamon and walnuts (if using) and spoon them evenly into the center of the apples. Drizzle with the extract and cover. Microwave the mixture on high 4 to 5 minutes, rotating $\frac{1}{4}$ turn after 2 minutes. Let the mixture stand for 2 minutes before serving.

Alternative Preparation Method #1: Substitute nutmeg for the cinnamon and maple extract for the vanilla.

Alternative Preparation Method #2: Substitute slivered almonds for the walnuts and almond extract for the vanilla.

For Dessert: Add $\frac{1}{2}$ teaspoon of honey to each apple center (this adds only 10 calories).

Cold Fruit Soup

*Don't forget this wonderful, easy recipe. You'll find it on page 292 with the other **Soups**.*

*Don't forget this wonderful, easy recipe. You'll find it on page 292 with the other **Soups**.*

VEGETARIAN, SUPERFAST

Fresh Blueberry Compote

For use in breakfasts, snacks, desserts—homemade (lower sugar) fruit on the bottom yogurt; easy fruit in a pinch for oatmeal; easy full-fruit, low-calorie dessert crumble. It's easy, versatile, and can be refrigerated for up to a week.

Servings: 5

Serving Size: ¼ cup

Volume: 1¼ cup

Prep Time: 3 minutes

Cook Time: 7 minutes

Total Time: 15 minutes

- 2 cups fresh or frozen blueberries (if frozen, do not thaw)
- 3 tablespoons honey
- ½ cup apple juice or wine
- ¼ cup water
- 1 cinnamon stick (or ½ teaspoon ground cinnamon)
- ¼ teaspoon ground ginger
- ½ teaspoon finely grated lemon zest

Wash the blueberries with a gentle spray of cool water and set aside to drain. Meanwhile, in a medium saucepan, combine the remaining ingredients. Bring just to a boil over medium-high heat, stirring until the sugar dissolves. Reduce the heat to simmer and add the blueberries. Allow mixture to simmer for 5 minutes uncovered. Remove the saucepan from the heat and cool slightly before serving. Refrigerate any leftovers.

SuperFoodsRx Spicy Pumpkin Butter

Servings: 8
Serving size: 3 tablespoons
Volume: 1½ cups

Prep Time: 7 minutes
Cook Time: 7 minutes
Total Time: 4 hours (meld time)

- 1 cup skim milk
- ⅓ cup orange juice
- 2 tablespoons cornstarch
- 1 egg
- ¼ cup firmly packed brown sugar
- ¾ cup cooked, mashed pumpkin or canned pumpkin
- ½ teaspoon pumpkin pie spice
- ½ teaspoon ground cinnamon

Place the milk in a microwave-safe bowl and microwave uncovered at high power for 3 minutes. Remove the bowl from the microwave oven and add the remaining ingredients. Stir the mixture with a wire whisk until all ingredients are completely combined. Cover and microwave the mixture on high power 4 minutes longer. Remove the bowl, uncover (careful, it will be hot!), and stir the mixture well. Allow the pumpkin butter to cool slightly, and then cover it and refrigerate for at least 4 hours. Use as a bread spread, fruit dip, or stir it into plain yogurt.

Option #1: Spread 3 tablespoons on 2 whole grain crackers (60–70 calories of crackers) as a snack.

Options #2: After the pumpkin mixture has cooled, spoon the following into individual serving dishes: ¼ cup of the Spicy Pumpkin Butter, topped with 1 tablespoon of the toasted chopped walnuts, and serve as a delicious dessert "pudding."

Option #3: Spread 2 tablespoons of the pumpkin butter with ¼ cup of the nonfat plain yogurt in a thin crepe (70–80 calories). Roll (jellyroll style) and enjoy.

Grilled Fruit Kabobs

Let your taste buds decide which option to select for dessert. Fresh from the farm, in-season produce can be grilled without the basting sauce.

Servings: 4

Serving size: 1 cup (2 kabobs)

Volume: 4 cups, makes 8 kabobs

Prep Time: 10 minutes

Cook Time: 5 minutes

Total Time: 15 minutes

Basting Sauce:
- 1 tablespoon freshly squeezed lime juice
- 1 tablespoon honey
- ½ teaspoon grated lime zest

Fruit Option #1: (Tropical)
- ¾ cup fresh pineapple, cut into 1½" cubes
- ¾ cup fresh cantaloupe, cut into 1½" cubes
- 1 banana (approximately 7"), thick sliced
- 6 whole strawberries, cored

Fruit Option #2: (Stone Fruit)
- 1 firm, ripe peach, pitted, and cut into 8 wedges
- 2 firm, ripe plums, pitted, and cut in half
- 1 firm, ripe apricot, pitted, and cut into 4 wedges
- 6 whole strawberries, cored

Preheat the grill at medium-high heat. Combine the lime juice, honey, and zest. Set the mixture aside. Thread assorted pieces of the fruit on the skewers. Spray each skewer—turning it to evenly coat—with the cooking spray for 2 seconds. Grill the kabobs 5 minutes until they are lightly browned, turning each to evenly cook. Baste the kabobs during the last minute of cooking with the lime mixture. Serve the kabobs warm.

Modern Ambrosia for One

This recipe is a cinch. I grew up on this one at home as a child . . . and here is the recipe for one serving! Okay, yes, back then we occasionally added a few marshmallows, but then we came to know better and upgraded to flaked coconut (optional, occasional) Add 1 tablespoon of unsweetened, flaked coconut—and that yields approximately 16 calories for another variation!

Servings: 1

Serving Size: 1 cup

Volume: 1 cup

Prep Time: 5 minutes

Total Time: 5 minutes

½ banana (3½"), sliced

2 teaspoons lemon juice—or better yet squeeze a thick wedge over banana slices

1 tablespoon chopped walnuts

½ navel orange, peeled and cut into segments

Drizzle the bananas with lemon juice and then swirl a bit to make sure all are coated (the lemon prevents browning). Add the chopped walnuts and oranges. Stir gently to coat and serve.

Variation 1: Use ½ (of a 10-ounce) can of mandarin oranges, drained and rinsed, as an alternative to the navel orange.

Variation 2: Use 1 large kiwi (or 2 small), peeled and cut into segments, in place of the orange for a contemporary color and flavor burst.

Vegetables and Other *without grain* Sides

Almond Green Beans

Newsflash: You don't have to cook green beans to death anymore! Try this recipe and see why!

Servings: 2

Serving Size: ½ cup

Volume: 1 cup

Prep Time: 5 minutes

Cook Time: 10 minutes

Total Time: 15 minutes

- ½ pound fresh green beans, snapped in equal lengths
- ½ tablespoon extra virgin olive oil
- ½ cup chopped red onion
- 1 small clove garlic, minced
- 2 tablespoons water
- ⅛ teaspoon sea salt
- 1 tablespoon slivered almonds, toasted

Place the green beans in steamer basket over boiling water. Cover and steam for 10 minutes. While the beans are steaming, heat the oil in a large skillet over medium heat. Add the onions and garlic. Sauté for 2 minutes, or just until the onions begin to brown slightly. Add the water, salt, and warm green beans, mixing gently. Transfer the beans to a serving container and garnish with toasted almonds. Serve hot.

Alternative Preparation Method: If fresh green beans are not available, use frozen loose-pack green beans. Prepare as instructed on package for steaming, and then follow directions above.

Broccoli and Cauliflower Salad

This is one of those dishes where the longer it sits, the better it gets. You'll find yourself loving this salad immediately and then experience a different flavor sensation after it has time to meld in the refrigerator. Either way is delicious!

Servings: 4

Serving Size: 1 cup

Volume: 4+ cups

Prep Time: 10 minutes

Cook Time: 4 minutes

Total Time: 14 minutes

2 cups broccoli florets

2 cups cauliflower florets

2 green onions, sliced

$1/4$ cup grated carrots

2 tablespoons extra virgin olive oil

1 tablespoon red wine vinegar

$1/8$ teaspoon dry mustard

$1/8$ teaspoon black pepper (3 good cranks of the pepper grinder)

Place the broccoli in steamer basket and put it over boiling water. Cover and steam the broccoli for 2 minutes. Remove the basket and rinse the broccoli with cold water to stop the cooking process. Drain he broccoli well on paper towels. Place the cauliflower in the steamer basket and repeat the process. When the vegetables are cool, place them in a serving bowl and add the onions and carrots. In a small bowl with a wire whisk, combine the oil, vinegar, mustard, and pepper. Pour the dressing over the vegetables. Serve the dish at room temperature or cold.

Note: This salad can be refrigerated up to 4 days or frozen for longer storage. If frozen, use within 1 month.

No Cook Vegetable Kabobs

Hit the garden or the farmer's market for these fresh vegetables and dinner becomes a feast!

Servings: 2
Serving size: About 1½ cups
Volume: 3 cups

Prep Time: 10 minutes
Total Time: 1 hour, 10 minutes

   8 cherry tomatoes
   1 large yellow summer squash, cut into 1" chunks
   1 large orange bell pepper, seeded and cut into 1½" wedges
   1 tablespoon garlic-flavored olive oil
   1 tablespoon balsamic vinegar
  ⅛ teaspoon black pepper (3 good cranks of the pepper grinder)
   8 fresh basil leaves
   2 cups shredded cabbage or chopped romaine

Place the tomatoes, squash, and bell pepper in a resealable plastic bag. Drizzle the vegetables with oil and vinegar, and then sprinkle evenly with pepper. Allow the vegetables to marinate 1 hour at room temperature. Alternately place the vegetables and basil leaves on 2 skewers. Place the cabbage or lettuce on chilled serving plates. Top with the vegetable skewers and drizzle leftover marinade evenly on top of each skewer.

Roasted Broccoli

You will never want to prepare broccoli another way after tasting the intensified flavor of it roasted. Use the same process for okra, bell peppers, carrots, and any type of squash. The amount of time roasted can be personal preference. Some like a longer roasting time than others, so play with it until you find your favorite.

Servings: 2
Serving size: ½ cup
Volume: 1¼ cups

Prep Time: 2 minutes
Cook Time: 10 minutes
Total Time: 12 minutes

$^1/_2$ pound broccoli florets (approximately 1+ cup)

$^1/_2$ tablespoon extra virgin olive oil

$^1/_4$ teaspoon sea salt

$^1/_8$ teaspoon black pepper (3 good cranks of the pepper grinder)

Preheat the oven to 400 degrees. Place the broccoli in a single layer on a baking sheet with sides. Sprinkle the tops as evenly as possible with the oil, salt, and pepper. Roast at least 10 minutes, turning the broccoli halfway through the roasting process. Remove from the oven and serve hot.

Alternative Preparation Method: Instead of using broccoli, substitute cauliflower or use a mixture of half and half for a lovely side dish.

Slow-Baked Tomatoes

Swallow your tongue delicious! The baking AND the extra virgin olive oil will help you get the most luscious lycopene from this treat, too.

Servings: 2	Prep Time: 2 minutes
Serving size: 1 tomato	Cook Time: 2 hours
Volume: 2 tomatoes	Total Time: 2 hours, 5 minutes

2 ripe fresh tomatoes

$1^1/_2$ teaspoons extra virgin olive oil

$^1/_8$ teaspoon black pepper (3 good cranks of the pepper grinder)

1 clove garlic, minced

1 tablespoon fresh basil, cut in strips

Preheat the oven to 325 degrees. Slice off the top of the tomatoes (including all of the core) and reserve for other uses. Place the tomatoes, cut side up on a baking sheet. Drizzle each tomato with half of the oil and sprinkle with half of the pepper. Bake for 2 hours, or until the tomatoes nearly collapse and begin to caramelize. Sprinkle with garlic halfway through the baking process. Remove the tomatoes from the oven and sprinkle the tops with basil strips. Serve warm or at room temperature.

Alternative Serving Suggestion: Top each tomato with 1 teaspoon of dry seasoned breadcrumbs 10 minutes before serving.

Steamed Carrots with Dill

Steaming preserves lots of vitamins and minerals in vegetables and is quick to boot. This recipe knows no season, so make it a regular on any menu.

Servings: 2

Servings size: About ½+ cup

Volume: 1¼ cups

Prep Time: 1 minute

Cook Time: 5 minutes

Total Time: 6 minutes

½ pound baby carrots (about 20 medium baby carrots)
1 teaspoon extra virgin olive oil
1 teaspoon fresh snipped dill
⅛ teaspoon black pepper (3 good cranks of the pepper grinder)

Place the carrots in a steamer basket over boiling water. Cover and steam for 5 minutes. Remove the carrots from the heat and transfer them to a serving bowl. Toss the carrots gently with the oil, dill, and pepper. Serve warm.

Honey Ginger Carrots

Servings: 2

Serving size: ¾ cup

Volume: 1½ cups

Prep Time: 2 minutes

Cook Time: 9 minutes

Total Time: 14 minutes

1½ cup carrots, sliced in ¼" coins (or approximately 20 baby carrots)
2 teaspoons honey
1 teaspoon ground ginger

Bring a small amount of water (enough to submerge carrots) to a boil and add the carrots. Boil the carrots for 5 to 6 minutes and drain. In the same pan, on medium-low heat, add the honey and ginger and stir to combine, add the carrots and warm for 2 to 3 minutes and serve. Serve warm, cold, or at room temperature.

Note: Recipe can easily be cut in half to serve one.

Sides *with grain*

....

Sweet Potato & Asparagus with Orange Glaze

This dish is lovely when served alongside a piece of grilled wild salmon, tuna, turkey breast, or chicken.

Servings: 2	Prep Time: 5 minutes
Serving Size: 2 cups	Cook Time: 14 minutes
Volume: 4 cups	Total Time: 2 hours, 20 minutes

- $\frac{1}{2}$ cup fresh orange juice
- Zest of 1 orange
- 1 tablespoon minced fresh ginger (from 1" of fresh ginger)
- 2 teaspoons low-sodium soy sauce
- 1 medium sweet potato (approximately 5" in length and 2" in diameter)
- 1 pound fresh asparagus, approximately 20 ($\frac{1}{2}$" diameter) spears or a 5" round bunch, washed, trimmed, and cut into thirds

In a small bowl, combine the orange juice, zest, ginger, and soy sauce. Mix well with a wire whisk and set aside.

Microwave the sweet potato until a fork can be inserted easily into the center. Depending on your microwave, this will take from 4 to 8 minutes. Slice into approximately $\frac{1}{4}$" thick slices. You should have around $1\frac{1}{2}$ cups.

Place the asparagus and potato in a shallow ovenproof dish that has been greased with cooking spray for 2 seconds. Cover with the sauce and refrigerate for at least 2 hours, turning occasionally, if possible.

Preheat the broiler. Broil 5 to 6 minutes, turning once halfway through, or until the asparagus is tender, being careful not to overcook. Serve immediately.

Tip: The sweet potato can also be steamed for 12 to 13 minutes if you prefer.

Variation: Glaze can be used on any vegetable. It is particularly good with sliced zucchini and yellow squash or partially cooked acorn squash rings.

Whole Wheat Pita Crisps

Servings: 2

Serving Size: 4 crisps

Volume: 8 crisps

Prep Time: 1 minute

Cook Time: 20 minutes

Total Time: 21 minutes

1 whole wheat pita (about 100 calories)

¼ teaspoon salt

Preheat the oven to 350 degrees. Cut the pita into 4 wedges, then separate the top from the bottom to form 8 pieces. Place in a single layer on a jellyroll pan and spritz with water. From 8" above, sprinkle the salt over all pieces. Bake 15 to 20 minutes, turning the pieces over once during baking. Cool on a wire rack.

Tip: An empty butter substitute spray bottle makes a handy water spritzer. Just wash out the container and the sprayer, and then fill with water. Test the sprayer until water runs clear and fresh. Label the bottle so there is no confusion!

Baked Sweet Potatoes

Simple, sweet, and satisfying! This can be a meal in itself when paired with a green salad or a substantial accompaniment to any protein.

Servings: 2

Serving Size: 1 potato

Volume: 2 potatoes

Prep Time: 1 minute

Cook Time: About 1 hour

Total Time: 1 hour

2 medium sweet potatoes (each 2" in diameter and 5" long)

Preheat the oven to 400 degrees. Wash the sweet potatoes and dry them with paper towels. Wrap each potato in a piece of aluminum foil and place in the center of the oven. Allow the potatoes to bake for about 1 hour. Remove the potatoes from the oven, unwrap, and serve immediately.

Confetti Salad

Want a unique twist to the ordinary salad everyone makes with leftover wild rice? We've got it!

Servings: 4

Serving Size: 1¼ cups

Volume: 5 cups

Prep Time: 7 minutes

Total Time: 7 minutes

1   (15-ounce) can black beans, drained and rinsed

¾   cup cooked wild rice

1   (5½-ounce) can whole kernel yellow corn, drained and rinsed

1   medium tomato, peeled and chopped

2   green onions, chopped

3   slices canned jalapeño peppers, minced

3   tablespoons tarragon vinegar

2   tablespoons extra virgin olive oil

1   tablespoon canned diced pimentos, drained

1   teaspoon prepared Dijon mustard

¼   teaspoon black pepper

1   tablespoon minced fresh chives (or 1 teaspoon dry)

In a serving bowl, combine the beans, rice, corn, tomatoes, and onions. In a small jar with a tight-fitting lid, combine the remaining ingredients except the chives. Cover and shake vigorously to blend. Pour the dressing over the bean mixture and stir gently. Top with fresh chives before serving. Serve over lettuce leaves, if desired.

Note: This salad can be made ahead of time, covered and refrigerated for up to 3 days.

Grilled Corn on the Cob

This is the side dish to enjoy all summer long when supplies of fresh sweet corn are at their peak. Always purchase corn in the morning right after harvest. Extended, warm storage causes the sugar to convert to starch. Truly sweet corn makes you feel as if you are eating dessert and no butter is required!

Servings: 2

Serving Size: 1 ear

Volume: 2 ears

Prep Time: 3 minutes

Cook Time: 10 minutes

Total Time: 28 minutes

2 (7") ears fresh sweet corn with husks and stalks intact

1 teaspoon fresh snipped parsley, chives, or thyme

Peel back the husks and remove silks from the corn. Remove all but a couple of layers of husks. Return two layers of husks to surround corn and place in a large pan of cold water. Allow the corn to soak for 15 minutes. Add to the soaking water two 6" pieces of cooking twine. Remove the corn from the water, pull back the husks and spray each ear with olive oil cooking spray for 2 seconds. Hold the corn by the stalk and turn the ear as you spray to evenly coat.

Sprinkle each ear with ½ teaspoon of fresh herbs. Return the husks to surround the corn. Tie the tops with the soaked cooking twine. Place the corn over medium-high heat on the grill for 10 minutes. Use the stalk as a handle for turning the corn every 2 minutes to evenly grill. Remove the corn from the grill, untie the twine and remove the husks and stalks. Serve immediately.

Homemade Tortilla Chips

Low salt, low fat, and low effort!

Servings: 2

Serving size: 8 chips

Volume: 16 chips

Prep Time: 1 minute

Cook Time: 7 minutes

Total Time: 8 minutes

2 (8") whole wheat tortillas (look for 60–80 calories versions if possible)

Preheat the oven to 325 degrees. Stack the tortillas on a cutting board. With a pizza cutter, cut the tortillas in half, then in half again. Place them on an ungreased baking sheet. Bake 3 to 4 minutes, then remove the chips from the oven and turn each wedge over. Return them to the oven and bake 3 minutes more, checking to make sure the chips don't turn too brown. Place the chips on a wire rack to completely cool. Store them in an airtight container and use within 1 week.

Citrus Apricot Couscous

Servings: 2

Serving Size: ⅓ cup

Volume: ⅔ cup

Prep Time: 2 minutes

Cook Time: 5 minutes

Total Time: 10 minutes

¼ cup whole wheat couscous

⅔ cup boiling water

1 tablespoon orange juice

2 tablespoons dried apricots, chopped

1 teaspoon grated orange zest

Place the couscous in a medium-size oven-safe bowl. Pour boiling water over the couscous and then add the orange juice, apricots, and orange zest. Stir, then cover and let stand for 5 minutes. Fluff the mixture with a fork and serve immediately.

Variation: Substitute lemon juice and zest for orange juice and zest.

Corn Salsa

A simple rendition of a side at a local Mexican restaurant that I like to frequent. Easy and delicious. Remember: Corn is a grain!

Servings: 2

Serving Size: ½ cup

Volume: 1 cup

Prep Time: 5 minutes

Total Time: 5 minutes unless allowed to meld

1 cup golden or yellow whole kernel corn (half of a 15-ounce can, defrosted frozen or fresh)

3 tablespoons red onion, diced

2 teaspoons fresh cilantro, coarsely chopped

1 tablespoon green or red bell pepper, chopped

2 teaspoons freshly squeezed lime juice

$\frac{1}{4}$ teaspoon ground red pepper

Combine all of the ingredients. This can be served immediately, but it's best if covered and refrigerated for several hours to allow flavors to meld.

Variation: Substitute flat leaf (Italian) parsley for cilantro.

Sandwiches, Pitas, Wraps, Tacos, Pizza

Salmon Taco with Mango & Avocado

Servings: 2

Serving Size: 1 taco (or 2 small)

Volume: 2 soft tacos (or 4 small)

Prep Time: 5 minutes

Cook Time: 5 minutes

Total Time: 10 minutes

$\frac{1}{2}$ pound (7–8 ounces) salmon fillet, skin removed, cut into $\frac{1}{4}$" strips

$\frac{1}{2}$ teaspoon ground cumin

$\frac{1}{4}$ avocado, peeled and cut into four $\frac{1}{4}$" strips

$\frac{1}{2}$ cup chopped mango

1 cup fresh baby spinach

2 tablespoons fresh tomato salsa

2 (8") whole grain tortillas (or 4 small soft or hard corn tortillas)

Sprinkle the salmon with cumin. Grease a sauté pan for 4 seconds with olive or canola cooking spray. Place the pan over medium-high heat. When it's hot, add the salmon and sauté 3 to 5 minutes or until it's opaque. Fill each tortilla with half of the salmon, 2 slices of avocado, $\frac{1}{4}$ cup of the mango, $\frac{1}{2}$ cup of the spinach and a tablespoon of salsa. Fold the tortilla into a roll and secure with a toothpick if necessary. Serve immediately.

Tip: Mango purchased in a jar in the fresh produce section is a quick and easy way to keep mango on hand.

Fresh and Light Tacos

Servings: 2

Serving Size: 2 tacos

Volume: 4 tacos

Prep Time: 10 minutes

Total Time: 10 minutes

1 cup canned black beans, drained and rinsed

1 cup tomatoes, chopped into $\frac{1}{2}$" dice

2 tablespoons red onions, chopped

2 teaspoons flat leaf parsley, finely chopped

$\frac{1}{2}$ teaspoon lime zest, finely minced

2 teaspoons freshly squeezed lime juice

1 teaspoon jalapeño peppers, minced

$\frac{1}{8}$ teaspoon garlic salt (2 shakes)

1 cup baby spinach leaves, chopped

1 cup Romaine lettuce, chopped

4 (8") soft corn tortillas

1 cup nonfat plain yogurt, strained to make Yogurt Cheese (see recipe *page 217*)

Combine the beans, tomatoes, onions, parsley, zest, lime juice, and peppers in a bowl and sprinkle with garlic salt. Stir gently but well to coat all ingredients with the lime juice. It can be used immediately or for a more intense flavor, cover and refrigerate the mixture for 3 or more hours.

When you're ready to serve it, combine the chopped spinach and romaine. Place a small handful of the lettuce mixture into a corn tortilla. Place a teaspoon of yogurt on top of the lettuce and spread it to cover the lettuce mixture. Add a scoop of the drained tomato/bean mixture on top of the lettuce. Add another small handful of lettuce to the taco and finish with another dollop of yogurt. Fold each tortilla into a roll and secure with toothpicks if necessary. Serve immediately.

Thin Crust Turkey Pita Pizza

Servings: 2

Serving size: 2 pizza rounds

Volume: 4 pizza rounds

Prep Time: 5 minutes

Cook Time: 8 minutes

Total Time: 15 minutes

- 2 whole wheat pita rounds
- 1 cup low-sodium pizza or pasta sauce
- 2 garlic cloves, minced
- 2 Roma tomatoes, diced
- ½ onion, diced
- ½ cup low-fat mozzarella cheese, shredded
- 6 ounces cooked, diced turkey breast
- 2 tablespoons fresh oregano, minced

Using a long serrated knife, split the pita bread in half so you have 4 rounds. Place the rounds on a baking sheet that has been lightly coated for 2 seconds with cooking spray. Toast very lightly with the inner part of the pita round facing up while the oven preheats to 350 degrees. In a small bowl, combine the pizza sauce and garlic. Spread ¼ cup of the sauce on each pita round. Top with ¼ of the diced tomatoes and onion, then ¼ cup of the cheese and 1½ ounces (¼) of the diced turkey. Sprinkle with ½ tablespoon of the oregano. Bake 8 minutes and remove the pizzas from the oven. Allow the pizzas to rest 2 minutes before cutting them into wedges and serving.

Option #1: Make it vegetarian with a twist: Instead of turkey or pizza sauce, puree 1 (10-ounce) can of drained garbanzo beans in a food processor until smooth. Stir in ½ tablespoon of olive oil, ½ tablespoon of lemon juice, ¼ teaspoon of red pepper, and ¼ teaspoon of black pepper. Mix well and spread the mixture on cut pita rounds or tortillas. Sprinkle diced Roma tomatoes and a mixture of fresh spinach and basil leaves (cut in slivers) on top. Heat as noted above.

Option #2: Substitute drained and crumbled tofu for mozzarella cheese or use ½ cup of each combined.

Variation: Substitute 4 (8") corn tortillas for the 2 whole wheat pita rounds. Prepare as directed above.

SuperFoodsRx Turkey Spinach Pita

Servings: 1

Serving Size: 1 pita sandwich

Volume: 1 pita sandwich

Prep Time: 3 minutes

Total Time: 3 minutes

1½ cups baby spinach

3 tablespoons Ginger Orange Dressing (see recipe *page 309*)

½ can (5.5 ounces) mandarin oranges, drained and rinsed (½–⅔ cup approximately)

3 ounces sliced turkey

⅔ whole wheat pita bread; cut off top third

Place the spinach in a large bowl. Toss with Ginger Orange Dressing and add the mandarin oranges. Place the sliced turkey in the bottom of the pita. Top with the spinach mixture and serve.

Variation: Serve as a spinach salad with turkey on top and pita bread cut into wedges and served on the side.

Note: Substitute equivalent amount of grilled, poached, or baked chicken for turkey.

Cold Vegetable Tortillas

Your refrigerator vegetable bin is full of fabulous ingredients for lunch. Just pick a color theme and wrap in a whole wheat tortilla. Feel free to use one of our sandwich spread options (see recipes pages 296–306) to enhance these combinations.

Servings: 1

Serving Size: 1 tortilla

Volume: 1 tortilla

Prep Time: 5 minutes

Total Time: 5 minutes

SEE ADDITIONAL SPREAD OPTIONS (recipes page 296–306)

1 (6–8") whole wheat tortilla (80–100 calories)

Green, orange, or red filling ingredients

Green Filling Ingredients:

4 (¼") slices seedless cucumbers, cut in half

4 (¼") Roasted Green Bell Pepper Rings, cut in half

1 (7") stalk celery or steamed asparagus, chopped

1 green onion (top only), chopped

¼ cup **Hummus** (see recipe page 301, or 1 serving other spread)

Red Filling Ingredients:

1 Roma tomato, diced

4 (¼") Roasted Red Bell Pepper Rings, cut in half

1 radish, cut in thin slices

4 (¼") red onion rings, cut in half

¼ cup **Garlic Lovers Dip** (see recipe page 299, or 1 serving other spread)

Orange Filling Ingredients:

¼ cup shredded carrots

4 (¼") Roasted Orange Bell Pepper Rings, cut in half

¼ cup Mashed Cooked Sweet Potatoes

1 tablespoon sunflower seeds, toasted

Lay the tortillas on serving plates. Spread either the hummus, Garlic Lovers Dip, or other spread on tortillas (for red or green); orange has the mashed sweet potatoes. Top each tortilla with half of the filling ingredients. Roll up the tortilla and hold together with toothpicks, if necessary. Slice the tortilla in half on the diagonal. Remove the toothpicks before serving.

Greek Salad Roll-Ups

A quick lunch doesn't have to be lackluster. This recipe proves it!

Servings: 2   Prep Time: 5 minutes

Serving Size: 1 roll-up   Total Time: 5 minutes

Volume: 2 roll-ups

- 2 6" whole wheat tortillas
- 1 cup spinach leaves
- 6 thin slices ($\frac{1}{8}$" thick) red onion
- 6 thin slices ($\frac{1}{8}$" thick) peeled cucumber
- 4 pitted black olives, sliced
- 4 cherry tomatoes, cut in half
- $\frac{1}{4}$ cup soy nuts
- 2 teaspoons extra virgin olive oil

Lay the tortillas on serving plates. Top each with half of the spinach, onions, cucumbers, olives, tomatoes, and soy nuts. Drizzle each top with 1 teaspoon of the oil. Roll up the tortilla and hold it together with toothpicks, if necessary. Microwave 15 seconds, then slice the tortilla in half on the diagonal. Remove the toothpicks before serving.

Tip: This is an easy recipe to make into a one-serving recipe. Practice simple math and you'll have a single sandwich OR make two and have one for tomorrow!

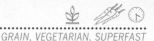

Grown-Up Peanut Butter Sandwiches

You've probably eaten peanut butter and jelly sandwiches most of your life. Now that you're an adult, put that jelly aside for healthier, more substantial peanut butter pairings. Try one of the following on your next sandwich and see how good it tastes not to be a kid anymore.

Servings: 1

Serving Size: 1 sandwich

Volume: 1 sandwich

Prep Time: 3 minutes

Total Time: 3 minutes

>   2 slices whole wheat bread
> 1½ tablespoons smooth peanut butter
>   ¼ teaspoon ground cinnamon (optional)

Select one of the following pairing options:

- ¼ cup sliced seedless purple grapes
- ¼ cup sliced strawberries
- ¼ cup sliced and pitted fresh cherries
- ¼ cup sliced and peeled strawberry guava
- ¼ cup sliced, seeded and peeled kiwi fruit
- ¼ cup sliced, seeded and peeled papaya
- 2 tablespoons grated apples
- 2 tablespoons grated carrots

Spread the peanut butter on one side of a whole wheat bread slice. Add the enhancement of your choice on top of the peanut butter. Top with the remaining piece of bread. Slice the sandwich on the diagonal and serve.

Hummus and Roasted Pepper Sandwich

Simply put . . . yummy!

Servings: 2   Prep Time: 3 minutes
Serving Size: 1 pita sandwich   Total Time: 3 minutes
Volume: 2 pita sandwiches

½ cup Hummus (see recipe *page 301*)
1 roasted bell pepper, thinly sliced
8 (⅛" thick) slices red onion
2 (6") rounds whole wheat pita bread

Cut a 1" slice off the pita bread and open it to expose the pocket. Place the cut slice in the pocket, and then spread ¼ cup of the hummus inside the pita bread. Place half of the roasted bell pepper and half of the onion slices inside each pita. Serve immediately. Refrigerate leftovers and use them within 1 week or freeze them for longer storage

Poached Salmon in Spinach Tortillas

A great leftover idea. Poach salmon the day before and enjoy for dinner. Use the extra for lunch the next day or freeze for later use.

Servings: 2   Prep Time: 4 minutes
Serving Size: 1 sandwich   Cook Time: 15 seconds
Volume: 2 sandwiches   Total Time: 5 minutes

2 (6") spinach tortillas (or 4 corn tortillas or 2 low-fat whole wheat tortillas)
2 (4–6") leaves watercress
6 ounces poached salmon steaks (half of recipe on *page 218*)
4 cherry tomatoes, quartered
1 teaspoon freshly squeezed lemon juice

Lay the tortillas on serving plates and top with the watercress. Mash the cold salmon into flakes and divide them evenly over the tortillas. Top each with 4 quarters of tomatoes and a sprinkling of lemon juice. Roll up the tortillas and secure them with toothpicks, if necessary. Microwave them on high for 15 seconds, and then cut them in half on the diagonal. Remove the toothpicks before serving.

GRAIN, VEGETARIAN

Roasted Vegetable Pita Sandwiches

Lunch is now a luxury thanks to this heavenly sandwich. Oven roasting brings intensity and depth to this quartet of fresh vegetables.

Servings: 2

Serving size: 1 pita sandwich

Volume: 2 pita sandwiches

Prep Time: 10 minutes

Cook Time: 45 minutes

Total Time: 55 minutes

- 2 cups broccoli or cauliflower florets
- 1 large beefsteak tomato, cut into 1" slices
- 1 zucchini, cut on the diagonal in 1" slices
- 1 bell pepper, seeded and cut into 8 pieces
- 1 tablespoon extra virgin olive oil
- 1 tablespoon fresh snipped chives
- 1 teaspoon garlic powder
- $\frac{1}{2}$ teaspoon black pepper
- 2 (6") rounds whole wheat pita bread

Preheat the oven to 350 degrees. Place the broccoli, tomatoes, zucchini, and peppers in a single layer on a large baking sheet lightly coated with cooking spray. Drizzle the vegetables with oil. Sprinkle with the chives, garlic, and pepper. Roast for 45 minutes or until the vegetables are golden brown and tender. Allow them to cool slightly. While the vegetables are cooling, cut a 1" slice off each pita round and open the pockets. Place the cut slices in the pockets, and then stuff each with half of the roasted vegetables. Drizzle each with $\frac{1}{2}$ tablespoon of the pan juices. Serve immediately.

Note: While you are roasting, prepare extra vegetables to refrigerate for other uses.

Thanksgiving Open-Faced Sandwich

Why enjoy these foods just once a year?

Servings: 1   Prep Time: 3 minutes

Serving Size: 1 open-faced sandwich   Total Time: 3 minutes

Volume: 1 open-faced sandwich

   2   tablespoons canned cranberry sauce
   2   tablespoons Yogurt Cheese (see recipe *page 217*)
   1   slice whole wheat bread
   3   ounces cooked turkey breast
   2   romaine lettuce leaves
   ¼   teaspoon black pepper

In a small bowl, combine the cranberry sauce and yogurt cheese, stirring until smooth. Spread the mixture on each side of the bread, and then top with the turkey, lettuce, and a sprinkling of black pepper. Slice the sandwich on the diagonal and serve.

Note: Cranberry "Mayonnaise" can be made ahead and refrigerated up to a week.

Tip: If you want to have the second slice of bread on this sandwich, use a 2-for-1 FlexPlan option! Keep bread to 80–100 calories.

Tofu "Eggless" Salad Sandwiches

A healthy, adult version of old-fashioned egg salad. You'll find it on page 228 with the other **Cold Entrées.**

Bean and Veggie Burrito

Servings: 1

Serving size: 1 burrito

Volume: 1 burrito

Prep Time: 5 minutes

Cook Time: 15 seconds

Total Time: 6 minutes

- 1 (6–8") whole wheat tortilla
- ½ cup black beans, no added salt
- ¼ cup chopped tomatoes
- ¼ cup fresh spinach, whole or chopped
- ½ medium green bell pepper, sliced
- 3 tablespoons mild Cheddar cheese, shredded
- 3 tablespoons Year Round Salsa (see recipe page 305) or Watermelon and Jalapeño Salsa (see recipe page 305) or commercial tomato salsa

Place the tortilla on a serving plate and layer it with the beans, tomatoes, spinach, and green peppers. Sprinkle it with cheese and spoon on the salsa. Roll the tortilla into a burrito by folding one end up ⅓ of the way, turning and rolling from the filling side across the burrito. Microwave the burrito for 15 seconds and serve immediately.

Variation: Two small corn tortillas can be substituted for the whole wheat tortilla

Pear, Feta, and Pecan Stuffed Pita

Servings: 1

Serving size: 1 pita

Volume: 1 pita

Prep Time: 6 minutes

Total Time: 6 minutes

$\frac{1}{2}$ pear, sliced

2 tablespoons crumbled feta cheese

2 tablespoons pecan halves or chopped

1 cup baby spinach

$\frac{1}{4}$ cup grated carrots

2 tablespoons Ginger Orange Dressing (see recipe *page 309*) or other SuperFoods approved dressing of your choice

$\frac{2}{3}$ pita (or equivalent approximately 80–100 calories)

In a small bowl, combine the pear slices, feta, pecans, spinach, and carrots. Drizzle with the vinaigrette, tossing well to coat the salad. Place the mixture in the pita and serve immediately.

Variation: Substitute a small sliced apple for pear and/or 1 to 2 tablespoons of shredded cheddar or goat cheese for feta. Substitute equal amounts of walnuts, almond slices, or pine nuts for pecan halves.

Hot Entrées

Broiled Salmon

Asian, Walnut Crusted, Lemon Herb, Cucumber Yogurt or Ginger Lime—Start with a couple of salmon fillets, then select the flavor option of your choice!

Servings: 2

Serving Size: 3 to 3$\frac{1}{2}$ ounces

Volume: 6 to 7 ounces

Time: Varies (see specific variations below)

2 (3–4 ounce raw) fresh salmon fillets, skinned

Asian Marinade Option

- 1 tablespoon low-sodium soy sauce
- 2 teaspoons sesame oil
- 1 tablespoon freshly squeeze lemon juice
- 1 tablespoon fresh chives, minced
- 1/4 teaspoon black pepper
- 2 lemon wedges

Place the salmon in a shallow baking dish. Combine the soy sauce, oil, lemon juice, chives, and pepper. Pour the mixture over the salmon and allow it to marinate at room temperature for 10 minutes. During the last 5 minutes of marinating, preheat the oven to 500 degrees. Place the baking dish in the oven and broil for 5 to 7 minutes or until the salmon is golden. When done, the salmon should flake with slight pressure from a fork. Garnish each fillet with a lemon wedge. Serve immediately.

Prep Time: 2 minutes (plus 10 minutes   Total Time: 19 minutes
to marinate)
Cook Time: 5 to 7 minutes

Walnut Crusted Option

- 1/8 cup finely chopped walnuts
- 1/4 cup fresh bread crumbs
- 1 tablespoon chopped fresh parsley
- 2 teaspoons extra virgin olive oil
- 1/8 teaspoon black pepper (3 good cranks of the pepper grinder)

Preheat the oven to 450 degrees. Combine the walnuts, crumbs, and parsley. Place the salmon fillets on a baking sheet greased for 2 seconds with cooking spray. Sprinkle the fillets evenly with the oil and pepper. Top with the walnut mixture, pressing it into the fillets. Bake 10 minutes or until the salmon flakes easily with a fork. Serve immediately.

Prep Time: 5 minutes   Total Time: 15 minutes
Cook Time: 10 minutes

Lemon Herb Option

 1 tablespoon fresh snipped dill
 1 tablespoon fresh minced parsley
 1 tablespoon fresh lemon juice
 1 teaspoon grated lemon zest
 1 clove garlic, minced
 2 teaspoons extra virgin olive oil
 ⅛ teaspoon black pepper (3 good cranks of the pepper grinder)

Preheat the oven to 450 degrees. Combine the dill, parsley, lemon juice and zest, and garlic. Place the salmon fillets on a baking sheet greased for 2 seconds with cooking spray. Sprinkle the fillets evenly with the oil and pepper. Top with the lemon herb mixture. Bake 10 minutes or until the salmon flakes easily with a fork. Serve immediately.

Prep Time: 5 minutes   Total Time: 15 minutes
Cook Time: 10 minutes

Cucumber Yogurt Option

 2 teaspoons extra virgin olive oil
 ¼ teaspoon garlic salt
 ⅛ teaspoon black pepper (3 good cranks of the pepper grinder)
 ½ cup plain nonfat yogurt
 1 small clove garlic, minced
 ¼ cup grated cucumber

Preheat the oven to 450 degrees. Place the salmon fillets on a baking sheet greased for 2 seconds with cooking spray. Sprinkle the fillets evenly with the oil, salt, and pepper. Bake 10 minutes or until the salmon flakes easily with a fork. While the fish bakes, in a small bowl combine the yogurt, garlic, and cucumber. Serve the cucumber-yogurt mix with the broiled fish.

Note: Cucumber sauce can be made ahead and refrigerated until ready to enjoy. Use within 5 days.

Prep Time: 5 minutes   Total Time: 15 minutes
Cook Time: 10 minutes

SUPERFAST

Ginger Lime Option

    2 teaspoons extra virgin olive oil
  1/8 teaspoon black pepper (3 good cranks of the pepper grinder)
    1 teaspoon freshly grated ginger
    1 tablespoon freshly squeezed lime juice
    1 teaspoon grated lime zest
    1 clove garlic, minced

Preheat the oven to 450 degrees. Place the salmon fillets on a baking sheet greased for 2 seconds with cooking spray. Sprinkle the fillets evenly with the oil and pepper. Combine the ginger, juice, zest, and garlic. Press the mixture evenly onto the top of each fillet. Bake 10 minutes or until the salmon flakes easily with a fork. Serve immediately.

Prep Time: 5 minutes   Total Time: 15 minutes
Cook Time: 10 minutes

Chicken Croquettes

Servings: 2

Serving Size: 2 croquettes (or 1 burger)

Volume: 4 croquettes, each 3" wide by
  1½" tall

Prep Time: 5 minutes

Cook Time: 15 minutes

Total Time: 20 minutes

1¼ cups cooked, diced chicken (6 ounces cooked)

½ cup soft whole grain bread crumbs

⅓ cup Yogurt Cheese (see recipe *page 217*)

1 green onion, finely chopped

1 teaspoon poultry seasoning

⅛ teaspoon black pepper (3 good cranks of the pepper grinder)

3 tablespoons dry whole grain bread crumbs (can be seasoned or plain)

2 lemon wedges

Paprika or cayenne pepper for garnish

Preheat the oven to 450 degrees. Combine the chicken, soft bread crumbs, yogurt cheese, onion, black pepper and poultry seasoning. Form the mixture into 4 croquettes. Place the dry crumbs in a shallow dish and coat the croquettes. Place them on an ungreased baking sheet and bake for 15 minutes. Serve the croquettes warm with lemon wedges and a sprinkling of paprika or cayenne pepper.

Note: If the mixture seems too wet (depending on the length of time the yogurt cheese has been made), add more soft bread crumbs. Bread crumbs are used in limited amounts as an *ingredient* in this recipe. You can make a **with** or **without** grain meal with this recipe.

Alternative Preparation Method: Substitute cooked turkey for chicken or drained, canned salmon.

Fast Option: Mix chicken, yogurt cheese, onion, poultry seasoning, and pepper together ahead of time. At the last minute, add soft bread crumbs and proceed as above.

Burger Option: Instead of forming 4 small croquettes, form 2 "burgers." Increase baking time to 30 minutes.

Ginger Grilled Turkey Tenderloin

Put your refrigerator and grill to work with this easy, yet delicious dinner option.

Servings: 2

Serving Size: 3 ounces

Volume: 6 ounces

Prep Time: 5 minutes

Cook Time: 20 minutes

Total Time: 2 hours, 25 minutes

- $1/2$ pound (7 ounces) turkey tenderloin
- 2 teaspoons low-sodium soy sauce
- 1 teaspoon freshly grated ginger
- 1 teaspoon rice wine vinegar
- $1/4$ teaspoon crushed red pepper flakes
- $1/2$ tablespoon peanut oil

Place the tenderloin in a shallow glass dish. Combine the remaining ingredients in a small jar with a tight-fitting lid. Shake vigorously until they are well combined. Pour the mixture over the tenderloin, cover, and refrigerate for at least 2 hours. Remove the tenderloin from the marinade and discard the marinade. Grill the tenderloin over medium-high heat for 5 minutes on each side. Cover and continue to cook for 10 minutes more or until the tenderloin has reached an internal temperature of 165 degrees. Cover loosely with aluminum foil and let it rest 10 minutes before slicing and serving.

Asian Stuffed Salmon Fillet

This dish can be baked or roasted in the oven or cooked on your grill.

Servings: 2

Serving Size: 3 ounces salmon and 1¼ cups vegetables

Volume: 7 ounces salmon and 2½ cups vegetables

Prep Time: 15 minutes

Cook Time: 20 minutes

Total Time: 35 minutes

- 1 teaspoon canola oil
- 1 baby bok choy, sliced into thin strips (rounds)
- 1 cup baby spinach
- ½ cup fresh bean sprouts
- ½ cup matchstick carrots (or 7–8 baby carrots cut in half or quarters lengthwise)
- 1 scallion, sliced thinly (using about ⅔ of the scallion)
- 1" fresh ginger, peeled and finely grated*
- 1 clove garlic, finely minced
- 2 teaspoons light soy sauce
- 7 ounces salmon fillet, skin removed
- 2 teaspoons honey
- 2 teaspoons Dijon mustard

Preheat the oven to 450 degrees. Heat the canola oil in a sauté pan over medium heat. Add all the vegetables, ginger, and garlic.

Cook until the vegetables are tender but firm, approximately 5 minutes. Add the soy sauce. Cook 2 to 3 minutes more.

Tear off 2 pieces of aluminum foil large enough to wrap one portion of salmon and seal it tightly. Cut the salmon through the center lengthwise so that you have 2 thinner slices. Lay 1 slice on the aluminum foil, top with half the vegetables and then cover with the other slice of salmon. Repeat this for the second portion.

In a small bowl, mix the honey and mustard. Brush the fish with the honey mustard. Wrap the fish in foil. Bake until the fish is flaky, approximately 20 minutes.

*Tip: Using a knife, after peeling, score your ginger with a line at approximately "1 inch" before grating and then easily grate on box back to the mark.

Variation: Use the vegetable mixture to stuff thin slices of turkey breast and cook as this recipe directs.

....

Pan Roasted Stuffed Turkey Breast with White Bean Sauce

Servings: 2

Serving size: 3 ounces cooked

Volume: 6 ounces

Prep Time: 15 minutes

Cook Time: 40 minutes

Total Time: 55 minutes

- 1 boneless, skinless turkey breast, aka Turkey London Broil, approximately 1/2 pound (7–8 ounces)
- 1 teaspoon minced garlic, approximately 1 clove
- 1/2 teaspoon dried oregano or 3 teaspoons fresh
- 1/2 teaspoon black pepper ground from a pepper grinder
- 2 tablespoons chopped roasted red peppers
- 3 cups bagged baby spinach, divided
- 8–10 cremini mushrooms, wiped clean and sliced
- 1 cup chopped fresh tomatoes, approximately 2 medium
- 1/2 cup low-sodium chicken stock
- 1 cup (canned) small white beans, drained and rinsed
- 1/2 teaspoon dry thyme or 3 teaspoons fresh
- 2 tablespoons chopped fresh basil or 1/2 teaspoon dry

Lay the turkey breast on a work surface. Using a long thin knife, carefully cut through the thicker side of the breast so you can unfold it to the outside and create a larger piece of breast. Rub the inside with the minced garlic, sprinkle with the oregano and grind enough black pepper to cover it. Sprinkle the roasted peppers over the seasoning. Top with 2 cups of the spinach. Roll the turkey breast and tie it at 2" intervals with cooking twine to hold the stuffing inside.

Spray extra virgin olive oil for 4 seconds in a 12-inch sauté pan. Heat the pan over medium heat and add the turkey. Brown the turkey on all sides. This will take approximately 5 minutes. Once browned, add the mushrooms, tomatoes, stock, beans, thyme, and basil to the pan. Bring the mixture to a boil and immediately turn the heat to low. Cover the pan and roast for approximately 25 minutes or until a meat thermometer registers an internal temperature of 160 degrees.

Remove the turkey from the pan and place it on cutting board. Let the turkey rest at least 5 minutes. Turn the pan back to high heat. Add the remaining cup of spinach and cook it while the turkey is resting.

Slice the turkey into ½"-thick slices. A serrated knife will make it easier to slice. Place some of the cooked spinach and sauce in the bottom of each plate and top with turkey.

Variation: During the cooking process, some of the beans can be mashed with a fork to create a thicker, creamier-style sauce.

....

Sicilian Style Stuffed Turkey Breast

This stuffing would also work nicely in boneless, skinless chicken breasts, pounded thin.

Servings: 2   Prep Time: 10 minutes
Serving Size: 2 cups   Cook Time: 25 minutes
Volume: 4 cups   Total Time: 35 minutes

- ½ cup plain dry whole wheat bread crumbs (or approximately 1 slice of bread toasted well and broken into crumbs)
- ⅛ teaspoon fine sea salt
- ⅛ teaspoon chili pepper or crushed red pepper flakes
- 1 clove garlic, minced
- 1 tablespoon raisins or dried mixed fruit bits
- 1 tablespoon chopped walnuts
- ½ cup fresh spinach leaves
- ½ cup dry white wine, divided
- 2 thin slices boneless skinless turkey breast, approximately 3–4 ounces each (also called turkey scaloppini)
- 2 large Roma tomatoes, diced (about 1 cup)
- ½ cup fresh basil leaves, chopped
- 1 teaspoon extra virgin olive oil

Preheat the oven to 375 degrees. Make a mixture with the bread crumbs, salt, chili pepper, garlic, raisins, walnuts, spinach, and $\frac{1}{4}$ cup of the white wine. Place half of the stuffing mixture on top of each of the turkey slices. Roll the slices and secure with toothpicks.

Place the tomato, basil, olive oil, and remaining $\frac{1}{4}$ cup of white wine in a baking dish large enough to hold the 2 rolled turkey breasts. Lay the turkey on top of this mixture. Turn the turkey to coat the outside with this mixture. Place seam side down and bake for 20 to 25 minutes. Serve the stuffed turkey with the sauce spooned on top.

Tip: Prepare a double batch of stuffing and freeze for later use.

Variations:

Sun Dried Tomato—Substitute sun-dried tomatoes for the raisins and Pignoli or pine nuts for the walnuts.

Asian Stuffed Turkey—Use the recipe from the Asian Stuffed Salmon but substitute thinly sliced turkey breast.

Note: This can be used in a ***with grains*** or ***without grains*** meal. The bread crumbs here are used as an ingredient in a small total amount and as part of the entree—not as the grain side.

Orange Flaxseed (or Sesame) Salmon

Servings: 2

Serving Size: 3 ounces

Volume: 6 ounces

Prep Time: 10 minutes

Cook Time: 10 minutes

Total Time: 50 minutes

$\frac{1}{2}$ cup fresh orange juice

1 tablespoon nonfat plain yogurt

1 teaspoon reduced-sodium soy sauce

$\frac{1}{2}$ teaspoon grated fresh ginger

1 small clove garlic, pressed

1 teaspoon white vinegar

$1\frac{1}{2}$ teaspoons fresh chives, chopped

2 salmon steaks ($3\frac{1}{2}$ ounces fresh or frozen)

3 tablespoons ground flaxseed or 5 tablespoons sesame seeds

Thin orange slices made into pinwheels for garnish

Mix together the orange juice, yogurt, soy sauce, ginger, garlic, vinegar, and chives in a glass pan until blended. Place the salmon steaks in the mixture and turn them to coat evenly. Cover and refrigerate the salmon for at least 30 minutes, but not more than 1 hour.

Remove the salmon steaks from the pan, letting the extra marinade drip back into the glass pan. Dip the steaks into either flaxseeds or sesame seeds. Heat a skillet over medium heat and place the steaks in the hot pan to cook. Turn them once, usually in about 5 minutes (for 1" thick steaks) and continue to cook on the other side. Pour the marinade the from glass pan into a small saucepan and heat it until it's just about boiling. Brush the steaks with the cooked marinade once on each side while cooking.

Remove the cooked salmon to a plate and drizzle it with the cooked marinade. Garnish the salmon with an orange pinwheel and serve immediately.

SUPERFAST

Great Northern Shrimp Salad

Use convenience products to make dinner . . . convenient!

Servings: 2

Serving size: 1 cup

Volume: 2¼ cups

Prep Time: 6 minutes

Cook Time: 6 minutes

Total Time: 12 minutes

- ½ (15-ounce) can Great Northern beans
- 2 teaspoons extra virgin olive oil
- 1 scallion, minced
- 1 clove garlic, minced
- 1 ripe tomato, peeled and diced
- 1½ teaspoons fresh oregano, chopped
- ¼ teaspoon black pepper
- ½ pound cooked salad shrimp
  - Crushed red pepper for garnish
  - Fresh oregano sprigs for garnish

Drain the beans in a colander over a liquid measuring cup. Rinse the beans with water and set them aside. Add enough water to the drained liquid to measure ¼ cup and set it aside.

Heat the oil in a large skillet over medium heat. When it is hot, add the scallion and garlic. Sauté 1 minute, and then add the reserved beans and drained liquid. Heat, stirring gently 3 minutes, and then add the tomatoes, oregano, and pepper. Cook 2 minutes more.

Meanwhile, place the salad shrimp in the colander that held the beans and run it under hot water for 30 seconds. Remove the bean mixture from the heat and divide it among the serving plates. Top with the warm salad shrimp. Garnish each plate with a sprinkling of crushed red pepper and a fresh oregano sprig. Serve immediately with a slice of whole wheat bread.

Note: Great Northern Shrimp Salad can be made ahead with the exception of adding the shrimp. Just gently reheat and add shrimp.

Alternative Serving Suggestion: Allow the bean mixture to cool, then cover and refrigerate. Serve cold and topped with cold shrimp.

Lemon Roasted Turkey

Turkey with zest (literally) and zing!

Servings: 2
Serving Size: 3 ounces
Volume: 6 ounces

Prep Time: 5 minutes
Cook Time: 25 minutes
Total Time: 2 hours, 30 minutes

- $\frac{1}{2}$ pound turkey tenderloin (7–8 ounces raw)
- 1 tablespoon freshly squeezed lemon juice
- $\frac{1}{2}$ tablespoon extra virgin olive oil
- $\frac{1}{4}$ teaspoon garlic salt
- $\frac{1}{8}$ teaspoon black pepper (3 good cranks of the pepper grinder)
- 1 tablespoon chopped fresh parsley
- 1 teaspoon grated lemon zest

Place the turkey in a shallow glass baking dish. Add the lemon juice and oil, making sure to coat all sides of the tenderloin. Cover and refrigerate for 2 hours.

Preheat the oven to 375 degrees. Place the turkey on the rack of a broiler pan that has been sprayed for 2 seconds with cooking spray. Pour any remaining marinade from the baking dish, along with 2 tablespoons of water into the bottom of the broiling pan. Rub the turkey with garlic salt and pepper. Roast the turkey 20–25 minutes or until an instant-read meat thermometer registers 165 degrees. Remove the turkey from the oven and sprinkle the top with parsley and zest. Cover the turkey loosely with aluminum foil and let it rest 10 minutes before slicing and serving.

Alternative Preparation Method: Instead of roasting the turkey, grill over medium-high heat, turning after 5 minutes to evenly brown on all sides. The turkey is done when an instant-read meat thermometer registers 165 degrees.

Lentil Meatballs

Versatile should probably be in the name of this recipe. The meatballs can easily transition from dinner to lunch to snack. They even make a unique addition on top of a green salad!

Servings: 2

Serving size: 5 meatballs (about 1" diameter) or 1 burger (3½" diameter by ¾" thickness)

Volume: 1½ cups; makes 10 meatballs or two 3½" diameter by ¾"-thick burgers

Prep Time: 15 minutes

Cook Time: 5 minutes

Total Time: 20 minutes

½ teaspoon extra virgin olive oil

¼ cup finely diced onion

½ teaspoon minced garlic

2 tablespoons finely chopped walnuts

1 cup Cooked Lentils (see recipe *page 219*)

2 tablespoons oil packed sun-dried tomatoes, drained, rinsed, and chopped

½ teaspoon snipped fresh sage (or ¼ teaspoon dry)

¼ teaspoon snipped fresh thyme (or ⅛ teaspoon dry)

Dry bread crumbs, as needed, up to ¼ cup max

Heat the oil in a large skillet over medium heat. Add the onions and garlic, stirring until the onions just begin to brown. Add the walnuts and continue to sauté for 4 minutes. Remove from the heat and allow to cool slightly.

Preheat the oven broiler. In a mixing bowl, combine the lentils, tomatoes, and herbs. Add the cooled onion mixture, stirring well. Using a tablespoon or melon baller, form meatballs. If the mixture is too moist, add dry bread crumbs.

Place the meatballs on the rack of a broiler that has been sprayed 2 seconds with cooking spray. Broil 2–3 minutes or until they are nicely browned. Remove the meatballs from the oven and rotate them. Return them to the oven and broil 2 minutes longer. Serve hot.

Alternative Preparation Method: Instead of meatballs, form the lentil mixture into three patties for lentil burgers. Simply double the broiling time.

Bread crumbs in this recipe are an ingredient and not as a *with*; enjoy this recipe as a *with* or *without* grains meal.

Papillote

(pah-pee-YOTE) Turkey/Chicken—Don't let the name of this recipe intimidate you—and now you'll sound oh, so sophisticated when you say and then serve this easy, delicious recipe. This cooking method allows both meat and vegetables to be prepared in paper-wrapped individual servings. It seals moisture in, so you've got a wonderfully juicy, tender entrée. Bonus: Cleanup is accomplished by just throwing away the parchment paper!

Servings: 2

Serving Size: 3 ounces turkey and ⅔ cup vegetables

Volume: 3 ounces turkey or chicken and ⅔ cup vegetables per serving.

Prep Time: 15 minutes

Cook Time: 10 minutes

Total Time: 25 minutes

2 (3–4-ounce each) portions turkey breasts or boneless, skinless chicken breasts
¼ teaspoon garlic salt
⅛ teaspoon black pepper (3 good cranks of the pepper grinder)
2 carrots, peeled and cut into ¼" rounds
8 sugar snap peas
1 red bell pepper, seeded and julienned
2 teaspoons pine nuts
2 tablespoons fresh basil leaves, cut in strips
2 teaspoons extra virgin olive oil

Preheat the oven to 400 degrees. Cut two pieces of parchment paper into 12-inch squares and place them on an ungreased baking sheet. Lightly grease one side of each piece of parchment for 2 seconds with cooking spray.

Place the meat on one half of the parchment and sprinkle each with half of the garlic salt and pepper. Top the meat with half of the carrots, peas, bell pepper strips, pine nuts, and basil. Drizzle each with a teaspoon of olive oil.

Seal the paper packets by folding the other half of the parchment over the ingredients. Make several pleats to close the edges by working around the packet. Fold the end edges under the packet and make sure it is sealed tightly. Bake for 10 minutes.

To serve, place the papillote on a serving plate and carefully cut a slit into each packet to expose the cooked meat and vegetables.

Alternative Preparation Method: Substitute 7 ounces of salmon for turkey or chicken.

You can also substitute green beans if sugar snaps are not available.

SUPERFAST IF YOU MARINATE IN ADVANCE

Peanut Glazed Shrimp

Marinate the shrimp before you head to work for a quick dinner that seems as if you spent the day preparing it!

Servings: 4

Serving size: 6 shrimp

Volume: 1 pound

Prep Time: 5 minutes

Cook Time: 4 minutes

Total Time: 2 hours, 9 minutes

- 1 pound raw large shrimp, shelled and deveined
- 3 tablespoons freshly squeezed lime juice, divided
- 1 tablespoon peanut oil
- ¼ cup peanut butter
- ¼ cup freshly squeezed orange juice
- 1 clove garlic, minced
- 1 teaspoon hot sauce

Place the shrimp in a resealable plastic bag. Combine 2 tablespoons of lime juice with the peanut oil. Refrigerate for at least 2 hours and up to 8 hours. Preheat the grill to medium heat. Skewer the shrimp and place them on the hot grill. Brush the shrimp with leftover lime mixture and grill for 2 minutes on each side. Combine the remaining ingredients in a small microwave-safe dish and whisk until smooth. Heat the mixture in a microwave oven on high for 15 seconds, and stir. Place the shrimp skewers on serving plates. Drizzle the shrimp with peanut sauce. Serve immediately.

Note: Shrimp can be served over any salad greens, cooked rice, or cooked whole wheat pasta.

Turkey (or Tofu) Meatballs

Forget what you know about high-fat, high-calorie, golf-ball sized meatballs. This healthy alternative is a tasty change of pace and perfect over pasta, in soup, or as an entrée.

Servings: 4

Serving size: 6, 1" meatballs

Volume: 24, 1" meatballs

Prep Time: 15 minutes

Cook Time: 20 minutes

Total Time: 35 minutes

NOTE: TOFU VERSION IS VEGETARIAN

- 1 pound ground turkey
- ¼ cup fine dry Italian seasoned bread crumbs
- ¼ cup ground walnuts
- 2 small cloves garlic, minced
- 2 tablespoons freshly squeezed lemon juice
- 1 tablespoon Dijon mustard
- 1 tablespoon dried parsley (or ¼ cup fresh)
- Cucumber Yogurt Sauce (see recipe on *page 266*)

Preheat the oven to 350 degrees. Lightly grease a jelly roll pan by spraying for 2 seconds with cooking spray. Set the pan aside. In a large bowl, mix all the ingredients together and shape into 1" meatballs. Place the meatballs on the prepared pan and bake for 20 minutes or until no longer pink. Turn the meatballs once to evenly brown during baking. Remove the meatballs from the oven and drain them on paper towels. Serve the meatballs at room temperature with Cucumber Yogurt Sauce.

Note: Turkey meatballs can easily be frozen. Place cooked meatballs in a single layer on a baking pan and freeze. When solid, transfer to a freezer container, label, and freeze. By freezing in this manner, you will be able to easily remove the amount needed from the freezer container because they will not clump. To reheat frozen meatballs, place in a preheated 350-degree oven for 15 minutes.

Alternative Preparation Method: Substitute 14 ounces of pressed firm tofu for the turkey and add 1 tablespoon of low-sodium soy sauce.

Turkey Meatloaf with Tomato Gravy

What's for dinner? An amazing meatloaf with plenty of flavor. What's for lunch tomorrow? An equally amazing meatloaf sandwich served on toasted whole wheat bread.

Servings: 4, cook once, eat twice or more (unless you share!)

Serving size: 1 slice—¼ of loaf

Volume: 4 cups

Prep Time: 15 minutes

Cook Time: 30 minutes

Total Time: 45 minutes

Meatloaf:

- ½ pound lean ground turkey
- ¼ pound hot ground turkey sausage
- ½ cup chopped onion
- 2 egg whites
- ¼ teaspoon black pepper

Gravy:

- 1 (14½ ounce) can diced tomatoes, drained
- 1 green onion, trimmed and sliced
- ¼ teaspoon garlic powder
- ¼ teaspoon black pepper

Grease the rack of a broiler pan with cooking spray for 2 seconds and set aside. Preheat the oven to 350 degrees. Combine the turkey, sausage, onions, egg whites, and pepper, mixing well. Place the meat mixture on the broiler rack and shape into a log. Place 2 tablespoons of water in the bottom of the broiler pan. Bake for 25–30 minutes or until the turkey loaf is firm (center temperature should read 165 degrees).

Meanwhile, puree all gravy ingredients in a food processor or blender. Transfer mixture to a small saucepan and cook over medium heat for 15 minutes, uncovered. Remove the pan from the heat and allow the mixture to cool slightly. During the final 10 minutes of cooking the meatloaf, glaze the top with the tomato gravy. Remove the meatloaf from the oven, cover it loosely with a tent of aluminum foil, and allow it to rest for 10 minutes before slicing. Cut the meatloaf into 4 equal slices.

Vegetable Kabobs with Shrimp or Tofu

Two taste variations use the same marinade!

Servings: 2

Serving size: Approximately 1+ cup (half recipe or two 8" kabobs)

Volume: 2¼ cups, makes four 8" kabobs

Prep Time: 20 minutes

Cook Time: 10 minutes

Total Time: 2 hours, 30 minutes

Marinade: *(can easily be doubled)*

- 3 tablespoons red wine vinegar
- 2 tablespoons extra virgin olive oil
- 2 cloves garlic, minced
- 1 teaspoon chopped fresh thyme
- ¼ teaspoon black pepper

Option #1:

- 6 large cherry tomatoes
- 6 medium-sized mushrooms
- 1 green or orange bell pepper, cut into 2" strips
- 2 medium-sized yellow summer squash, cut into 1" chunks
- 1 small eggplant, cut into 1½" cubes
- 12 large shrimp, shelled and deveined (do not marinate)

Option #2:

- ⅔ pound extra firm light tofu, cut into 1½" cubes
- 2 medium-sized zucchini, cut into 1" chunks
- 1 medium onion, cut into wedges
- 1 sweet potato, peeled and cut into 1½" cubes and parboiled 7 minutes

Prepare the marinade by combining all of the ingredients in a small jar with a tight-fitting lid. Shake the jar vigorously to combine. Place the vegetables in a small baking dish. Pour the marinade over the vegetables (and the tofu for option #2), cover and allow them to marinate at least 2 hours or overnight.

Do not marinate the shrimp (option #1). Spear the marinated vegetables and tofu or shrimp on skewers in a mixed sequence. Grill them over medium heat or broil for 10 minutes, turning every couple of minutes to cook evenly. Baste, if desired with leftover marinade. Serve hot.

Note: After preparation, Vegetable Kabobs can also be removed from the skewers and served over salad greens, cooked wild or brown rice, cooked couscous, or cooked whole wheat pasta.

Tofu Stir Fry

Servings: 1

Serving Size: 2 cups

Volume: 2 cups

Prep Time: 5 minutes

Cook Time: 4 minutes

Total Time: Overnight + 9 minutes

4–5 ounces firm or extra-firm tofu

2 teaspoons extra virgin olive oil or grapeseed oil

$\frac{1}{2}$ cup onion, coarsely chopped

1 clove garlic, crushed

1 teaspoon Italian seasoning

$\frac{1}{4}$ teaspoon black pepper

$\frac{3}{4}$ cup broccoli florets

$\frac{3}{4}$ cup chopped fresh tomato, seeded if desired

1 cup fresh spinach (loosely chopped or whole baby spinach leafs)

Hot couscous

Freeze the tofu (overnight is convenient) and then defrost* it and cut into 1" cubes. In a large skillet, heat the olive oil over medium-high heat. When hot, add the onions, garlic, seasoning, pepper, and tofu. Stir-fry for 1 minute. Add the broccoli and stir-fry an additional 2 minutes. Add the tomatoes and spinach and stir-fry 1 minute more. Serve immediately over the couscous.

Alternative Preparation Methods: Substitute $\frac{1}{2}$ cup frozen spinach for the fresh. Add with the broccoli and proceed as directed. Halved cherry or teardrop tomatoes can be substituted for chopped tomatoes.

*Tip: Freezing the tofu before slicing and stir-frying helps with the texture so it stays together better in the high-heat cooking process.

Grilled Salmon with Yogurt Dill Drizzle

Servings: 1

Serving size: 3 ounces

Volume: 3 ounces

Prep Time: 5 minutes

Cook Time: 5 minutes

Total Time: 10 minutes

4–5 ounce salmon steak

  2 teaspoons extra virgin olive oil

  2 tablespoons nonfat plain yogurt

  $\frac{1}{8}$ teaspoon prepared or fresh horseradish

  $\frac{1}{8}$ teaspoon fresh snipped dill

Rub the salmon steak with 1 teaspoon of the olive oil on each side to prevent sticking. Grill the salmon over medium-hot coals for 2 minutes on each side or until the salmon is done and flakes easily with a fork. Meanwhile, in a small bowl, whisk together the yogurt, horseradish, and dill. Transfer the salmon to a serving plate and drizzle it with sauce in a zigzag pattern. Serve immediately.

Soups

DEPENDING ON THE OPTION SELECTED, CAN BE VEGETARIAN

SuperFoodsRx SoupBase

Here you are: the soup of many faces, many flavors, many SuperNutrients. With a single SuperFoodsRx SoupBase, you have 12 unique and tasty soups to create! And when you get familiar with a soup recipe that is great for you, you'll enjoy it again and again and again in your weight-managing, health-promoting diet!

Servings: Depends on option selected
(listed below each option)

Serving Size: Depends on option selected
(listed below each option)

Volume: Depends on option selected
(listed below each option)

Prep Time: 15 minutes

Cook Time: 2 hours, 15 minutes

Total Time: 2 hours, 30 minutes

3 cups peeled and diced turnips or potatoes
1 cup diced carrots (about 15 baby carrots)
1 cup diced onions
1 cup diced celery
1 cup diced red bell peppers
6 cups water
$\frac{1}{4}$ cup minced fresh parsley (Italian or curly leaf)
2 cloves garlic, minced
$\frac{1}{2}$ teaspoon freshly ground black pepper

Lightly grease a large stockpot with a bottle of spray oil (olive, grapeseed, or canola) for 4 seconds. Place over the pot over medium heat. When it's hot, add the turnips, carrots, onions, celery, and red peppers. Sauté for 15 minutes, stirring often. Add the water, parsley, garlic, and pepper. Bring the mixture to a boil, cover, reduce the heat and simmer for 2 hours. Use this as a soup base for any of the following options.

Note: Potatoes in this SuperFoods SoupBase are great sources of potassium and vitamin C and help to create the easy base you will use again and again. As an ingredient, you can use this recipe any time in a *with grains* **or** *without grains* meal.

Option #1: For **Garbanzo Vegetable Soup**, during the last 30 minutes of cooking the SuperFoods SoupBase, add 2 (15-ounce) cans of drained and rinsed low-sodium garbanzo beans, 1 (28-ounce) can of undrained diced tomatoes, $1\frac{1}{2}$ tablespoons of balsamic vinegar and 1 cup of water. Add more water if necessary.

Variations: You can use $4\frac{1}{2}$ cups of chopped fresh raw tomatoes for equivalent calories of a 28-ounce can. You can use $3\frac{1}{2}$ cups of home-cooked garbanzo beans instead of canned.

Servings: 6   Volume: 12 cups
Serving Size: 2 cups

Option #2: For **Lentil Vegetable Soup**, during the last hour of cooking the SuperFoods SoupBase, add 2 tablespoons of minced fresh chives, 2 teaspoons of ground red pepper, and 1 cup of water. In the last 20 minutes of cooking, add 2 (15-ounce) cans of low-sodium lentils. Add more water if necessary.

Variation: You can use 3 cups of home-cooked Lentils (double or triple recipe on page 219) with no salt added for comparable calories.

Servings: 4
Serving Size: 2²/₃+ cups

Volume: 11½ cups

Option #3: For a **Spicy Vegetable Soup**, during the last hour of cooking, add 3 cups of low-sodium vegetable juice, 1 tablespoon of dried no-salt Italian seasoning, ½ teaspoon of paprika or ground red pepper, and 1½ teaspoons of hot sauce. Add more water if necessary.

Note: You can enjoy this also as a **SuperNutrient Booster**—1 cup (page 327).

Servings: 4
Serving size: 2¾ cups
Volume: 11 cups

Option #4: For an **Italian Vegetable Soup,** during the last 30 minutes, add 2 cups of stewed tomatoes (one 15-ounce can), 2 teaspoons of dried oregano, 2 teaspoons of dried basil, and 6 ounces (approximately ⅓ of a 16-ounce bag or ⅔ of an 8-ounce bag) of dried pasta. Add approximately 2 cups or more water if necessary.

Servings: 6
Serving size: 2 cups

Volume: 12 cups
🌱 Grain

Option #5: For **Seafood Gumbo**, substitute oyster or clam juice for all or part of the 6 cups water in the SoupBase. During the last 45 minutes of cooking, add 1 cup of brown rice (dry.) During the last 30 minutes of cooking, add 1 (10-ounce) package of frozen cut okra, ¾ pound of frozen shucked oysters or clams (or a combination), 1 tablespoon of Cajun seasoning, 1 tablespoon of prepared horseradish, 1 tablespoon of hot sauce, and 1½ cups of water to the soup. Add more water if necessary. Heat thoroughly and serve with a garnish of cayenne pepper.

Tip: If you want to add leftover cooked brown rice, quinoa, etc., add 2 cups of cooked grains in the last 10 minutes of cooking to reheat thoroughly.

Servings: 6
Serving size: 2 cups

Volume: 12 cups
🌱 Grain

Option #5b:

To make this soup an equivalent *without grain* meal, add 2 cups (15-ounce) can) of white beans within the last 30 minutes of cooking and omit the brown rice.

Option #6: For **Oriental Vegetable Soup**, during the last 30 minutes of cooking, add 3 cups of bok choy (sliced on the diagonal), 1 cup of snow peas, 1 tablespoon of rice wine vinegar, 1 cup of sliced shitake mushrooms, $\frac{1}{2}$ cup of sliced water chestnuts, and 1 cup of water. Add more water if necessary. Garnish with Chinese noodles (approximately $\frac{1}{3}$ cup each serving).

Servings: 6   Volume: 12 cups
Serving size: 2 cups

Option #7: For **Tortellini Vegetable Soup**, during the last 30 minutes of cooking, add $1\frac{1}{2}$ cups of frozen cut green beans, 1 bay leaf, 1 (15-ounce) can of undrained diced tomatoes, and 2 cups of water. Add 3 cups of refrigerated, cooked or fresh spinach tortellini to the soup 10 minutes before serving. Add more water if necessary.

Alternate: 2 to 3 cups fresh diced tomatoes can be added instead of canned for comparable calories.

Servings: 6   Volume: 15 cups
Serving size: $2\frac{1}{2}$ cups   ⚘ Grain

Option #8: For **Mexican Chowder,** when the water is added for the Super-Foods SoupBase, add 2 ($14\frac{3}{4}$-ounce) cans of whole kernel corn, 2 (4-ounce) cans of chopped green chiles, 1 teaspoon of ground cumin, 1 teaspoon of chili powder, and 1 additional cup of water to the soup. Add more water if necessary. Garnish each serving with 3 sprigs of fresh cilantro (9 total).

Servings: 6   Volume: 12 cups
Serving size: 2 cups   ⚘ Grain

Option #9: For **Turkey Vegetable Soup**, during the last 30 minutes of cooking, add $1\frac{1}{2}$ pounds of cooked and diced turkey breast meat, 1 tablespoon of fresh rosemary, 1 tablespoon of fresh thyme, 1 (15-ounce) can of undrained diced tomatoes, $1\frac{1}{2}$ cups of washed spinach leaves, and 2 cups of water to the soup. Add more water if necessary.

Alternate: You can use 2 to 3 cups of diced fresh tomatoes instead of canned.

Servings: 5
Serving size: $2^2/_3$ cups
Volume: about 14 cups

Option #10: For **Chili**, allow the soup base to cool completely, and then puree the mixture in blender. Return to the stockpot and add 12 ounces of cooked ground turkey, 1 (15-ounce) can of drained and rinsed red kidney beans, 1 tablespoon of chili powder, and 1 (28-ounce) can of undrained diced tomatoes. Cook over medium heat for 45 minutes and add more water if necessary. Serve with hot sauce.

Servings: 6
Serving size: 2 cups for entree soup

1 cup for side soup
Volume: 13 cups

Option #11: For **Edamame Vegetable Soup**, place 3 cups of shelled edamame in a saucepan filled with 2 quarts of boiling water for 6 minutes. Drain in a colander over a bowl and allow the edamame to cool for 10 minutes. Place the edamame and 1 cup of reserved, strained cooking water in a blender and puree until smooth. Add to the soup base during the last 15 minutes of cooking. Add more reserved, strained cooking water if necessary.

Servings: 5
Serving size: Approximately 2 cups

Volume: $10^1/_2$ cups

Option #12: For **Tofu Vegetable Soup**, cut 12 ounces of firm tofu into small cubes and toss them with $1^1/_2$ tablespoons of curry powder. During the last 5 minutes of cooking, add the tofu cubes. Cover and serve the soup hot with a garnish of fresh parsley. Add more water if necessary.

Servings: 4
Serving size: $2^1/_3$ cups

Volume: $9^1/_2$ cups

Soup Garnish Option #1: Ladle the soup into a serving bowl and garnish with a dollop of drained yogurt cheese.

Soup Garnish Option #2: Garnish the finished soup servings with 1 tablespoon of grated carrots.

Sweet Potato Soup

This soup should be married to fall and winter menus. It is as beautiful as it is delicious. Spice it up, if you want, with a dash of cayenne pepper and a garnish of fresh cilantro leaves.

Servings: 4

Serving size: 1½ cups

Volume: 5¾ cups

Prep Time: 10 minutes

Cook Time: 50 minutes

Total Time: 1 hour

½ tablespoon extra virgin olive oil

1 medium onion, peeled and cut into dice

2 cloves garlic, minced

2 (7") celery stalks, sliced

1 (8") carrot stick, peeled and sliced

1 teaspoon fresh grated ginger

½ teaspoon ground cumin

4 cups water

2 medium sweet potatoes, peeled and diced

2 tablespoons freshly squeezed lemon juice

1 tablespoon Roasted Pumpkin Seeds for garnish (see recipe *page 291*)

In a stockpot, heat the oil over medium heat. Add the onions, garlic, celery, and carrots. Cook for 4 to 5 minutes or until the vegetables begin to slightly brown. Add the ginger, cumin, water, and sweet potatoes. Stir well and cover the pot. Allow the soup to cook 45 minutes or until the sweet potatoes are tender. Add the lemon juice. Using an immersion blender (see note), puree the soup. Ladle into warmed soup bowls and garnish the soup with roasted pumpkin seeds.

Note: If you do not have an immersion blender, allow the soup to cool slightly. Then puree in batches in a blender. Return to the soup pot and gently reheat.

Tip: This soup freezes well. Allow to cool completely, ladle into freezer containers, label and freeze. Use within 3 months.

Turkey Meatball Soup

This version of Italian Wedding Soup is destined to be served frequently at your house from now on!

Servings: 2

Serving size: 2 cups

Volume: 4 cups

Prep Time: 15 minutes

Cook Time: 20 minutes

Total Time: 35 minutes

- 3 cups water
- 2 Roma tomatoes, diced
- 1 large carrot, peeled and grated
- 1 (7") celery stalk, chopped
- 1 cup fresh spinach, chopped
- ½ cup diced onions
- 2 cloves garlic, minced
- 1 teaspoon fresh chopped oregano
- ¼ teaspoon black pepper
- ½ recipe (12 total) Turkey Meatballs, cooked (see recipe *page 280*)
- 2 tablespoons dry couscous
- ¼ cup grated carrots for garnish

Place a large soup pot over medium heat and add the water, tomatoes, carrots, celery, spinach, onions, garlic, oregano, and pepper. Allow the mixture to come to a boil, and then reduce the heat to a simmer. Add the cooked meatballs and couscous. Cover and simmer for 10 minutes, stirring frequently and adding more water if necessary. Serve in warm soup bowls and garnish with the grated carrots.

Note: Serve as a *with grains* meal (couscous) along with a Small SuperFoodsRx side salad (see recipe page 233) or remove the couscous from the recipe and serve as a *without* grains meal accompanied by No Cook Vegetable Kabobs (see recipe page 244).

Turkey Pumpkin Chili with Roasted Pumpkin Seeds

Servings: 8
Serving Size: 1 cup
Volume: 8 cups

Prep Time: 10 minutes
Cook Time: 55 minutes
Total Time: 65 minutes

- 2 tablespoons extra virgin olive oil
- 1 large onion, chopped (about 1½ cups)
- 1 large green bell pepper, cut into ½" dice
- 2 cloves garlic, peeled and crushed
- 3 cups low-fat, low-sodium chicken or turkey stock
- 3 tablespoons no-salt chili powder
- 1 (28-ounce) can low sodium canned diced tomatoes
- 1¼ pounds ground turkey breast
- 2 cups cubed fresh pumpkin or butternut squash, steamed until fork tender
- 2 tablespoons chopped fresh cilantro
- 1 (16-ounce) can white beans, drained and rinsed
  Roasted pumpkin seeds (see recipe below)

Heat the oil in a large saucepan over medium heat. When the pan is hot, add the onions and sauté for 8 minutes or until they are lightly browned. Add the bell peppers and garlic, and sauté 5 more minutes.

Add the stock, chili powder, tomatoes, and turkey. Bring the chili to a boil and quickly reduce to a simmer. Cook for 20 minutes or until the turkey is done. Stir in the pumpkin, cilantro, and beans, and cook 5 minutes. Serve immediately.

To roast pumpkin seeds: Preheat the oven to 300 degrees. Remove the seeds right from the pumpkin, scraping away as much flesh and strings as possible, but do not rinse the seeds. Spread the seeds on a cookie sheet that has been lightly greased with cooking spray for 2 seconds. Bake for approximately 45 minutes, stirring halfway through the roasting process.

Note: This chili freezes well. Place in individual plastic containers and freeze. Thaw in the refrigerator and reheat prior to serving.

Alternative Preparation Method: Instead of fresh pumpkin or butternut squash, equivalent amounts of frozen butternut squash, fresh or frozen sweet potatoes, fresh sliced carrots, or chopped orange bell peppers can be substituted.

Cold Fruit Soup

Keep an open mind here! Not all soups have to be savory and served hot. This soup will cool you off on warm spring, summer, and Indian summer days.

Servings: 2   Prep Time: 10 minutes

Serving Size: 1+ cups   Total Time: 1 hour, 10 minutes

Volume: 2½ cups

1 cup honeydew melon, peeled, seeded, and diced
1 cup cantaloupe, peeled, seeded, and diced
1 cup seedless watermelon, diced
⅓ cup water
2 tablespoons nonfat plain yogurt
¼ teaspoon grated lemon zest
Fresh mint sprigs for garnish

Place all the ingredients in a food processor or blender and puree until smooth. Adjust the thickness with more or less water. Refrigerate for at least 1 hour to allow the flavors to meld. Pour the soup into chilled soup bowls and garnish with mint sprigs.

Alternative Preparation Method #1: Instead of honeydew, cantaloupe, and watermelon, substitute 3 cups of peeled, seeded, and sliced peaches, apricots, or nectarines. Substitute ½ teaspoon of ground cinnamon for the lemon zest. Garnish each serving with 5 fresh blueberries.

Alternative Preparation Method #2: Substitute 3 cups of sliced kiwis or hulled and capped fresh strawberries for honeydew, cantaloupe, and watermelon. Garnish each serving with a fresh mint sprig.

Four-Bean Chili

Cook once, eat twice! Dedicate an afternoon to letting this chili cook and you'll enjoy it for dinner now and again later since it freezes beautifully.

Servings: 4

Serving Size: Approximately 1¼ cups

Volume: 5¼ cups

Prep Time: 10 minutes

Cook Time: 3 hours, 30 minutes

Total Time: 3 hours, 40 minutes

¼ cup dried kidney beans

¼ cup dried pinto beans

¼ cup dried Great Northern beans

¼ cup dried chickpeas

1 teaspoon dried oregano

1 teaspoon cumin seeds, toasted

1 bay leaf

1 teaspoon extra virgin olive oil

½ cup diced onion

1 clove garlic, minced

1 medium bell pepper, diced

1 teaspoon chili powder

½ teaspoon ground coriander

½ teaspoon red pepper flakes

¼ cup red wine vinegar

1 cup diced tomatoes, fresh or canned (drained, if using canned)

Place the dried beans in a large stockpot with a quart of water. Bring to a boil and cook for 2 minutes over medium heat. Turn off the heat and cover the pot. Allow the beans to soak for 1 hour. Drain and rinse the beans thoroughly. Return the beans to the stockpot, adding the oregano, cumin seeds, bay leaf, and 6 cups of fresh water. Bring the mixture to a boil and reduce the heat to medium. Simmer for 2 hours, stirring occasionally and checking the water amount, adding more as needed. Remove and discard the bay leaf.

During the last 10 minutes of cooking, heat the oil in a large skillet over medium heat. Sauté the onions, garlic, and bell peppers for 7 minutes. Add the remaining ingredients and heat through. Add the vegetable mixture to the bean mixture and cook for 30 minutes more.

Remove the pot from the heat and allow the chili to cool slightly. Divide the chili, placing half in a freezer-safe container. When it's completely cool, label the container and freeze. Serve the remaining chili immediately.

GRAIN

Turkey Sausage and Tortellini Soup

Once you taste this soup, you'll crave it regularly, so go ahead and make sure to keep the supplies for it in your kitchen!

Servings: 2

Serving Size:

Volume: 3¼ cups

Prep Time: 5 minutes

Cook Time: 2 hours, 10 minutes

Total Time: 2 hours, 15 minutes

3 ounces fully cooked smoked turkey sausage, thinly sliced
1 cup pre-shredded coleslaw mix
½ cup loose-pack frozen cut green beans or Italian-style green beans
1 (14½-ounce) can Italian-style stewed tomatoes, undrained
2 cups water
¼ (9-ounce) package refrigerated mushroom-filled tortellini
   Grated carrots for garnish

Place the sausage, coleslaw mix, green beans, tomatoes, and water in a stockpot. Bring the mixture to a boil and reduce the heat to a simmer. Cover and cook 2 for hours, stirring occasionally and adding more water as needed. Stir in the tortellini, cover, and cook 10 minutes more. Ladle the soup into serving bowls and sprinkle the tops with grated carrots. Serve immediately.

Tuscan Bean Soup

Use dried beans and you've got aromatherapy from the kitchen. Use canned and you've got dinner in a flash. Either way, this soup is divine!

Servings: 4

Serving Size: 1¼ cups

Volume: 5 cups

Prep Time: 5 minutes

Cook Time: 1 hour, 40 minutes

Total Time: 2 hours, 45 minutes

¾ cup dried cannellini beans (yields approximately 2 cups)
2 tablespoons extra virgin olive oil, divided
1 medium onion, peeled and sliced
2 cloves garlic, peeled and chopped
½ tablespoon fresh snipped sage (or scant 1 teaspoon dry)
Fresh sage leaves for garnish

Place the dried beans in a stockpot with a quart of water. Bring the beans to a boil and cook for 2 minutes over medium heat. Turn off the heat and cover. Allow the beans to soak for 1 hour. Drain and rinse the beans thoroughly. Return the beans to the stockpot and cover them with 3 cups of fresh water. Bring them to a boil and reduce the heat to medium. Simmer for 30 to 40 minutes or until the beans are done, skimming away any foam that develops.

During last 10 minutes of cooking, heat the oil in a large skillet over medium heat. Add the onions and garlic, stirring constantly. Cook for 3 to 4 minutes or until the onions are nicely browned. Add the entire contents of the skillet to the beans and remove from heat. With an immersion blender (see note), puree the soup, adjusting the thickness with water. Stir in the minced sage, cover and let stand for 10 minutes before serving. Ladle two 1¼-cup servings into the soup bowls. Garnish with fresh sage leaves and serve warm. Allow the remaining half of the soup to cool. Pour the soup into a shallow freezer container, label, and freeze.

Note: If you do not own an immersion blender, allow the soup to cool slightly. Puree it in batches in a blender. Return half of the soup to the stockpot and gently reheat. Allow the remaining soup to completely cool and freeze.

Alternative Preparation Method: Instead of dried cannellini beans, use a 15½-ounce can of drained and rinsed beans. Begin the recipe with the second paragraph of instructions and heat the mixture until hot.

Spreads, Dips, Salsas

Black Bean & Mango Salsa

Salsas make wonderful condiments or side dishes to simply prepared foods. You can create many variations of a salsa by changing the fruit or vegetables used in them.

Servings: 2

Serving Size: 1/3 cup

Volume: 2/3 cups

Prep Time: 5 minutes

Total Time: 5 minutes

- 1/2 cup black beans, drained and rinsed
- 1/4 cup chopped mango
- 1 teaspoon seeded and finely minced jalapeño pepper (see tip below)
- 1 tablespoon minced scallion
- 1 tablespoon freshly squeezed lime juice
- 1 tablespoon chopped fresh cilantro

Mix all of the ingredients together. Serve the salsa as a condiment alongside your favorite foods, such as grilled salmon or turkey, or as a snack with whole grain crackers.

Tip: Wear rubber gloves when mincing the jalapeño so that you don't get the capsaicin on your hands.

Creamy Spinach Dip

This recipe makes a very flavorful and really healthy low-fat dip or spread that your guests will not believe is so good for them!

Servings: 4

Serving size: ⅓-cup serving

Volume: 1½ cups

Prep Time: 5 minutes

Total Time: 8 minutes

1 cup fresh baby spinach
2 cloves garlic, minced
1 tablespoon minced shallot
2 tablespoons grated Parmigiano-Reggiano
½ cup fresh basil
1 cup nonfat cottage cheese (see note below)

Place the spinach, garlic, shallots, Parmigiano-Reggiano, and basil in a food processor. Process to a paste-like consistency. With the motor running, add the cottage cheese. Process until smooth. Cover and refrigerate the dip until ready to use.

Note: You can substitute yogurt cheese or strained, Greek-style yogurt (either fat-free or 2%) for the cottage cheese.

Tip: Best when made a day ahead.

Variation: For Onion Garlic Dip, eliminate the Parmigiano-Reggiano and basil and add 2 tablespoons dried onion flakes.

Smoked Salmon Spread

This can be prepared up to 2 days ahead.

Servings: 4 servings

Serving size: ½ cup (Snack serving size: ⅓ cup)

Volume: 2 cups

Prep Time: 3 minutes

Total Time: 5 minutes

½ cup sliced hearts of palm (canned)
1 lemon, juiced, divided
2 tablespoons minced shallot
4 ounces smoked salmon, roughly chopped
¼ cup fresh dill or 1 tablespoon dried dill
1 cup nonfat plain yogurt

Place the hearts of palm, juice of half the lemon, shallots, salmon, and dill in a food processor fitted with the steel blade. Pulse until the mixture is finely minced. Add the yogurt and pulse until the mixture is evenly blended and creamy. Taste for seasoning and add the remaining lemon juice if desired. Serve with vegetables such as broccoli and tomatoes or whole grain crackers

Variation: For Tuna Spread, substitute 4 ounces of low-sodium canned tuna in spring water (drained) for the salmon. Use yogurt cheese for a thicker, creamier spread.

Yogurt Banana Strawberry Spread

This spread is wonderful when served for breakfast on whole grain bread, waffles or pancakes or with whole grain chips or vegetables for a quick pick-me-up snack.

Servings: 5

Serving Size: ¼ cup

Volume: 1¼ cups

Prep Time: 5 minutes

Total Time: 5 minutes

$^1/_2$ cup nonfat plain yogurt or yogurt cheese

$^1/_2$ cup chopped fresh strawberries

$^1/_2$ cup chopped banana, slightly mashed (4–5 inches)

$^1/_4$ cup chopped walnuts

Place all of the ingredients in a small bowl and gently mix. This is best made several hours ahead so that flavors can blend

Variation: Use 1 cup of your favorite fruit such as sliced blueberries or sliced grapes.

···

VEGETARIAN, SUPERFAST

Garlic Lover's Dip (and Sandwich Spread)

A bean-based dip for snacking or spread for pita sandwiches.

Servings: 6

Serving Size: $^1/_4$ cup

Volume: Approximately 1$^1/_2$ cups

Prep Time: 5 minutes

Total Time: 5 minutes

2   cloves garlic

1   (15-ounce) can Great Northern beans, drained and rinsed

2   tablespoons freshly squeezed lemon juice (include pulp with juice for extra flavor)

$^1/_8$ teaspoon kosher salt

$^1/_8$ teaspoon freshly ground pepper (3 good cranks of the pepper grinder)

2   tablespoons nonfat plain yogurt

Zest of one lemon, divided

Place the peeled garlic cloves in a food processor bowl and process until they are finely chopped. Add the beans and pulse until they are chopped, stopping to scrape down the sides as needed. Add the lemon juice, salt, pepper, yogurt, and half of the lemon zest. Pulse until the entire mixture is mixed. Do not over process. Refrigerate the mixture until needed and serve it with the remaining lemon zest as garnish. If the product thickens, thin it with a small amount of additional yogurt.

Great Northern Bean Dip

Servings: 8
Serving Size: ¼ cup
Volume: 2 cups

Prep Time: 5 minutes
Total Time: 5 minutes

  1 (15½ ounce) can Great Northern beans, drained and rinsed
  1 tablespoon extra virgin olive oil
  2 tablespoons freshly squeezed lemon juice
2½ teaspoons minced garlic
  ¼ teaspoon salt
  ¼ teaspoon pepper

Place the beans in the bowl of a food processor. Add the remaining ingredients and pulse until smooth. Scrape the bowl as necessary to incorporate ingredients. Serve this immediately or cover and refrigerate up to 2 days.

"Brocco-Mole"

Stand facing the food processor and in a flash you've got a great-tasting substitute for guacamole!

Servings: 5
Serving Size: ¼ cup
Volume: 1¼ cups

Prep Time: 15 minutes
Cook Time: 10 minutes
Total Time: 2 hours, 25 minutes

  1 tablespoon extra virgin olive oil
  2 cups finely chopped onion
  1 clove garlic, minced
  ¾ cup chopped broccoli florets
  1 small green bell pepper, chopped
  ½ cup finely chopped zucchini
  1 tablespoon freshly squeezed lime juice

1 tablespoon chopped fresh parsley
¼ teaspoon garlic salt
¼ teaspoon black pepper
1 tablespoon toasted sesame seeds for garnish

In a large skillet, heat the oil over medium heat and add the onion and garlic. Cook for about 2 minutes or until the onions soften, but don't turn brown. Add the broccoli and cook another for 4 minutes. Add the bell pepper and zucchini and cook for 4 minutes more. Remove the skillet from the heat and add the lime juice, parsley, salt, and pepper. Allow the mixture to cool slightly. Transfer the vegetables to a food processor or blender and puree until smooth. Adjust the consistency by adding a tablespoon or two of water if necessary. Place the mixture in a serving bowl, cover and refrigerate for at least 2 hours. Just before serving, garnish it with toasted sesame seeds. Serve with homemade pita crisps (see page 248), crackers, or raw vegetables.

VEGETARIAN

Hummus

Servings: 8

Serving size: ¼ cup

Volume: 2 cups

Prep Time: 5 minutes

Total Time: 20 minutes

1 (14-ounce) can low-sodium garbanzo beans, drained and rinsed
2 cloves garlic, minced
2 tablespoons freshly squeezed lemon juice
2 tablespoons water
2 tablespoons extra virgin olive oil
¼ teaspoon ground coriander

Place the garbanzo beans, garlic, lemon juice, water, oil, and coriander in a food processor and puree. Adjust the thickness with more or less water. Allow the flavors to meld at least 15 minutes or refrigerate for later use. Use the hummus as a dip for Homemade Tortilla Chips (see recipe page 251). Garnish, if desired, with chopped roasted bell pepper and onions.

"Refried" Beans

Okay, we tricked you! These delicious beans will taste like they were fried, but they aren't. The slow cooker does practically all the work for you. Use it as a sandwich spread as well as a tasty side dish. Pressed for time? Open a 16-ounce can of low-fat refried beans as a quick substitute.

Servings: 11

Serving size: $\frac{1}{4}$ cup

Volume: $2\frac{3}{4}$ cups

Prep Time: 5 minutes

Cook Time: 10 hours

Total Time: 18 hours

$\frac{1}{2}$ pound dried pinto beans ($1\frac{1}{8}$ cup dry)

$\frac{1}{2}$ cup diced onions

$\frac{1}{2}$ tablespoon chili powder or adobo seasoning

$\frac{1}{2}$ teaspoon garlic powder

Place the beans in slow cooker and cover them with 6 cups of water. Allow them to sit, covered overnight. Drain and cover the beans again with 6 cups of fresh water. Cook the beans on low for 10 hours, or until they are soft. During the last hour of cooking, add the onions. Drain the beans, but reserve the cooking water. Add the seasonings and mash the beans with a potato masher or on the low speed of a hand mixer. Adjust the thickness with cooking water.

When the bean mixture has cooled, place a heaping tablespoon into each compartment of clean ice cube trays and freeze. When hard, transfer the frozen cubes of refried beans to a freezer container. This makes it convenient to use later for a sandwich spread by simply thawing a cube or two. Larger quantities can also be frozen to use as a side dish.

Roasted Pepper Puree

This spread will make you ask, "Mayonnaise who?"

Servings: 10

Serving size: 2 tablespoons (⅛ cup)

Volume: 1¼ cups

Prep Time: 15 minutes

Cook Time: 15 minutes

Total Time: 30 minutes

- 2 large orange, red, or green bell peppers
- 1 tablespoon fresh snipped herbs (basil, chives, oregano, thyme, tarragon, or parsley)
- 1 small clove garlic, minced
- ⅛ teaspoon black pepper (3 good cranks of the pepper grinder)
- 1 tablespoon extra virgin olive oil
- 1 tablespoon water

Preheat the broiler. Place the whole peppers on a baking sheet and put it in the oven. Turn on the oven light to watch the peppers closely or crack the oven door. Turn the peppers frequently so the outer skins blacken evenly. Remove the peppers from the oven and place them in a large resealable plastic bag. Close the bag and allow the peppers to stand for 15 minutes. Remove the peppers and slip off the outer skins. Allow the peppers to cool, and then cut them open and remove the white pith and seeds.

Place the roasted peppers, garlic, pepper, oil, and water in a food processor and process until smooth. Adjust the thickness with water. Cover and refrigerate the puree until you are ready to use it.

Salsa Bean Dip

Food should always look as good as it tastes. This recipe is a great example of that philosophy. It looks beautiful enough to carry to a picnic or tailgating party. It's also perfect to serve at a patio party of your own, with no guilt!

Servings: 4   Prep Time: 5 minutes

Serving size: ½ cup   Total Time: 10 minutes

Volume: 2 cups

- 2 green onions, trimmed and cut into 4 pieces
- 1 clove garlic, peeled
- ¼ teaspoon ground cumin
- 1 (1- ounce) can low-sodium cannellini beans, drained and rinsed
- 2 tablespoons water
- ¼ cup medium hot or hot salsa (see recipe pages 305–306)
  Fresh cilantro sprigs for garnish

Place the green onions, garlic, and cumin in the bowl of a food processor and coarsely chop the mixture. Add the beans and water, and process until it is smooth.

To make 4 individual servings: Divide the bean mixture between 4 small, shallow serving bowls. Use a rubber spatula to smooth the top evenly. Spoon a quarter of the salsa into center of each bean dish. Pull the point of a wooden pick through the salsa toward the edge of the dish to create a starburst design. Cover and refrigerate 1 bowl to enjoy within the next 5 days. Garnish the remaining bowl with fresh cilantro sprigs and serve with Homemade Tortilla Chips—8 per serving. (See recipe page 251).

Alternate Serving Method: Spread the bean mixture into 1 shallow dish. Continue as above and serve at room temperature with a double recipe of homemade tortilla chips.

Alternative Preparation Method: Salsa may also be stirred into the bean mixture. Or puree the salsa with the bean mixture for a great sandwich spread.

Watermelon & Jalapeño Salsa

Similar to tomato salsa, but with a sweet and spicy twist!

Servings: 2

Serving Size: About 1/4 cup

Volume: 1/2+ cup

Prep Time: 5 minutes

Total Time: 5 minutes

- 1/2 cup seedless watermelon, cut into 1/2" pieces
- 1 teaspoon seeded and finely minced jalapeño pepper
- 1 tablespoon minced scallion
- 1 tablespoon freshly squeezed lime juice
- 1 tablespoon chopped fresh mint

Mix all of the ingredients together. Serve as a condiment alongside your favorite foods, such as grilled salmon or turkey, or as a snack with whole grain crackers.

Year-Round Salsa

Who says salsa is only good during the summer months? With this recipe, you can enjoy salsa every season. The instructions are the same for all versions. Just mix together and serve at room temperature. Pair with Homemade Tortilla Chips (see recipe page 251).

Servings: 3 to 4

Serving size: 1/2 cup

Volume: Varies and is listed below each salsa

Prep Time: 5 minutes

Total Time: 5 minutes

Spring Salsa:

- 4 medium ripe greenhouse tomatoes, chopped
- 1 (4 ounce) can diced green chilies, drained
- 1/4 cup chopped onion
- 1/4 cup fresh snipped cilantro
- 1/4 teaspoon black pepper

Volume: 1 1/2 cups

Summer Salsa:

- 3 medium ripe tomatoes, chopped and drained (use Heirloom varieties)
- 1 clove garlic, minced
- ¼ cup chopped onion
- 1 tablespoon fresh snipped oregano
- 2 fresh jalapeño peppers, diced

Volume: 1-¼ cups

Late Summer Salsa:

- 1 bell pepper, minced
- 4 medium ripe tomatoes, chopped, seeded, and drained (use slicing varieties)
- ½ cup chopped onions
- 1 clove garlic, minced
- 4 small green chili peppers, chopped fine with stems and seeds removed
- 1 teaspoon fresh snipped oregano

Volume: 1½ cups

Fall Salsa:

- 1½ cups canned tomatillos, drained
- ¼ cup diced onions
- 1 clove garlic, minced
- 2 jalapeño peppers, seeded and diced
- ¼ cup snipped fresh cilantro

Volume: 1½ cups

Winter Salsa:

- 2 cups canned, diced tomatoes, drained
- 1 (4 ounce) can diced green chilies, drained
- ½ teaspoon garlic powder
- ½ teaspoon dried crushed oregano
- ¼ teaspoon chili powder

Volume: 2¼ cups

Salad Dressings and Marinades

You can use any of the SuperFoodsRx dressings interchangeably! Stick w
tablespoons (a couple allow up to 3 tablespoons maximum; see below). Homemade dressings are so easy to make and are a major upgrade nutritionally—
while saving you lots of calories and chemicals—in your diet and your life.

Basic SuperFoodsRx "Vinaigrette" Dressing with Variations

A collaboration from our SuperFoods Kitchen! Classic Vinaigrette is 3 parts oil to 1 part vinegar. Our recipe has cut the calories from the oil by adding some water and additionally changing the ingredients to provide variety. Replacing some of the vinegar or acid with fruit juices also provides interest and preparing it ahead of time will enhance flavor. Additional vinaigrette can be refrigerated for several days, providing convenience.

Versatile "vinaigrettes" can be used as salad dressing, marinades for salmon, turkey or vegetables, and as a condiment that you can drizzle over your protein or vegetables.

Servings: 5
Serving Size: 2 tablespoons
Volume: ²/₃ cup (10 tablespoons)

Prep Time: 3 minutes
Total Time: 3 minutes

- 3 tablespoons orange, lemon or lime juice
- 3 tablespoons water
- 2 tablespoons red or white wine vinegar
- 2 tablespoons extra virgin olive oil
- 1 tablespoon Dijon mustard
- 1 teaspoon honey
- ⅛ teaspoon sea salt
- ⅛ teaspoon black pepper (3 good cranks of the pepper grinder)

Whisk all of the ingredients together or shake them in a jar with a tight-fitting lid. Use immediately or store in the refrigerator.

Alternative Preparation Methods

1. **Rosemary Garlic Dressing:** Add a teaspoon of finely minced garlic and $\frac{1}{2}$ teaspoon chopped fresh rosemary or $\frac{1}{8}$ teaspoon dried rosemary to basic recipe. Increase water to 4 tablespoons.

2. **Celery Chive Dressing:** Add $\frac{1}{4}$ teaspoon celery seeds and 1 teaspoon fresh snipped chives or $\frac{1}{4}$ teaspoon dried chives to basic recipe. Increase water to 4 tablespoons.

3. **Basil Garlic Dressing:** Add 1 teaspoon chopped fresh basil leaves or $\frac{1}{4}$ teaspoon dried basil and 1 teaspoon minced garlic to basic recipe. Increase water to 4 tablespoons.

4. **Lemon Dressing:** Use lemon juice and add 1 teaspoon grated lemon zest to the basic recipe.

5. **Orange Dressing:** Use orange juice and add 1 teaspoon grated orange zest to the basic recipe.

6. **Lime Dressing:** Use lime juice and add 1 teaspoon grated lime zest to the basic recipe.

7. **Pomegranate Dressing:** Replace juice with pomegranate juice.

8. **Blueberry Dressing:** Place $\frac{1}{4}$ cup fresh blueberries (about 12) in a blender and add all remaining ingredients for basic dressing, using lemon juice and increasing the amount to 4 tablespoons. Blend until blueberries are finely chopped and dressing is smooth. Thin with additional water if desired.

Asian Inspired Red Pepper Sesame Dressing

Servings: 6   Prep Time: 3 minutes

Serving Size: 2 tablespoons   Total Time: 3 minutes

Volume: ²/₃ cup

- ¼ cup rice wine vinegar
- 1 tablespoon light soy sauce
- 1 tablespoon hot chili sesame oil (regular sesame oil can be used but add 1 teaspoon ground red pepper)
- 1 tablespoon grapeseed or canola oil
- ½ cup (½ small bunch) scallions, sliced about ¼" thick

Whisk all of the dressing ingredients together in bowl large enough to hold the salad ingredients.

This accompanies the **Asian Inspired Broccoli Salad** (see recipe *page 230*) or other salads, or use as a marinade.

Ginger Orange Dressing

Servings: 4   Prep Time: 3 minutes

Serving Size: 3 tablespoons   Total Time: 3 minutes

Volume: ¾ cup

- ½ cup plain low-fat or nonfat yogurt
- ¼ cup fresh orange juice
- 1 tablespoon freshly grated ginger
- ⅓ cup chopped scallions or green onions

Whisk all ingredients together. Serve with **Turkey Spinach Pita** (see recipe *page 256*) or on other salads.

Honey Mustard Salad Dressing

Servings: 5½   Prep Time: 5 minutes

Serving Size: Approximately 3 tablespoons   Total Time: 5 minutes

Volume: 1 cup

⅔   cup plain nonfat or low-fat yogurt

2   tablespoons honey

1½ teaspoons dry mustard (or 1 tablespoon Dijon prepared mustard)

1   teaspoon apple cider vinegar

Whisk together all of the ingredients in a small bowl. Cover and chill until serving time.

Alternative Preparation Method: Substitute ⅔ cup of yogurt cheese for the yogurt.

Cucumber Yogurt Sauce

For those evenings when you just aren't in the mood for a tomato-based sauce.

Servings: 2   Prep Time: 5 minutes

Serving size: ⅓ cup   Total Time: 20 minutes

Volume: ⅔ cup

¼   cup finely chopped cucumber (can be grated if desired)

½   cup plain nonfat yogurt

½   teaspoon finely chopped parsley

1   tablespoon freshly squeezed lime juice

⅛   teaspoon garlic salt

⅛   teaspoon black pepper (3 good cranks of the pepper grinder)

Whisk all of the ingredients together in a medium bowl. Cover the bowl and let if stand for 15 minutes before using it. Or make it up to 2 days in advance, and then cover and refrigerate it. When you are ready to use it, allow the sauce come to room temperature for 15 minutes before serving. Yield: ⅔ cup.

Serving Suggestion: Goes beautifully with Turkey (or Tofu) Meatballs (recipe page 280)

Watermelon & Jalapeño salsa

(See recipe page 305). Vegetable and fruit salsas are great options for topping salads, fish and poultry.

Year Round Salsa

(See recipe page 305) This chunky and flavorful salsa is a delicious alternative to thin dressings.

VEGETARIAN, SUPERFAST

Tangy Tomato Dressing

Great over a green spinach salad sprinkled with toasted pine nuts.

Now I said nothing is "free" on this diet, but if I had to make an exception this would be one. This dressing contains 33 calories in 2 tablespoons. You could practically drink it! But don't—it's a terrific salad dressing as recommended.

Servings: 8
Serving Size: 2 tablespoons
Volume: 1 cup

Prep Time: 5 minutes
Total Time: 15 minutes

½ cup diced fresh tomatoes or canned diced tomatoes, drained
1 tablespoon red wine vinegar
2 tablespoons extra virgin olive oil
1 tablespoon chopped fresh chives

1   small clove garlic, minced

½   tablespoon freshly squeezed lemon juice

½   tablespoon hot sauce

½   cup water

Place all of the ingredients in a blender. Pulse the mixture first, then puree until it's smooth. Adjust the thickness with more or less water. Allow the flavors to meld about 10 minutes before using.

Refrigerate the leftovers.

Tofu Herb Dressing

Excellent with baby greens, as an enhancement for raw broccoli, cauliflower, carrots, bell peppers, tomatoes, or served with grilled fish or turkey.

Servings: 8   Prep Time: 5 minutes

Serving size: 2 tablespoons   Total Time: 15 minutes

Volume: 1 cup

4   ounces firm silken tofu

1   small clove garlic, minced

¼   cup freshly squeezed lemon juice

1   tablespoon snipped fresh herbs (basil, oregano, tarragon, thyme, or dill)

1   tablespoon white wine vinegar

1   tablespoon extra virgin olive oil

1   tablespoon finely minced onion

⅛   teaspoon black pepper (3 good cranks of the pepper grinder)

½   cup water

Place all of the ingredients in a blender. Pulse the mixture first, then puree until it's smooth. Adjust the thickness with more or less water. Allow the flavors to meld about 10 minutes before using. Refrigerate the leftovers.

Bakery Items, Sweets, Desserts

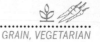

Dark Chocolate Chip Cookies

A special treat that can be made and frozen and baked off a couple at a time. Treats can be nutrient dense, too—and there's portion control built into the "practice" of eating a delicious homemade cookie.

Servings: 21

Serving size: 2 cookies (FlexPlan Flex option)

Volume: 42 cookies (approximately 2" diameter, ¾" tall per cookie)

Prep Time: 15 minutes

Cook Time: 15 minutes

Total Time: 30 minutes

2¼ cups whole wheat flour

1 teaspoon baking soda

1 teaspoon baking powder

¼ cup butter, softened

¼ cup applesauce

4 teaspoons honey

2 large eggs, beaten

¾ teaspoon ground cinnamon

1 teaspoon pure vanilla extract

⅔ cup dark chocolate chips

⅔ cup regular oats

Preheat the oven to 375 degrees. In a large bowl, combine the flour, baking soda, and baking powder. Cut in the butter. Add the applesauce, honey, eggs, cinnamon, and vanilla. Cream together until the dough is well mixed. Add the chips and oats. With a teaspoon, drop the cookies (1" diameter balls) on a baking sheet and slightly spread them out. Bake for 12–15 minutes or until lightly browned. Remove the cookies from the oven and cool on a baking sheet for 5 minutes before transferring them to a wire rack. Cool the cookies completely before storing them in airtight containers.

Variation: Instead of oats, substitute an equal amount of toasted, coarsely chopped walnuts.

Oatmeal Cinnamon Bars

Servings: 24

Serving size: 1 bar

Volume: 24 squares (2¼" x 2¼" squares, 1¼" tall

Prep Time: 15 minutes

Cook Time: 25 minutes

Total Time: 40 minutes

  2 cups rolled oats

1½ cups whole wheat flour

  1 teaspoon ground cinnamon

  1 teaspoon baking powder

 ¼ cup granulated sugar

 ½ cup brown sugar

 ½ teaspoon salt

  1 cup cinnamon applesauce

 ½ cup vegetable oil

Preheat the oven to 350 degrees. Combine the oats, flour, cinnamon, baking powder, sugars, and salt. Add the applesauce and oil. Stir just until blended. Pour the batter into a lightly greased 13" x 9" baking dish. Bake for 20–25 minutes or until the bars are set in the center. Allow the cake to cool on a wire rack before cutting it into bars.

Pumpkin Dessert Crepe with Yogurt Sauce

Servings: 4

Serving Size: 2 crepes

Volume: 8 dessert crepes

Prep Time: 20 minutes

Cook Time: 15 minutes

Total Time: 35 minutes

Filling:

$^3/_4$ cup pureed pumpkin (approximately half a 15-ounce can; not pie filling)

1 tablespoon maple syrup

$^1/_2$ teaspoon pumpkin pie spice

In a medium bowl, combine all of the filling ingredients together, mixing well. Cover and chill for up to 2 hours.

Yogurt Sauce:

$^1/_2$ cup plain nonfat yogurt

2 teaspoons honey

Stir all of the ingredients until the honey is incorporated. Allow the sauce to stand for 10 minutes at room temperature. Stir it again. Then cover and chill the sauce until needed.

Crepe Recipe:

$^1/_2$ cup 2% Milk

2 eggs

$^1/_2$ cup unbleached all-purpose flour

$^1/_4$ teaspoon salt

Place all of the ingredients in a blender and mix until they are well blended. Place the covered blender in the refrigerator for at least $^1/_2$ an hour to allow the flour to be fully absorbed. The mixture should have the consistency of a medium cream after cooling.

To Cook Crepes:

Preheat a 6" or 8" crepe or fry pan. Lightly grease the pan with spray canola or grapeseed oil (3 seconds). Stir the batter after retrieving it from the refrigerator. (If it's too thick, add a small amount of water and stir). Place the pan over medium to medium-high heat. With one hand, pour 1½ to 2 ounces of the batter into the center of the pan, and with the other hand quickly rotate the pan so that the batter evenly forms a very thin pancake covering the entire bottom of the pan. After cooking for about ½ a minute, gently lift the edge of the crepe with the tines of a fork and check the cooked side for a light golden brown color. When the color is reached, gently lift the crepe edge from the pan with the fork, grasp the edge with your fingers and gently turn the crepe over. Allow it to cook for another 10 to 15 seconds. Slide the finished crepe onto a flat plate and continue. This recipe will make 6 to 8 crepes depending on the size of the pan and thickness of the crepe.

To assemble crepes:

Once all of the crepes are made, remove the filling and yogurt sauce from the refrigerator. Take a crepe from the top of the stack and lay it flat with the first-cooked side down. Place 3 tablespoons of the pumpkin mixture in the center of the crepe. Fold one side over the filing, and then the other. Turn the crepe so that the seam side is down on the plate. Gently flatten the crepe so that the filling is evenly distributed, with a little filling showing at the open ends. Repeat with the second crepe for serving.

Stir the yogurt sauce. With the crepes side by side on the individual serving plate, pour 2 tablespoons of yogurt sauce over the center of the crepes, allowing some to pool onto the plate. Garnish with a sprinkling of ground cinnamon if desired.

Alternative Preparation Method: Substitute ¼ cup of light ricotta for the yogurt.

Chocolate Tofu Mousse

Servings: 6

Serving size: ⅓ cup

Volume: 2¼ cups

Prep Time: 10 minutes

Cook Time: 1 minute maximum

Total Time: 10 minutes plus 1 hour to chill

- ½ cup semisweet chocolate chips
- ¼ cup soy milk
- 1 package silken tofu (lightly firm), crumbled
- 2 tablespoons honey

  Whole strawberries for garnish or dipping

Place the chocolate chips and soy milk in a microwave-safe bowl. Melt in the microwave oven on high for 30 seconds. Stir to combine the ingredients. If necessary, repeat the heating until the chocolate chips are completely melted. Set the mixture aside to cool.

Place the tofu and honey in a blender or food processor container. Add the melted chocolate. Blend until it's completely smooth, scraping down the sides of the container. Transfer the mousse to individual serving bowls, and then cover and refrigerate for at least 1 hour before serving. Garnish with strawberries and serve.

Blueberry Compote Crumble

Servings: 5

Serving size: About ¼ cup

Volume: 6 cups

Prep Time: 5 minutes

Cook Time: 5 minutes

Total Time: 10 minutes

1 recipe Blueberry Compote (see recipe *page 238*)

½ cup dry oats

¼ cup chopped walnuts

1 tablespoon brown sugar

1 tablespoon butter

Spoon the compote immediately into 5, dessert-sized ramekins or an 8" x 8" baking dish (coat the dish with grapeseed or canola spray for 4 seconds). Preheat the oven to 375 degrees. Combine the oats (quick or old-fashioned), walnuts, brown sugar, and butter. Evenly distribute the oat mixture over the top of the Blueberry Compote. Bake for 5 minutes and serve warm.

Variation: For 1 serving, use approximately ¼ cup of the compote, 1 tablespoon of oats, ½ teaspoon of brown sugar, 2 teaspoons of chopped walnuts, and ½ teaspoon of butter. Follow the instructions using 1 dessert-sized ramekin.

SuperFoodsRx Blueberry Muffin with Walnuts

This muffin is a portable meal in itself. It is packed full of hearty SuperFoods such as oatmeal, walnuts, and blueberries with an added punch from the whole grain flour and dried fruits.

Servings: 12 muffins

Serving Size: 1 muffin (2½ ounces)

Volume: 5 cups batter, 12 (2½-ounce) muffins

Prep Time: 15 minutes

Cook Time: 20 minutes

Total Time: 35 minutes

½ cup unsweetened applesauce

½ cup plain nonfat yogurt

2 large egg whites

1 large egg

1 teaspoon pure vanilla extract

2 tablespoons pure maple syrup

½ cup whole wheat flour

½ cup unbleached all-purpose flour

1 cup old-fashioned oats

1 tablespoon baking powder

1 teaspoon baking soda

1 teaspoon ground cinnamon

¼ cup dried fruit such as blueberries or cherries

½ cup chopped walnuts

1½ cups fresh or frozen blueberries (if frozen, do not thaw)

Preheat the oven to 400 degrees. Place muffin liners/papers in the pan and set aside.

Mix the applesauce, yogurt, egg whites, egg, vanilla, and maple syrup together in a large bowl until smooth.

Mix the whole wheat flour, all-purpose flour, oats, baking powder, baking soda, cinnamon, dried fruit, and walnuts together. Add the blueberries so that they are coated with dry ingredients. (This will keep the blueberries evenly distributed through the batter.)

Add the dry mixture to the wet ingredients and mix gently, just until the dry ingredients are moistened. Divide the batter among 12 regular muffin cups. Bake for 15 to 20 minutes or until the tops are dry and golden. Turn the muffins onto a wire rack. Cool and enjoy!

SuperFoodsRx Pumpkin Walnut Muffins

No need to wait until the fall months to enjoy this scrumptious muffin. Bake a batch, freeze them and enjoy any time of the year.

Servings: 12 muffins

Serving Size: 1 muffin (2½ ounces)

Volume: 5 cups batter, 12 (2½ ounce) muffins

Prep Time: 15 minutes

Cook Time: 20 minutes

Total Time: 35 minutes

- 1 cup unbleached all-purpose flour
- 1 cup wheat bran
- 1 teaspoon baking powder
- ½ teaspoon baking soda
- ¼ teaspoon salt
- ¼ teaspoon ground cinnamon
- ¼ teaspoon ground nutmeg
- 1 egg, lightly beaten
- 1 cup plain nonfat yogurt
- 4 tablespoons butter, melted
- 3 tablespoons light brown sugar
- 1 cup canned pumpkin or pumpkin puree
- ¼ cup finely chopped walnuts

Preheat the oven to 350 degrees. Fill a 12-muffin tin with baking cups and it set aside. In a large bowl, combine the flour, wheat bran, baking powder, baking soda, salt, cinnamon, and nutmeg. Make a well in the center.

In a separate bowl, beat together the egg, yogurt, melted butter, sugar, pumpkin, and walnuts. Pour into the well of dry ingredients and mix the batter just until the ingredients are combined. Evenly distribute the batter among the muffin cups. Bake for 15 to 20 minutes or until a toothpick inserted in the center comes out clean. Remove the muffins from the pan and allow them to cool on a wire rack.

Note: Place completely cooled leftover muffins in resealable plastic freezer bag, label and freeze. Frozen muffins should be used within 3 months. Either thaw at room temperature for 30 minutes or microwave on defrost and enjoy.

SuperNutrient Boosters

Commercial, store-bought options certainly come in handy for travel and to keep the office stocked for when you're in a pinch, but I think you'll agree that making your own is actually really rewarding and very tasty. I like to call them by their color: Red, Green, Blue, and Orange. And talk about SuperFoodsRx SuperNutrients—this is your daily insurance. Culinary expert Tammy Algood developed these recipes for SuperFoodsRx dieters like you. After many, many taste tests, here are the best of the best. Cheers!

Commercial Options for You:

Serving size: 6 ounces (¾ cup)

- R.W. Knudsen Family™ Very Veggie® Low Sodium Vegetable Cocktail
- V8® Low Sodium Vegetable Juice
- Trader Joe's Garden Medley Low Sodium
- Evolution™ Essential Greens
- Evolution™ Organic V
- Evolution™ Carrot Celery Beet

SuperNutrient Booster
Red—Cooked

Tangy Tomato Vegetable Juice

Not quite as fast as our uncooked version, but just as tasty! Cook up a batch and you've got enough for the work week!

Servings: 5

Serving Size: 1 cup

Volume: 5 cups

Prep Time: 5 minutes

Cook Time: 30 minutes

Total Time: 45 minutes

- 4 large fresh, ripe beefsteak tomatoes (or a 28-ounce can whole tomatoes, undrained)
- 2 (7") stalks celery, sliced
- ½ cup diced red bell peppers
- 2 green onions, trimmed and sliced
- 4 cups water, divided
- 2 cloves garlic, minced
- 6 sprigs fresh basil
- 6 sprigs fresh oregano or flat leaf parsley
- ¼ teaspoon black pepper
- 1 teaspoon hot sauce

Peel, core and quarter the tomatoes. Seed the tomatoes, if desired. Place the tomatoes, celery, bell peppers, onions, 2 cups of water (decrease to 1½ cups if using canned tomatoes), and garlic in a medium saucepan. Place over medium heat, and then cover and allow it to simmer 30 minutes. Remove the pan from the heat, uncover and allow the mixture to cool.

Transfer the mixture to a blender and add the remaining 2 cups of water, basil, oregano, black pepper, and hot sauce. Process the mixture until smooth. Adjust the consistency with more or less water. Serve at room temperature, over ice or chilled.

Note: This juice can be strained if a thinner juice is desired.

SuperNutrient Booster
Red—No Cook

Easy Tomato Veggie Juice

This juice is a real morning eye-opener both in color and flavor. When prepared extra thin, it can double as a broth base for vegetable soup. Cut the water to a ½ cup and it becomes the soup.

Servings: 3   Prep Time: 5 minutes

Serving size: 5+ ounces (just over ½ cup)   Total Time: 5 minutes

Volume: 2 cups

- 1 (15 ounce) can whole tomatoes, undrained
- 1 (7") stalk celery, thinly sliced
- ¼ cup diced red bell peppers
- 1 green onion, trimmed and thinly sliced
- 6 sprigs fresh basil, oregano or curly leaf parsley
- 2 cranks black pepper
- 1½ cups cold water

Place all of the ingredients in a blender and process until smooth. Adjust the consistency with additional water. Serve it over ice or as is.

Optional Seasonings: For a bit of kick, add ¼ teaspoon of red pepper flakes, Worcestershire sauce, cayenne pepper, or hot sauce to the blender.

SuperNutrient Booster Green—No Cook

Go Green!

Servings: 4

Serving Size: 6 ounces (¾ cup)

Volume: 3 cups

Prep Time: 5 minutes

Total Time: 5 minutes

- 1 large Granny Smith apple (or 2 small), washed, cored, and seeded (not peeled)
- 1 7" stalk celery, thinly sliced
- 1 2" slice peeled fresh ginger
- 6 springs curly leaf parsley
- 1 cup water
- ¾ cup soy milk
- ¼ cup freshly squeezed orange or lemon juice
- 2 handfuls (about 1½ cups) fresh spinach leaves, washed and patted dry

Place all of the ingredients in a blender and process until smooth. Adjust the consistency with additional water. Serve it over ice or as is.

Alternative Preparation Method: Add half of a banana to the blender if desired and reduce the serving size to 4 to 5 ounces or just over ½ cup.

SuperNutrient Booster
Blue—No Cook

"It's Good to be Blue" Bevvy

One taste of this drink and you'll be singing the blues for all the right reasons!

Servings: 4

Serving size: ½ cup

Volume: 2 cups

Prep Time: 3 minutes

Total Time: 3 minutes

1½ cups fresh or frozen blueberries (if frozen, do not thaw)

¾ cup soy milk

¼ cup nonfat plain yogurt

1 teaspoon freshly squeezed lemon juice

1 teaspoon honey

4 ice cubes

Place all of the ingredients in a blender and process until smooth. Adjust the consistency with cold water.

Note: Recipe can easily be doubled or tripled. Store unused portions in the refrigerator with a tight-fitting lid. Shake vigorously before serving and use within 3 days.

SuperNutrient Booster Orange—Cooked

Carrot Charger

Need a bit of an energy boost? Here's your solution!

Servings: 5

Serving Size: 2-ounce "shooter"—use a sake cup or shot glass!

Volume: 1¼ cups

Prep Time: 5 minutes

Cook Time: 15 minutes

Total Time: 20 minutes

    6 medium carrots, peeled and sliced
    ½ orange bell pepper, seeded and sliced
    1 cup water
    ½ cup fresh apple cider
    1 tablespoon honey
    ½ teaspoon freshly grated ginger
    ¼ teaspoon ground nutmeg

In a small saucepan, place the carrots, bell pepper, and water over medium-high heat. Cover and cook for 15 minutes. Remove the pan from the heat, but do not drain the water. Uncover the pan and allow the mixture to cool. Transfer the carrot mixture and remaining ingredients to a blender. Process until it's smooth. Adjust the consistency with cold water or ice cubes.

Note: Recipe can easily be doubled or tripled. Store the unused portions in the refrigerator in a container with a tight-fitting lid. Shake vigorously before serving and use within 3 days.

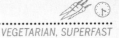

SuperNutrient Booster Yogurt & Fruit Smoothie

Perfect for those mornings when you feel like something a bit more substantial than your RED. The sweetness comes only from the fruit here!

Servings: 1

Serving size: 5 ounces or just over ½ cup

Volume: 5 ounces or just over ½ cup

Prep Time: 5 minutes

Total Time: 5 minutes

¼ cup nonfat, plain yogurt

⅓ cup sliced fruit (strawberries, cherries, watermelon, strawberry guava, papaya)

2 ice cubes

Blend all of the ingredients in a food processor or blender until smooth. Adjust the thickness with water. Serve immediately.

Additional SuperFoodsRx recipe alternatives to your RED, GREEN, BLUE and ORANGE SuperNutrient Boosters:

- **SuperFoodsRx Spicy Vegetable Soup**—Option #3 (see recipe *page 286*)

    Serving size for SuperNutrient Booster: 1 cup

- **Sweet Potato Soup** (see recipe *page 289*)

    Serving size for SuperNutrient Booster: ½ to ¾ cup

Superfoods on the Table *Super Fast*

15-Minute SuperFast ⏱
SuperFoods Recipes

Protein Salads—Make it a habit to pre-chop servings of raw vegetables and refrigerate. Dinner simply becomes a matter of arranging the salad. Pair any of our 14 salad options (see page 234) with 3 ounces of leftover grilled, roasted, or baked turkey or skinless chicken breast, or salmon to make yourself an entrée salad. The meat can be chopped or sliced and arranged attractively on the plate. Pair with a serving of homemade vinaigrette (see page 307).

SuperFast SuperFoodsRx Entrée Recipes:

- Asian Inspired Broccoli Salad
- Bean and Veggie Burrito
- Broccoli & White Beans with Crushed Red Pepper
- Broiled Salmon
- Chicken Salad with Thyme, Walnuts & Grapes
- Cold Vegetable Tortillas
- Confetti Salad
- Fresh and Light Tacos
- Great Northern Shrimp Salad
- Greek Salad Roll-Ups
- Grilled Salmon with Yogurt Dill Drizzle
- Grown-Up Peanut Butter Sandwiches
- Hummus and Roasted Pepper Sandwich
- Layered Turkey (or Chicken) Salad
- Marvelous Mediterranean Salad
- Pear, Feta, and Pecan Stuffed Pita
- Peanut Glazed Shrimp (if you marinate in advance)
- Poached Salmon in Spinach Tortillas

- Salmon Taco with Mango & Avocado
- Stuffed Tuna Salad Tomatoes
- SuperFoodsRx Turkey Spinach Pita
- SuperFoodsRx Salads
- Thanksgiving Open-Faced Sandwich
- Thin Crust Turkey Pita Pizza
- Tofu "Eggless" Salad Sandwiches
- Tofu Stir Fry (freeze tofu in advance)
- Vegetarian Bean Chili (can)—5-minute meal
- Don't forget soups—once made, they're a snap to reheat out of the refrigerator!

SuperFast Breakfasts—*You can also have Breakfast for Lunch or Dinner*

Add a side from column D of the "Trades" table on page 208 to turn any of the following into a healthy and nutritious, complete lunch or dinner.

- Egg Frittata with Cherry Tomatoes, Spinach & Cheese
- "Eggsellent" Spinach, Mushroom & Onion Scramble
- Fruit Delight Smoothie
- Pumpkin "Julius" Smoothie

Other SuperFast SuperFoodsRx Recipes:

- All Season Fruit Salad
- Almond Green Beans
- Asian Inspired Red Pepper Sesame Dressing
- Baked Apples
- Black Bean & Mango Salsa

- Blueberry Compote Crumble
- Broccoli and Cauliflower Salad
- Citrus Apricot Couscous
- Corn Salsa
- Chocolate Tofu Mousse
- Creamy Spinach Dip
- Crunchy Coleslaw
- Fresh Blueberry Compote
- Garlic Lover's Dip (and Sandwich Spread)
- Ginger Orange Dressing
- Grilled Fruit Kabobs
- Great Northern Bean Dip
- Honey Ginger Carrots
- Honey Mustard Dressing
- Modern Ambrosia for One
- Roasted Broccoli
- Salsa Bean Dip
- Smoked Salmon Spread
- Steamed Carrots with Dill
- SuperFoodsRx SuperNutrient Boosters
- SuperFoodsRx "Vinaigrette" Dressings
- Tangy Tomato Dressing
- Tofu Herb Dressing
- Watermelon & Jalapeño Salsa
- Year Round Salsa
- Yogurt Banana Strawberry Spread

Select SuperFoodsRx Diet–Friendly Brand Name Shopping List

Sodium Alert—Be especially aware of sodium when you shop for these foods in your supermarket:

- Snack foods: especially crackers, chips, and nuts
- Soups
- Frozen meals
- Beans
- Pasta sauces
- Sauces
- Dips
- Salad Dressings
- Marinades
- Seasonings

To Get You Started

Here are some SuperFoodsRx Diet–friendly brand name items of special interest to guide you as you shop smart.*

In addition to lots of fresh whole foods, here are some of the foods that you might be looking for in order to round out your *SuperFoodsRx Diet*. There are lots of options available to you today. I'm giving you just a few to get the ball

*Because name brand foods, packaging, and ingredients change frequently, be sure to examine the package at the store for accurate nutritional information. These guidelines and throughout the SuperFoodsRx Diet should help guide you to the best choices regardless of brand.

rolling—look for these or similar items that fit the guidelines and your personal tastes.

Low-Sodium Tomato Products

Pasta Sauce
- ☐ Vons O® Organic Mushroom Pasta Sauce, Tomato Basil Pasta Sauce
- ☐ Francis Coppola® Mammarella Organic Arrabbiata, Organic Pomodoro Basilico
- ☐ Classico® Organic Tomato Herbs & Spices
- ☐ Safeway Select Mushroom & Onion Pasta Sauce
- ☐ Safeway Select Red Bell Pepper

Tomatoes
- ☐ Del Monte® Diced Tomatoes No Salt Added
- ☐ Eden® Organic Crushed Tomatoes No Salt Added
- ☐ Vons O® Organics Tomato Paste
- ☐ Contadina® Tomato Paste
- ☐ Contadina® Crushed Tomatoes with Roasted Garlic
- ☐ Progresso® Tomato Puree
- ☐ Hunt's® Organic Diced Tomatoes
- ☐ Safeway Crushed Tomatoes in Puree

Salsa
Look for:
- • About 10–15 calories per 2 tablespoons and <200 mg sodium
- ☐ Safeway Select Brand Salsas (various flavors and heat)
- ☐ Desert Pepper Trading Company® Peach Mango Salsa
- ☐ Santa Fe Packing Co.® (various flavors and heat)

Low-Sodium Canned Soups

Look for (per 1 cup serving—most cans are considered 2 cups):
- • SuperFoods—it's easy in soups!

- **Best:** No added salt varieties OR Less than 350 milligrams of sodium per cup, 8 ounces.
  - **OK:** No more than 480 milligrams sodium.
  - Avoid the cream or high total, or saturated fats (>2 g), per serving.
- ☐ Health Valley® No Salt Added Line: Organic Black Bean, Organic Vegetable, Organic Minestrone, Organic Potato Leek, Organic Tomato
- ☐ Health Valley® Fat Free Minestrone, 14 Garden Vegetable
- ☐ Amy's® Organic Soups Light in Sodium: Butternut Squash, Tomato Bisque, Chunky Tomato Bisque, Minestrone, Lentil Vegetable, Lentil, Split Pea, Spicy Chili, Medium Chili
- ☐ Walnut Acres® Organic Split Pea Soup
- ☐ Progresso® 50% Less Sodium Garden Vegetable, Chicken Noodle
- ☐ Healthy Choice® Chicken Tortilla Soup, Garden Vegetable
- ☐ Campbell's® Select Healthy Request Savory Chicken and Long Grain Rice, Mexican Style Chicken Tortilla
- ☐ Campbell's® Chunky Healthy Request Vegetable
- ☐ Healthy Choice® Old Fashioned Chicken Noodle, Chicken with Rice, Healthy Choice Country Vegetable

Low-Sodium Canned Beans

Look for per ½ cup serving:

- You can find canned beans with 35 milligrams or less per serving— seek them out!
- Aim for less than 150 mg per sodium per ½ cup (maximum 220 mg)
- Always drain and rinse your beans—especially if sodium is higher.
- ☐ Eden Foods® Organic Aduki, Black, Black Eyed, Black Soybeans, Butter, Cannellini, Great Northern, Kidney, Navy, Pinto, Small Red
- ☐ Goya® Low Sodium black, pinto, kidney, pink beans and garbanzo
- ☐ Trader Joe's Cannellini Beans

- ☐ Vons O® Organic Black Beans, Garbanzo Beans
- ☐ Amy's® Organic Soups Light in Sodium: Refried Black Beans, Refried Traditional Beans

Grains—Pasta, Tortillas, Bread

Look for:

- Whole grain—'whole' is first on the ingredients
- 2 or more grams fiber per serving
- Low sodium varieties

Pasta

- ☐ Ronzoni® Healthy Harvest Whole Wheat Blend Pasta Spaghetti Style
- ☐ Barilla® Plus Thin Spaghetti
- ☐ Vons O® Organics Whole Wheat Spaghetti
- ☐ Vons O® Organics Penne Rigate
- ☐ Nature's Path Organic Whole Grain & Flax+ Penne, 14-Ounce Bags

Tortillas/Tacos

- ☐ Mission® White Corn Taco Shells (small)
- ☐ Vons® White Corn Taco Shells (small)
- ☐ Vons® Jumbo Taco Shells
- ☐ Santa Fe Tortilla Company® Carb Chopper Wheat Tortillas
- ☐ Mission® Soft White Corn Tortillas
- ☐ Mission® Yellow Corn Tortillas
- ☐ La Tortilla Factory® Whole Wheat Low-Carb/Low-Fat Tortillas Large Size
- ☐ La Tortilla Factory® Whole Wheat Low-Carb/Low-Fat Tortillas Original Flavor

Bread

Look for:

- 80–100 calories per slice

- ☐ Ezekiel 4:9®—7 Sprouted Grains, Sesame, Cinnamon Raisin
- ☐ Milton's® Healthy Whole Grain Plus
- ☐ O Organics® Whole Wheat
- ☐ Eating Right™ Reduced Sodium Whole What Cracked Oat Bread
- ☐ Oroweat®—Whole Wheat & Honey, 12 Grain, Honey Fiber Whole Grain
- ☐ Sara Lee® Mr. Pita 100% Whole Wheat

Cereal/Oats

Cold Cereal

Look for:

- 4 or more grams fiber per serving (8 or more is better)
- Maximum 10 grams sugar
- Whole grains
- According to Nutrient Facts on box: ¾ cup serving not more than 150 calories; 1 cup serving not more than 190 calories

- ☐ Kashi® GOLEAN®
- ☐ Nutritious Living Hi-Lo™
- ☐ Nature's Path® Optimum PowerFlax®—Soy-Blueberry
- ☐ Cascadian Farm® Great Measure
- ☐ Cascadian Farm® Raisin Bran
- ☐ Barbara's® Multigrain Shredded Spoonfuls
- ☐ Cheerios®
- ☐ Post® Shredded Wheat
- ☐ Post® Shredded Wheat Biscuits
- ☐ Cascadian Farm® Organic Clifford Crunch
- ☐ Uncle Sam® with Mixed Berries

Oatmeal and Instant Hot Cereal

- ☐ McCann's® Instant Irish Oatmeal—regular
- ☐ Mother's® 100% Natural Rolled Oats

- ☐ Old Fashioned Quaker® Oats 100% Whole Grain
- ☐ Kashi® GOLEAN® Hearty All Natural Instant Hot Cereal—Truly Vanilla, Honey & Cinnamon
- ☐ Kashi® Heart to Heart™ Instant Oatmeal—Apple Cinnamon, Raisin Spice, Golden Brown Maple
- ☐ Quaker® Instant Oatmeal—Regular Flavor
- ☐ Quaker® Simple Harvest All Natural Instant Multigrain Hot Cereal Oat Wheat Barley
- ☐ Uncle Sam® Instant Oatmeal

Crackers

Look for:

- Whole grain—'whole' is first on the ingredients
- 2 or more grams fiber per serving
- Low sodium varieties

- ☐ AkMak® 100% Whole Wheat Stone Ground Sesame Cracker
- ☐ Hain Pure Foods® Wheatettes
- ☐ Wasa® Oats Crispbread, Hearty Crispbread, Light Rye, Fiber Crispbread, Crisp'n Light 7 Grain
- ☐ Kavli®—All Natural Whole Grain Crispbread, Hearty Thick Crispbread
- ☐ RyKrisp
- ☐ Ryvita®—Dark Rye, Light Rye, Sesame Rye, Rye & Oat Bran
- ☐ Milton's® All Natural Whole Wheat Baked Crackers
- ☐ Health Valley® Whole Wheat Crackers
- ☐ Nabisco® Triscuit Low Sodium, Reduced Fat

SuperNutrient Boosters (Commercial Options)

Look for:

- 50–80 calories per 8 ounces
- 2 or more SuperFoods (minimum 2–3 vegetables/fruits combined)

- Low sodium varieties
- ☐ R.W. Knudsen Family™ Very Veggie® Low Sodium Vegetable Cocktail
- ☐ V8® Low Sodium Vegetable Juice
- ☐ Trader Joe's Garden Medley Low Sodium
- ☐ Evolution™ Essential Greens
- ☐ Evolution™ Organic V
- ☐ Evolution™ Carrot Celery Beet

Salad Dressings

Look for:

- 40–60 calories in 2 tablespoons dressing
- Natural ingredients
- Watch the sodium and dilute with water, vinegar or juice
- ☐ Annie's Naturals® Raspberry Vinaigrette Low Fat-Low Sodium
- ☐ Consorzio® Raspberry & Balsamic Fat-Free Dressing
- ☐ Annie's Naturals® Low-Fat Gingerly Vinaigrette
- ☐ Annie's Naturals® Goddess Dressing (90 calories—dilute)
- ☐ Spectrum Naturals® *Nonfat* and *Low Fat* Dressings—Creamy Dill, Creamy Garlic, Honey Dijon, Porcini Mushroom Vinaigrette, Provencal Garlic Lover's, Sweet Onion & Garlic, Sweet Onion & Garlic, Toasted Sesame, Zesty Italian
- ☐ Newman's Own® Light Italian Dressing
- ☐ Newman's Own® Light Raspberry & Walnut Vinaigrette (70 calories—dilute)
- ☐ Newman's Own® Light Balsamic Vinaigrette (higher sodium—use 1 tablespoon dressing and dilute)
- ☐ Ken's® Steakhouse Lite Olive Oil Vinaigrette
- ☐ Vons O® Organic Light Balsamic Dressing
- ☐ Maple Grove Farms® Fat Free Balsamic Vinaigrette

Canned and Vacuum-Packed Fish and Chicken

Look for:

- 3 ounce containers (for convenience at work and travel) as well as larger sizes
- Options that are plain packed in water, or low calorie natural sauce
- For salmon: make sure it's wild salmon
- For tuna: look for chunk light plain or packed in water
- For chicken: look for plain or packed in water

☐ Chicken of the Sea® Skinless Boneless Pink Salmon in Water (3 ounce tuna cups, 3 pack)

☐ Bumble Bee® Premium Wild Pink Salmon (pouch and cans)

☐ Chicken of the Sea® Premium Smoked Alaskan Pacific Salmon Wild Caught (pouch)

☐ Deming's® Red Sockeye Wild Alaska Salmon (can)

☐ Safeway™ Alaska Pink Salmon Wild Caught (can)

☐ Hormel® Premium Chunk Breast of Chicken in Water 98% Fat Free

☐ Hormel® Chicken in Water

☐ Starkist® Chunk Light Tuna in water (pouch)

☐ Starkist® Low Sodium Chunk Light Tuna in water (can)

☐ Bumble Bee® Premium Light Tuna in Water (3 ounce pouch)

☐ Bumble Bee® Chunk Light Tuna in Water—Plain and "Touch of Lemon" ™ (3 ounce cans and additional sized)

☐ Chicken of the Sea® Premium Chunk Light Tuna in water (3 ounce cans, 2 pack)

☐ Valley Fresh® Premium Chunk White Chicken (pouch)

☐ Valley Fresh® Premium Chunk White Chicken in water (3 ounce cans)

☐ Yankee Clipper® Sardines in Tomato Sauce, Mustard Sauce, Lemon Sauce

☐ Yankee Clipper® Sardines in Mustard Sauce

☐ Snow's® Minced Clams in Clam Juice

Energy Bars

Look for:

- 120–150 calories per bar (preferred)
- *Less than:* 15 grams sugar, 150 mg sodium, 35% fat
- Try for 2 grams fiber or more per bar (some have only 1 gram and are OK if other criteria are met)
- Whole grains, real ingredients—aim for especially the SuperFoods

☐ Kashi® TLC: Trail Mix, Honey Almond Flax, Peanut Peanut Butter, Cherry Dark Chocolate

☐ Cascadian Farm® Organic Chewy Granola Bars: Fruit & Nut, Harvest Berry, Multi Grain, Chocolate Chip

☐ Clif® Z Bars for Kids (assorted)—Peanut Butter (preferred), Chocolate Chip, Chocolate Brownie

☐ Luna® Tea Cakes: Berry Pomegranate, Vanilla Macadamia, Orange Blossom

☐ SOYJOY™ Bars: Raisin Almond, Apple, Berry, Mango Coconut

Tea

Green

☐ Choice® Organic Teas

☐ Yogi Tea® Green

☐ Mighty Leaf® Organic Green Teas: Tropical Green, Hojicha

☐ Numi® Organic Green Tea

☐ Salada® 100% Green Tea

☐ Good Earth® Green Tea Blend with Lemongrass

☐ Bigelow® Green Tea: plain, peach, mint, lemon, variety pack

☐ Stash® Chai Green, Premium Green

☐ Tazo® China Green Tips, Zen

☐ Lipton® Green

☐ Twinings® Green

☐ Celestial Seasonings® Green: Authentic, Honey Lemon Ginseng,

Blueberry Breeze, Raspberry Gardens, Antioxidant Green, Decaf Mint Green, Decaf Mandarin Orchard Green

Black (various)

- ☐ Choice® Organic
- ☐ Yogi Tea®
- ☐ Numi® Organic
- ☐ Stash®
- ☐ Tazo®
- ☐ Celestial Seasonings®
- ☐ Twinings®
- ☐ Lipton®
- ☐ Bigelow®
- ☐ Red Rose®

Soymilk

Look for:

- No more than 10 grams of sugar per serving; ≤ 7 is better.
- The unsweetened varieties also. They are lightly sweet and tasty with less sugar and more protein for equal volume.

- ☐ Silk®
- ☐ Soy Dream®
- ☐ West Soy®
- ☐ VitaSoy®
- ☐ Organic Eden Soy®
- ☐ Pacific Soy®
- ☐ Trader Joe's

Seasonings

Look for:

- Sodium: <150 mg, preferably none.
- Watch out for occasional corn syrup solids or MSG

☐ The Spice Hunter® Salt Free Italian Seasoning 100% Organic, Salt Free Herbs de Provence 100% Organic, Salt Free Barbecue Grill Spice, Red Pepper (Ground Cayenne) 100% Organic, Arrowroot (ground)

☐ Lizzie's Kitchen® Herbes de Provence, Garden Vegetable

☐ Spice Islands® Salt Free Seasoning Citrus Herb, Mediterranean Seasoning, Fines Herbs, Garlic Herb Blend, Rosemary Garlic Blend

☐ McCormick® Salt Free All Purpose, Salt Free It's A Dilly®

☐ Mrs. Dash®—Any of the 9 Seasoning Blends or 4 Grilling Blends

☐ Various others: cinnamon, pumpkin pie spice, oregano, thyme, turmeric, garlic, cumin, parsley, sage, rosemary, mint, mustard, cayenne (ground red pepper), dill, orange peel, etc.

☐ Almond extract, pure vanilla extract

Your SuperFoodsRx Diet Shopping List

SuperFoods Category 1

- Pumpkin
- Oats (whole grains)
- Walnuts (nuts, seeds, nut butters)
- Ground flaxseed, wheat germ
- Tea–green and black

SuperFoods Category 2

- Beans
- Salmon (chunk light tuna)
- Soy (tofu, soymilk, beans)
- Turkey (chicken)
- Yogurt

SuperFoods Category 3

- Blueberries
- Broccoli
- Oranges
- Spinach
- Tomatoes

Vegetables (choose ≥4) fresh and frozen

- Artichokes+
- Asparagus+
- Avocado+
- Beans (green or string)*
- Beets
- Bell peppers–orange*, red, green
- Bok choy*
- Broccoli*
- Brussels sprouts*
- Butternut squash*
- Cabbage*
- Carrots*
- Cauliflower*
- Celery
- Cucumber
- Greens—kale, mustard, turnip, Swiss chard*
- Jicama
- Kale*
- Leeks+
- Mushrooms
- Onions, scallions, shallots+
- Peas (green or snap)
- Potatoes
- Pumpkin*
- Radishes

- Romaine lettuce*
- Spinach*
- Squash
- Sweet potatoes/yams*
- Tomatoes*
- Turnips

Fruit (choose ≥4) fresh and frozen

- Apples+
- Apricots
- Bananas
- Blueberries*
- Boysenberries*
- Cantaloupe
- Cherries*
- Grapefruit*
- Grapes (purple or green)*
- Guava+
- Honeydew
- Kiwi+
- Lemon*
- Mandarin oranges*
- Mango
- Oranges*
- Papaya*
- Peaches
- Pears+
- Japanese persimmons*
- Pineapple+
- Pomegranate+
- Raisins+
- Raspberries*
- Strawberries*
- Tangerines*
- Dried fruits—blueberries, raisins, apricots, cranberries, dates, figs, cherries, currants+

Protein Foods and Nuts

- Black beans*
- Garbanzo beans*
- Kidney beans*
- Lentils*
- Pinto beans*
- Soybeans (edamame)*
- Beans other: _____
- Turkey*
- Chicken*
- Salmon*
- Chunk light tuna*
- Shrimp
- Other fish: _____
- Tofu*
- Tempeh*
- Veggie burgers

* SuperFood or Sidekick
+ Newer SuperFood or Sidekick

GRAINS ("WHOLE")	FATS/NUTS/ CONDIMENTS	DAIRY/CALCIUM
• Bread	• Nuts (any variety—no or low sodium)	• Soy milk (enriched)
• Cereal	• Seeds—sesame, sunflower, pumpkin	• 1% milk
• Couscous*	• Natural peanut butter*	• Rice milk (enriched)
• Brown rice*	• Almond butter (other nut butters)*	• Yogurt (low fat or nonfat)*
• Corn*	• Extra virgin olive oil*	• Cottage cheese
• Dinner rolls	• Organic canola oil*	• Low-fat cheese
	• Butter	• Snack-sized cheese
• Grains: barley, rye, millet, bulgur wheat, amaranth, quinoa, kamut, spelt, triticale*	• Salad dressing—SuperFoodsRx–approved varieties	MISCELLANEOUS/ PANTRY
• Pasta	• Butter	• Whole wheat flour
• Pita	• Trans-free spread	• Honey+
• Whole grain crackers	• Mustard	• Organic cane sugar
• Baked tortilla chips	• Vinegar (balsamic and variety)	• Low sodium soups
• Tortillas	• _____	• Healthy snacks
• Lite popcorn/yellow	• _____	• Beverages—tea, water, soda water, coffee
• Corn tortillas	• _____	• Tea—green or black
• Ground flaxseed	• _____	• Dark chocolate+
• Wheat germ	• _____	• Organic cocoa
• _____	• _____	• Salt-free seasonings
• _____	• _____	• _____
	• _____	• _____
	• _____	• _____

SuperFood or Sidekick
+ Newer SuperFood or Sidekick

SuperFoodsRx Diet Shopping List Planning Guide

In planning your week ahead, list any meals and specific recipes or additional items you will need.

Other Fresh: _____   *Other Fridge:* _____
_____   _____
_____   _____
_____   _____
_____   _____

Other Frozen: _____   *Other Pantry:* _____
_____   _____
_____   _____
_____   _____
_____   _____

Meal/Recipe: _____   *Meal/Recipe:* _____
Ingredients: *Ingredients:*

Meal/Recipe: _____   *Meal/Recipe:* _____
Ingredients: *Ingredients:*

Meal/Recipe: _____   *Meal/Recipe:* _____
Ingredients: *Ingredients:*

References

Introduction

1. Michels KB & Wolk A. (2002) A prospective study of variety of healthy foods and mortality in women. *International Journal of Epidemiology*, 31(4), 847-854.

2. Cox DJ, Kovatchev BP, Gonder-Frederick LA, Summers KH, McCall A, Grimm KJ & Clark WL. (2005). Relationships between hyperglycemia and cognitive performance among adults with type 1 and type 2 diabetes. *Diabetes Care*, 28(1), 71-77.

3. Levine M, Conry-Cantilena C, Wang Y, Welch RW, Washko PW, Dhariwal KR, Park JB, Lazarev A, Graumlich JF, King J, & Canitlena LR. (1996). Vitamin C pharmacokinetics in healthy volunteers: evidence for a recommended dietary allowance. *Proceedings of the National Academy of Sciences USA*, 93(8), 3704-3709.

CHAPTER 1: SuperNutrients for Super Weight Loss

1. Canene-Adams K, Lindshield BL, Wang S, Jeffery EH, Clinton SK & Erdman JW Jr. (2007). Combinations of tomato and broccoli enhance antitumor activity in dunning r3327-h prostate adenocarcinomas. *Cancer Research*, 67(2), 836-843.

2. St-Onge MP. Dietary fats, teas, dairy, and nuts: potential functional foods for weight control? (2005). *American Journal of Clinical Nutrition*, 81(1), 7-15.

3. Block G. (2004). Foods contributing to energy intake in the US: data from NHANES III and NHANES 1999–2000. *Journal of Food Composition and Analysis*, 17(3-4), 439-447.

Nearly one-third of the calories in the US diet come from junk food, researcher finds. *UC Berkeley News* (June 2004). Retrieved June 20, 2007 from http://www.berkeley.edu/news/media/releases/2004/06/01_usdiet.shtml

4. Anderson RA & Polansky MM. (2002). Tea enhances insulin activity. *Journal of Agricultural and Food Chemistry*, 50(24), 7182-7186.

5. Cooper R, Morre DJ & Morre DM. (2005). Medicinal benefits of green tea: Part I. Review of non-cancer health benefits. *Journal of Alternative and Complementary Medicine*, 11(3), 521-528.

6. Shixian Q, VanCrey B, Shi J, Kakuda Y & Jiang Y. (2006). Green tea extract thermogenesis-induced weight loss by epigallocatechin gallate inhibition of catechol-O-methyltransferase. *Journal of Medicinal Food*, 9(4), 451-458.

7. Rumpler W, Seale J, Clevidence B, Judd J, Wiley E, Yamamoto S, Komatsu T, Sawaki T, Ishikura Y & Hosoda K. (2001). Oolong tea increases metabolic rate and fat oxidation in men. *Journal of Nutrition*, 131(11), 2848-2852.

8. Westerterp-Plantenga MS, Lejeune MP, & Kovacs EM. (2005) Body weight loss and weight maintenance in relation to habitual caffeine intake and green tea supplementation. *Obesity Research*, 13(7), 1195-1204.

Rumpler W, Seale J, Clevidence B, Judd J, Wiley E, Yamamoto S, Komatsu T, Sawaki T, Ishikura Y & Hosoda K. (2001). Oolong tea increases metabolic rate and fat oxidation in men. *Journal of Nutrition*, 131(11), 2848-2852.

9. Dulloo AG, Duret C, Rohrer D, Girardier L, Mensi N, Fathi M, Chantre P & Vandermander J. (1999). Efficacy of a green tea extract rich in catechin polyphenols and caffeine in increasing 24-h energy expenditure and fat oxidation in humans. *American Journal of Clinical Nutrition*, 70(6), 1040-1045.

Dulloo AG, Seydoux J, Girardier L, Chantre P & Vandermander J. (2000). Green tea and thermogenesis: interactions between catechin-polyphenols, caffeine and sympathetic activity. *International Journal of Obesity and Related Metabolic Disorders*, 24(2), 252-258.

Kao YH, Hiipakka RA & Liao S. (2000). Modulation of endocrine systems and food intake by green tea epigallocatechin gallate. *Endocrinology*, 141(3), 980-987.

Kao YH, Hiipakka RA & Liao S. (2000). Modulation of obesity by a green tea catechine. *American Journal of Clinical Nutrition*, 72(5), 1232-1234.

Murase T, Nagasawa A, Suzuki J, Hase T & Tokimitsu I. (2002). Beneficial effects of tea catechins on diet-induced obesity: stimulation of lipid catabolism in the liver. *International Journal of Obesity and Related Metabolic Disorders*, 26(11), 1459-1464.

10. Anderson RA & Polansky MM. (2002). Tea enhances insulin activity. *Journal of Agricultural and Food Chemistry*, 50(24), 7182-7186.

11. Rumpler W, Seale J, Clevidence B, Judd J, Wiley E, Yamamoto S, Komatsu T, Sawaki T, Ishikura Y & Hosoda K. (2001) Oolong tea increases metabolic rate and fat oxidation in men. *Journal of Nutrition*, 131(11), 2848-2852.

Murase T, Nagasawa A, Suzuki J, Hase T & Tokimitsu I. (2002). Beneficial effects of tea catechins on diet-induced obesity: stimulation of lipid catabolism in the liver. *International Journal of Obesity and Related Metabolic Disorders*, 26(11), 1459-1464.

12. Han LK, Takaku T, Li J, Kimura Y & Okuda H. (1999). Anti-obesity action of oolong tea. *International Journal of Obesity and Related Metabolic Disorders*, 23(1), 98-105.

13. du Toit R, Volsteedt Y & Apostolides Z. (2001) Comparison of the antioxidant content of fruits, vegetables and teas measured as vitamin C equivalents. *Toxicology*, 166(1-2), 63-69.

14. Canoy D, Wareham N, Welch A, Bingham S, Luben R, Day N & Khaw KT. (2005). Plasma ascorbic acid concentrations and fat distribution in 19,068 British men and women in the European Prospective Investigation into Cancer and Nutrition Norfolk cohort study. *American Journal of Clinical Nutrition*, 82(6), 1203-1209.

15. Johnston CS (2005). Strategies for healthy weight loss: from vitamin C to the glycemic response. *Journal of the American College of Nutrition*, 24(3), 158-165.

16. Naylor GJ, Grant L & Smith C. (1985). A double blind placebo controlled trial of ascorbic acid in obesity. *Nutrition and Health*, 4(1), 25-28.

17. Hun CS, Hasegawa K, Kawabata T, Kato M, Shimokawa T & Kagawa Y. (1999). Increased uncoupling protein2 mRNA in white adipose tissue, and decrease in leptin, visceral fat, blood glucose, and cholesterol in KK-Ay mice fed with eicosapentaenoic and docosahexaenoic acids in addition to linolenic acid. *Biochemical and Biophysical Research Communication*, 259(1), 85-90.

18. Huang XF, Xin X, McLennan P & Storlien L. (2004). Role of fat amount and type in ameliorating diet-induced obesity: insights at the level of hypothalamic arcuate nucleus leptin receptor, neuropeptide Y and pro-opiomelanocortin mRNA expression. *Diabetes, Obesity & Metabolism*, 6(1), 35-44.

19. Wang H, Storlien LH & Huang XF. (2002). Effects of dietary fat types on body fatness, leptin, and ARC leptin receptor, NPY, and AgRP mRNA expression. *American Journal of Physiology, Endocrinology and Metabolism*, 282(6), E1352-E1359.

20. Hill, AM, Buckley, JD, Murphy KJ & Howe, PRC. (2007). Combining fish-oil supplements with regular aerobic exercise improves body composition and cardiovascular disease risk factors. *American Journal of Clinical Nutrition*, 85(5), 1267-1274.

21. Heaney RP (2003). Normalizing calcium intake: projected population effects for body weight. *Journal of Nutrition*, 133(1), 268S-270S.

22. Lin YC, Lyle RM, McCabe LD, McCabe GP, Weaver CM & Teegarden D. (2000). Dairy calcium is related to changes in body composition during a two-year exercise intervention in young women. *Journal of the American College of Nutrition*, 19(6), 754-760.

23. Zemel, MB, Richards J, Mathis S, Milstead A, Gebhardt L & Silva E. (2005). Dairy augmentation of total and central fat loss in obese subjects. *International Journal of Obesity*, 29(4), 391-397.

24. Zemel MB. (2003). Mechanisms of dairy modulation of adiposity. *Journal of Nutrition*, 133(1), 252S-256S.

25. Zemel MB. (2005). The role of dairy foods in weight management. *Journal of the American College of Nutrition*, 24(6 Suppl.), 537S-546S.

26. Shapses SA & Riedt CS. (2006). Bone, body weight, and weight reduction: what are the concerns? *Journal of Nutrition*, 136(6), 1453-1456.

27. Bowen J, Noakes M & Clifton PM. (2004). A high dairy protein, high-calcium diet minimizes bone turnover in overweight adults during weight loss. *Journal of Nutrition*, 134(3), 568-573.

Layman DK & Walker DA. (2006). Potential Importance of Leucine in Treatment of Obesity and the Metabolic Syndrome. *Journal of Nutrition*, 136(1 Suppl), 319S-323S.

28. Megías-Rangil I, García-Lorda P, Torres-Moreno M, Bullo M & Salas-Salvado J. (2004) [Nutrient content and health effects of nuts.] *Archivos Latinoamericanos de Nutrición*, 54(2 Suppl 1), 83-86.

29. Sabaté, J. (1999). Nut consumption, vegetarian diets, ischemic heart disease risk, and all-cause mortality: evidence from epidemiologic studies. *American Journal of Clinical Nutrition*, 70 (3 Suppl), 500S-503S.

30. Sabaté J. (2003). Nut consumption and body weight. *American Journal of Clinical Nutrition*, 78(3 Suppl), 647S-650S.

31. Coates AM & Howe PR. (2007). Edible nuts and metabolic health. *Current Opinion in Lipidology*, 18(1), 25-30.

32. Sabaté J. (2003). Nut consumption and body weight. *American Journal of Clinical Nutrition*, 78(3 Suppl), 647S-650S.

33. Bes-Rastrollo M, Sabaté J, Gómez-Gracia E, Alonso A, Martinez JA & Martínez-González MA. (2007). Nut consumption and weight gain in a Mediterranean cohort: The SUN study. *Obesity* (Silver Spring), 15(1), 107-116.

34. Rajaram S & Sabaté J. (2006). Nuts, body weight and insulin resistance. *British Journal of Nutrition*, 96(Suppl 2), S79-S86.

35. Sacks FM, Lichtenstein, Van Horn L, Harris W, Kris-Etherton P, & Winston M: the American Heart Association Nutrition Committee. (2006). Soy Protein, Isoflavones, and Cardiovascular Health: An American Heart Association Science Advisory for Professionals from the Nutrition Committee. *Circulation*, 113(7), 1034-1044.

Desroches S, Mauger JF, Ausman LM, Lichtenstein AH & Lamarche B. (2004). Soy protein favorably affects LDL size independently of isoflavones in hypercholesterolemic men and women. *Journal of Nutrition*, 134(3), 574-579.

Sagara M, Kanda T, NJelekera M, Teramoto T, Armitage L, Birt N, Birt C, & Yamori Y. (2004). Effects of dietary intake of soy protein and isoflavones on cardiovascular disease risk factors in high risk, middle-aged men in Scotland. *Journal of the American College of Nutrition*, 23(1), 85-91.

36. Trock BJ, Hilakivi-Clark L & Clarke R. (2006). Meta-analysis of soy intake and breast cancer risk. *Journal of the National Cancer Institute*, 98(7), 459-471.

Potter JD & Steinmetz K. (1996). Vegetables, fruit and phytoestrogens as preventive agents. *IARC Scientific Publications*, 139, 61-90.

37. Zhang X, Shu XO, Li H, Yang G, Li O, Gao YT & Zheng W. (2005). Prospective cohort study on soyfood consumption and risk of bone fracture among postmenopausal women. *Archives of Internal Medicine*, 165(16), 1890-1895.

Messina M, Ho S & Alekel DL. (2004). Skeletal benefits of soy isoflavones: a review of the clinical trial and epidemiologic data. *Current Opinion in Clinical Nutrition and Metabolic Care*, 7(6), 649-658.

Lydeking-Olsen E, Beck-Jensen JE, Setchell KD & Holm-Jensen T. (2004). Soymilk or Progesterone for prevention of bone loss —a 2 year randomized, placebo-controlled trial. *European Journal of Nutrition*, 43(4), 246-257

Ho SC, Woo J, Lam S, Chen Y, Sham A & Lau J. (2003). Soy protein consumption and bone mass in early postmenopausal Chinese women. *Osteoporosis International*, 14(10), 835-842.

38. Davis J, Higginbotham A, O'Connor T, Moustaid-Moussa N, Tebbe A, Kim YC, Cho KW, Shay N, Adler S, Peterson R & Banz W. (2007). Soy protein and isoflavones influence adiposity and development of metabolic syndrome in the obese male ZDF rat. *Annals of Nutrition & Metabolism*, 51(1), 42-52.

Azadbakht L, Kimiagar M, Mehrabi Y, Esmaillzadeh A, Padyab M, Hu FB, & Willett WC. (2007). Soy inclusion in the diet improves features of the metabolic syndrome: a randomized crossover study in postmenopausal women. *American Journal of Clinical Nutrition*, 85(3), 735-741.

39. Potter JD & Steinmetz K. (1996). Vegetables, fruit and phytoestrogens as preventive agents. *IARC Scientific Publications*, 139, 61-90.

American Dietetic Association, Dietitians of Canada. (2003). Position of the American Dietetic Association and Dietitians of Canada: Vegetarian Diets. *Journal of the American Dietetic Association*, 103(6), 748-765.

40. Azadbakht L, Kimiagar M, Mehrabi Y, Esmaillzadeh A, Padyab M, Hu FB, & Willett WC. (2007). Soy inclusion in the diet improves features of the metabolic syndrome: a randomized crossover study in postmenopausal women. *American Journal of Clinical Nutrition*, 85(3), 735-741.

41. Grundy SM, Cleeman JI, Daniels SR, Donato KA, Eckel RH, Franklin BA, Gordon DJ, Krauss RM, Savage PJ, Smith SC, Spertus JA & Costa F. (2005). *Diagnosis and Management of the Metabolic Syndrome: An American Heart Association/National Heart, Lung, and Blood Institute* Scientific Statement: Executive Summary. Circulation, 112, e285-e290.

42. Deibert P. (2004). Weight loss without losing muscle mass in pre-obese and obese subjects induced by a high-soy-protein diet. *International Journal of Obesity and Related Metabolic Disorders*, 28(10), 1349-1352.

43. Anderson JW, Luan J & Høie LH. (2004). Structured weight-loss programs: meta-analysis of weight loss at 24 weeks and assessment of effects of intervention intensity. *Advances in Therapy*, 21(2), 61-75.

44. McCarty MF. (1999). Vegan proteins may reduce risk of cancer, obesity, and cardiovascular disease by promoting increased glucagon activity. *Medical Hypotheses*, 53(6), 459-485.

45. Velasquez MT & Bhathena SJ. (2007). Role of dietary soy protein in obesity. *International Journal of Medical Sciences*, 4(2), 72-82.

46. Zhang HM, Chen SW, Zhang LS & Feng XF. (2006). [Effects of soy isoflavone on low-grade inflammation in obese rats] [abstract] *Zhong Nan Da Xue Xue Bao Yi Xue Ban*, 31(3), 336-339.

47. Papanikolaou Y, Fulgoni SA, Fulgoni VL, Kelly RM & Rose SF. (2006). Bean consumption by adults is associated with a more nutrient dense diet and a reduced risk of obesity. Presented at the Federation of the American Societies for Experimental Biology (FASEB) conference in San Francisco, April 2006.

48. Yao M & Roberts SB (2001). Dietary energy density and weight regulation. *Nutrition Reviews*, 59(8 Pt 1), 247-258.

49. Crujeiras AB, Parra D, Abete I & Martínez JA. (2007) A hypocaloric diet enriched in legumes specifically mitigates lipid peroxidation in obese subjects. *Free Radical Research,* 41(4), 498-506.

50. Weigle DS, Breen PA, Matthys CC,Callahan HS, Meeuws KE Burden VR & Purnell JQ. (2005). A high-protein diet induces sustained reductions in appetite, ad libitum caloric intake, and body weight despite compensatory changes in diurnal plasma leptin and ghrelin concentrations. *American Journal of Clinical Nutrition,* 82(1), 41-48

51. Zhang Y, Guo K, Leblanc RE, Loh D, Schwartz GJ & Yu YH. (2007). Increasing dietary leucine intake reduces diet-induced obesity and improves glucose and cholesterol metabolism in mice via multi-mechanisms. *Diabetes,* 56(6), 1647-1654.

52. Sun X & Zemel MB. (2007). Leucine and calcium regulate fat metabolism and energy partitioning in murine adipocytes and muscle cells. *Lipids,* 42(4), 297-305.

53. Nielsen SJ & Popkin BM. (2004). Changes in beverage intake between 1977 and 2001. *American Journal of Preventive Medicine,* 27 (3), 205-210.

54. Bermudez O. (2005). Consumption of sweet drinks among American adults from the NHANES 1999–2000. [Abstract # 839.5]. Presented at the Federation of the American Societies for Experimental Biology (FASEB) conference in San Diego, California, April 2005.

55. Flood JE, Roe LS & Rolls BJ. (2006). The effect of increased beverage portion size on energy intake at a meal. *Journal of the American Dietetic Association,* 106(12), 1984-1990.

56. Rolls BJ, Roe LS & Meengs JS. (2004). Salad and satiety: energy density and portion size of a first-course salad affect energy intake at lunch. *Journal of the American Dietetic Association,* 104(10), 1570-1576.

57. Ello-Martin JA, Roe LS & Ledikwe JH . (2007). Dietary energy density in the treatment of obesity: a year-long trial comparing 2 weight-loss diets. *American Journal of Clinical Nutrition,* 85(6), 1465-1477.

58. Davis JN, Hodges VA & Gillham MB. (2006). Normal-weight adults consume more fiber and fruit than their age- and height-matched overweight/obese counterparts. *Journal of the American Heart Association,* 106(6), 833-840.

59. Ledikwe JH, Blanck HM, Khan LK, Serdula MK, Seymour JD, Tohill BC & Rolls BJ. (2006). Low-energy-density diets are associated with high diet quality in adults in the United States. *Journal of the American Dietetic Association,* 106(8), 1172-1180.

Newby PK. (2006). Examining energy density: comments on diet quality, dietary advice, and the cost of healthful eating. *Journal of the American Dietetic Association,* 106(8), 1166-1169.

60. Davis JN, Hodges VA & Gillham MB. (2006). Normal-weight adults consume more fiber and fruit than their age- and height-matched overweight/obese counterparts. *Journal of the American Heart Association,* 106(6), 833-840.

61. Liu S, Willett WC, Manson JE, Hu FB, Rosner B & Colditz G. (2003). Relation between changes in intakes of dietary fiber and grain products and changes in weight and development of obesity among middle-aged women. *American Journal of Clinical Nutrition,* 78(5), 920-927.

62. Burton-Freeman B, Davis PA & Schneeman BO. (2002). Plasma cholecystokinin is associated with subjective measures of satiety in women. *American Journal of Clinical Nutrition,* 76(3), 659-667.

63. Yao M & Roberts SB. (2001). Dietary energy density and weight regulation, *Nutrition Reviews,* 59(8 Pt 1), 247-258.

64. Bazzano LA, Song Y, Bubes V, Good CK, Mason JE & Liu S. (2005). Dietary intake of whole and refined gran breakfast cereals and weight gain in men. *Obesity Research,* 13(11), 1952-1960.

65. Melanson KJ, Angelopoulos TJ, Nguyen VT, Martini M, Zukley L, Lowndes J, Dube TJ, Fiutem JJ, Yount BW & Rippe JM. (2006). Consumption of whole-grain cereals during weight loss: effects

on dietary quality, dietary fiber, magnesium, vitamin B-6, and obesity. *Journal of the American Dietetic Association*, 106(9), 1380-1388.

CHAPTER 2: Before You Begin . . . .

1. Centers for Disease Control. Retrieved June 1, 2007, from: http://www.cdc.gov

Flegal KM, Carroll MD, Ogden CL & Johnson CL. (2002). Prevalence and trends in obesity among U.S. Adults, 1999-2000. *JAMA*, 288(14), 1723-1727.

Ogden CL, Carroll MD, Curtin LR, McDowell MA, Tabak CJ & Flegal KM. (2006) Prevalence of Overweight and Obesity in the United States, 1999-2004. *JAMA*, 295(13), 1539-1555.

2. Ello-Martin JA, Ledikwe JH & Rolls BJ. (2005). The influence of food portion size and energy density on energy intake: implications for weight management. *American Journal of Clinical Nutrition*, 82(1 Suppl), 236S-241S.

3. Wing RR, Tate DF, Gorin AA, Raynor HA & Fava JL. (2006). A self-regulation program for maintenance of weight loss. *New England Journal of Medicine*, 355 (15), 1563-1571.

4. Mazzali G, Di Francesco V, Zoico, E, Fanitn F, Zamboni G, Benati C, Bambara V, Negri M, Bosello O & Zamboni M. (2006). Interrelations between fat distribution, muscle lipid content, adipocytokines, and insulin resistance: effect of moderate weight loss in older women. *American Journal of Clinical Nutrition*, 84(5), 1193-1199.

Manson JE, Willett WC, Stampfer MJ, Colditz GA, Hunter DJ, Hankinson SE, Hennekens CH & Speizer FE. (1995). Body weight and mortality among women. *New England Journal of Medicine*, 333(11), 677-685

CHAPTER 3: The SuperFoodsRx SlimDown

1. Song WO, Chun OK, Obayashi S, Cho S & Chung CE.. (2005). Is consumption of breakfast associated with body mass index in US adults? *Journal of the American Dietetic Association*, 105(9), 1373-1382.

2. Potter JD & Steinmetz K. (1996). Vegetables, fruit and phytoestrogens as preventive agents. *IARC Scientific Publications*, 139, 61-90.

3. Rolls BJ, Roe LS & Meengs JS. (2004). Salad and satiety: energy density and portion size of a first-course salad affect energy intake at lunch. *Journal of the American Dietetic Association*, 104(10), 1570-1576.

4. Su LJ & Arab L. (2006). Salad and raw vegetable consumption and nutritional status in the adult US population: results from the Third National Health and Nutrition Examination Survey. *Journal of the American Dietetic Association*, 106(9), 1394-1404.

5. Jordan HA, Levitz LS, Utgoff KL & Lee HL. (1981). Role of food characteristics in behavioral change and weight loss. *Journal of the American Dietetic Association*, 79(1), 24-29.

6. Rolls BJ, Roe LS, Beach AM & Kris-Etherton PM. (2005). Provision of foods differing in energy density affects long-term weight loss. *Obesity Research*, 13(6):1052-1060

7. Mattes R. (2005). Soup and satiety. *Physiology & Behavior*, 83(5), 739-747.

8. Liu S, Willett WC, Manson JE, Hu FB, Rosner B & Colditz G. (2003). Relation between changes in intakes of dietary fiber and grain products in weight and development of obesity among middle-aged women. *American Journal of Clinical Nutrition*, 78(5), 920-927.

9. Benton D, Slater O, & Donohoe RT. (2001). The influence of breakfast and a snack on psychological functioning. *Physiology & Behavior*, 74(4-5), 559-571.

10. Streit, KJ, Stevens NH, Stevens VJ & Rossner J. (1991). Food Records: A Predictor and Modifier of Weight Change in a Long-Term Weight Loss Program. *Journal of the American Dietetic Association*, 9(2), 213-216

11. Phelan S, Wyatt HR, Hill JO & Wing RR. (2006). Are the Eating and Exercise Habits of Successful Weight Losers Changing? *Obesity*, 14, 710-716.

Wing RR & Phelan S. (2005). Long-term weight loss maintenance. *American Journal of Clinical Nutrition*, 82(1), 222S-225S.

12. McManus K, Antinoro L & Sacks F. (2001). A randomized controlled trial of a moderate-fat, low-energy diet compared with a low fat, low-energy diet for weight loss in overweight adults. *International Journal of Obesity and Related Metabolic Disorders*, 25(10), 1503-1511.

13. Brunstrom, JM & Mitchell GL. (2006). Effects of distraction on the development of satiety. *British Journal of Nutrition*, 96(4), 761-769.

CHAPTER 4: The SuperFoodsRx Prep and Practice Week

1. Bray GA, Nielsen SJ & Popkin BA. (2004). Consumption of high-fructose corn syrup in beverages may play a role in the epidemic of obesity. *American Journal of Clinical Nutrition*, 79(4), 537-543.

Economic Research Service, United States Department of Agriculture. U.S. Consumption of Caloric Sweeteners, Table 52—High fructose corn syrup: estimated number of per capita calories consumed daily, by calendar year (1970-2005). Retrieved June 1, 2007, from http://www.ers.usda.gov/Briefing/Sugar/data/table52.xls

2. Nielsen SJ & Popkin BM. (2004). Changes in beverage intake between 1977 and 2001. *American Journal of Preventive Medicine*, 27 (3), 205-210.

3. Guthrie JF & Morton JF. (2000). Food sources of added sweeteners in the diets of Americans. *Journal of the American Dietetic Association*, 100(1), 43-51.

U.S. Department of Health and Human Services, U.S. Department of Agriculture. (2005). *Dietary guidelines for Americans, 2005*. Washington (DC): U.S. Department of Health and Human Services, U.S. Department of Agriculture.

4. Block G. (2004). Foods contributing to energy intake in the US: data from NHANES III and NHANES 1999–2000. *Journal of Food Composition and Analysis*, 17(3-4), 439-447.

5. DiMeglio DP & Mattes, RD. (2000). Liquid versus solid carbohydrate: effects on food intake and body weight. *International Journal of Obesity and Related Metabolic Disorders*, 24(6), 794-800.

6. Tucker, KL, Morita K, Qiao, N, Hannan MT, Cupples LA & Kiel DP. (2006). Colas, but not other carbonated beverages, are associated with low bone mineral density in older women: The Framingham Osteoporosis Study. *American Journal of Clinical Nutrition*, 84(4), 936-942.

7. Fowler SP. (2005). *65th Annual Scientific Sessions, American Diabetes Association, San Diego, June 10-14, 2005* [Abstract 1058-P]. University of Texas Health Science Center School of Medicine, San Antonio.

8. Davidson TL & Swithers SE. (2004). A Pavlovian approach to the problem of obesity. *International Journal of Obesity and Related Metabolic Disorders*, 28(7), 933-935.

9. Larsson SC, Bergkvist L & Wolk A (2006). Consumption of sugar and sugar-sweetened foods and the risk of pancreatic cancer in a prospective study. *American Journal of Clinical Nutrition*, 84(5), 1171-1176.

10. Darmon N, Darmon M, Maillot M & Drewnowski A. (2005). A nutrient density standard for vegetables and fruits: nutrients per calorie and nutrients per unit cost. *Journal of the American Dietetic Association*, 105(12), 1881-1887.

11. Sobal J & Wansink B. (2007). Kitchenscapes, tablescapes, platescapes, and foodscapes. *Environment and Behavior*, 39(1), 124-142.

12. Hetherington MM. (2007). Cues to overeat: psychological factors influencing overconsumption. Symposium on 'Molecular mechanisms and psychology of food intake.' *Proceedings of the Nutrition Society*, 66(1), 113-123.

13. Wansink B, van Ittersum K & Painter JE. (2006). Ice cream illusions bowls, spoons, and self-served portion sizes. *American Journal of Preventive Medicine*, 31(3), 240-243.

14. Popkin BM, Armstrong LE, Bray GM, Caballero B, Frei B & Willett WC. (2006). A new proposed guidance system for beverage consumption in the United States. *American Journal of Clinical Nutrition*, 83(3), 529-542.

15. Nielsen SJ & Popkin BM. (2004). Changes in beverage intake between 1977 and 2001. *American Journal of Preventive Medicine*, 27(3), 205-210.

16. Guthrie JF & Morton JF. (2000). Food sources of added sweeteners in the diets of Americans. *Journal of the American Dietetic Association*, 100(1), 43-51.

U.S. Department of Health and Human Services, U.S. Department of Agriculture. (2005). *Dietary guidelines for Americans, 2005*. Washington (DC): U.S. Department of Health and Human Services, U.S. Department of Agriculture.

17. Stookey J. (2006). Children's Hospital & Research Institute Oakland. Retrieved June 20, 2007, from http://www.childrenshospitaloakland.org/about/press_releases/Waterweightloss.asp Presented at Annual meeting of the Obesity Society Oct 24, 2006.

18. Sawka MN, Burke LM, Elchner ER, Maughan RJ, Montain SJ & Stachenfeld NS. (2007). American College of Sports Medicine position stand: Exercise and Fluid Replacement. *Medicine & Science in Sports & Exercise*, 39(2): 377-390.

Panel on Dietary Reference Intakes for Electrolytes and Water, Standing Committee on the Scientific Evaluation of Dietary Reference Intakes. (2004). The National Academies, Food and Nutrition Board. (2004). Dietary Reference Intakes for Water, Potassium, Sodium, Chloride, and Sulfate. USA: The National Academies Press.

19. Boschmann M, Steiniger J, Hille U, Tank J, Adams F, Sharma AM, Klaus S, Luft FC & Jordan J. (2003). Water-Induced Thermogenesis. *Journal of Clinical Endocrinology & Metabolism*, 88(12), 6015-6019.

20. Streit KJ, Stevens NH, Stevens VJ & Rossner J. (1991). Food Records: A Predictor and Modifier of Weight Change in a Long-Term Weight Loss Program. *Journal of the American Dietetic Association*, 9(2), 213-216.

CHAPTER 5: The SuperFoodsRx FlexPlan

1. Kamel HK. (2003). Sarcopenia and Aging. *Nutrition Reviews*, 61(5 Pt 1), 157-167.

2. Thompson, DL, Rakow J & Perdue SM. (2004). Relationship between Accumulated Walking and Body Composition in Middle-Aged Women. *Medicine & Science in Sports & Exercise*, 36(5), 911-914.

3. Phelan S, Wyatt HR, Hill JO & Wing RR. (2006). Are the Eating and Exercise Habits of Successful Weight Losers Changing? *Obesity* (Silver Spring), 14(4), 710-716.

4. Wing RR & Phelan S. (2005). Long-term weight loss maintenance. *American Journal of Clinical Nutrition*, 82(1): 222S-225S.

5. Luo CX, Jiang J, Zhou QG, Zhu XJ, Wang W, Zhang ZJ, Han X, & Zhu DY. (2007). Voluntary exercise-induced neurogenesis in the postischemic dentate gyrus is associated with spatial memory recovery from stroke. *Journal of Neuroscience Research*, 85(8), 1637-1646.

6. Pereira AC, Huddleston DE, Brickman AM, Sosunov AA, Hen R, McKhann GM, Sloan R, Gage FH, Brown TR & Small SA. (2007). An in vivo correlate of exercise-induced neurogenesis in the adult dentate gyrus. *Proceedings of the National Academies of Sciences USA*, 104(13), 5638-5643.

7. Binzen CA, Swan PD & Manore MM. (2001). Postexercise oxygen consumption and substrate use after resistance exercise in women. *Medicine & Science in Sports & Exercise*, 33(6), 932-938.

8. Feigenbaum MS & Pollock ML. (1999). Prescription of resistance training for health and disease. *Medicine & Science in Sports & Exercise*, 31(1), 38-45.

9. Calorie equivalents from:

Nieman DC. (2003). *Exercise Testing and Prescription*, New York: McGraw Hill. 2003.

Ainsworth BE, Haskell WL, Leon AS, Jacobs DR Jr, Montoye HJ, Sallis JF, & Paffenbarger RS Jr. (1993). Compendium of physical activities: classification of energy costs of human physical abilities. *Medicine & Science in Sports & Exercise*, 25(1), 71-80.

Ainsworth BE, Haskell WL, Whitt MC, Irwin ML, Swartz AM, Strath SJ, O'Brien WL, Bassett DR Jr, Schmitz KH, Emplaincourt PO, Jacobs DR Jr & Leon AS. (2000). Compendium of physical activities: and update of activity codes and MET intensities. *Medicine & Science in Sports & Exercise*, 32(9 Suppl), S498-S504.

CHAPTER 6: The SuperFoodsRx LifePlan

1. Jordan HA, Levitz LS, Utgoff KL & Lee HL. (1981). Role of food characteristics in behavioral change and weight loss. *Journal of the American Dietetic Association*, 79(1), 24-29.

2. Wing RR, Tate DF, Gorin AA, Raynor HA & Fava JL. (2006). A self-regulation program for maintenance of weight loss. *New England Journal of Medicine*, 355(15), 1563-1571.

3. Yudkin JS, Kumari M, Humphries SE & Mohamed-Ali V. (2000). Inflammation, obesity, stress and coronary heart disease: is interlueukin-6 the link? *Atherosclerosis*, 148(2), 209-214.

4. Davidson RJ, Kabat-Zinn J, Schumacher J, Rosenkranz M, Muller D, Santorelli SF, Urbanowski F, Harrington A, Bonus K & Sheridan JF. (2003). Alterations in brain and immune function produced by mindfulness meditation. *Psychosomatic Medicine*, 65(4), 564–570.

National Institutes of Medicine, NCCAM, Retrieved June 21, 2007, from http://nccam.nih.gov/health/backgrounds/mindbody.htm#heal

5. Steptoe A, Gibson EL, Vuononvirta R, Williams ED, Hamer M, Rycroft JA, Erusalimsky JD & Wardle J. (2007). The effects of tea on psychophysiological stress responsivity and post-stress recovery: a randomised double-blind trial. *Psychopharmacology* (Berl), 190(1), 81-89.

6. Patel SR, Malhotra A, White DP, Gottlieb DJ & Hu FB. (2006). Association between reduced sleep and weight gain in women. (2006). *American Journal of Epidemiology*, 164(10), 947-954.

Trenell MT, Marshall NS & Rogers NL. (2007). Sleep and metabolic control: waking to a problem? *Clinical and Experimental Pharmacology & Physiology*, 34(1-2), 1-9.

7. Copinschi G. (2005). Metabolic and endocrine effects of sleep deprivation. *Essential Psychoparmacology*, 6(6), 341-347.

Spiegel K, Leproult R & Van Cauter E. (1999). Impact of sleep debt on metabolic and endoctrine function. *Lancet*, 354(9188), 1435-1439.

8. Patel SR, Malhotra A, White DP, Gottlieb DJ & Hu FB. (2006).Association between reduced sleep and weight gain in women. *American Journal of Epidemiology*, 164(10), 947-954.

9. Gangwisch JE, Malaspina D, Boden-Albala B & Heymsfield SB. (2005). Inadequate sleep as a risk factor for obesity: analyses of the *NHANES I. Sleep*, 28(10), 1289-1296.

10. Gangwisch JE, Malaspina D, Boden-Albala B & Heymsfield SB. (2005). Inadequate sleep as a risk factor for obesity: analyses of the *NHANES I. Sleep*, 28(10), 1289-1296.

11. Van Cauter E, Holmback U, Knutson K, Leproult R, Miller A, Nedeltcheva A, Pannain S, Peneve P, Tasali E & Spiegel K. (2007). Impact of sleep and sleep loss on neuroendocrine and metabolic function. *Hormonal Research*, 67(Suppl 1), 2-9.

Copinschi G. (2005). Metabolic and endocrine effects of sleep deprivation. *Essential Psychopharmacology*, 6(6), 341-347.

Nilsson PM, Rööst M, Engström G, Hedblad B & Berglund G. (2004). Incidence of diabetes in middle-aged men is related to sleep disturbances. Diabetes Care, 27(10), 2464-2469.

12. Spiegel K, Tasali E, Penev P & Van Cauter E. (2004). Brief communication: Sleep curtailment in healthy young men is associated with decreased leptin levels, elevated ghrelin levels, and increased hunger and appetite. Annals of Internal Medicine, 141(11), 846-850.

Copinschi G. (2005). Metabolic and endocrine effects of sleep deprivation. *Essential Psychopharmacology*, 6(6), 341-347.

13. Copinschi G. (2005). Metabolic and endocrine effects of sleep deprivation. *Essential Psychopharmacology*, 6(6), 341-347.

14. Copinschi G. (2005). Metabolic and endocrine effects of sleep deprivation. *Essential Psychopharmacology*, 6(6), 341-347.

Knutson KL, Spiegel K, Penev P & Van Cauter E. (2007). The metabolic consequences of sleep deprivation, *Sleep Medicine Reviews*, 11(3), 163-178.

Spiegel K, Leproult R & Van Cauter E. (1999). Impact of sleep debt on metabolic and endocrine function. *Lancet*, 354(9188), 1435-1439.

15. Naska A, Oikonomou E, Trichopoulou A, Psaltopoulou T & Trichopoulos D (2007). Siesta in healthy adults and coronary mortality in the general population. *Archives of Internal Medicine*, 167(3), 296-301.

16. Keystone Center. (2006, June). Keystone forum on away-from-home foods—final report. Retrieved June 20 2007, from http://www.keystone.org/spp/documents/Forum_Report_FINAL_5-30-06.pdf

17. Oliver G & Wardle J. (1999) Perceived effects of stress on food choice. *Physiology & Behavior*, 66(3), 511-515.

The SuperFoodsRx Diet Recipe Credits

The SuperFoodsRx Kitchen Chefs

The team of culinary experts invited to develop recipes for *The SuperFoodsRx Diet* were chosen not only because they are the best at what they do, but they also truly understand the stress of today's busy households and demanding lifestyles. Each member of the culinary team—Tammy Algood, Barbara Seelig Brown, and Barbara Snow—brings experience and expertise in creating healthy and easy recipes made with readily available ingredients in a short amount of time! A tall order— accomplished with creativity and pizazz. Each provided innovative, tasty, and nutritionally appropriate recipes that were all tested, analyzed, revised, and retested to ensure SuperFoodsRx dieters' long-term interests and long-term success. Tammy Algood oversaw the recipe development process for *The SuperFoodsRx Diet*.

Specific Recipe Contributions by the SuperFoodsRx Kitchen:

Barbara Seelig Brown

Asian Inspired Broccoli Salad
Asian Inspired Red Pepper Sesame Dressing
Asian Stuffed Salmon Fillet
Basic SuperFoodsRx "Vinaigrette" Dressing
    With 8 Variations
Black Bean & Mango Salsa
Broccoli & White Beans with Crushed Red
    Pepper
Chicken Salad with Thyme, Walnuts & Grapes
Creamy Spinach Dip
Pan Roasted Stuffed Turkey Breast with White
    Bean Sauce

Poached Chicken
Salmon Taco with Mango & Avocado
Sicilian Style Stuffed Turkey Breast
Smoked Salmon Spread
Stuffed Tuna Salad Tomatoes Basic Tuna
    Salad, Blueberry Walnut Tuna Salad,
    Curried Tuna Salad
Sweet Potato & Asparagus with Orange Glaze
Turkey Pumpkin Chili with Roasted Pumpkin
    Seeds
Watermelon & Jalapeño Salsa
Yogurt Banana Strawberry Spread

Barbara Snow

Fresh and Light Tacos
Garlic Lover's Dip
Ginger Orange Dressing
SuperFoodsRx Granola
Great Northern Bean Dip

Orange Flaxseed (or Sesame) Salmon
Pumpkin Dessert Crepe with Yogurt Sauce
SuperFoodsRx Turkey Spinach Pita
Thin Crust Turkey Pita Pizza
Whole Wheat Pita Crisps

Tammy Algood

All-Season Fruit Salad
Almond Green Beans
Baked Apples
Baked Sweet Potatoes
Blueberry Compote Crumble
Broccoli and Cauliflower Salad
"Brocco-Mole"
Broiled Salmon: Asian, Walnut Crusted, Lemon
     Herb, Cucumber Yogurt or Ginger Lime
Carrot Charger
Chicken Croquettes
Chocolate Tofu Mousse
Cold Fruit Soup
Cold Vegetable Tortillas
Confetti Salad
Cooked Lentils
Crunchy Coleslaw
Cucumber Yogurt Sauce
Easy Tomato Veggie Juice
Four Bean Chili
Fresh Blueberry Compote
Ginger Grilled Turkey Tenderloin
Go Green!
Grilled Corn on the Cob
Grilled Fruit Kabobs
Grown Up Peanut Butter Sandwiches
Hummus
Dark Chocolate Chip Cookies
Great Northern Shrimp Salad
Greek Salad Roll-Ups
Homemade Tortilla Chips
Hummus and Roasted Pepper Sandwich
"It's Good To Be Blue" Bevvy
Lemon Roasted Turkey
Lentil Meatballs
No Cook Vegetable Kabobs
Oatmeal Cinnamon Bars
Papillote
Peanut Glazed Shrimp
Poached Salmon
Poached Salmon in Spinach Tortillas
Pumpkin Julius Smoothie
"Refried" Beans
Roasted Broccoli
Roasted Pepper Puree
Salsa Bean Dip
Roasted Vegetable Pita Sandwiches

Slow Baked Tomatoes
Spicy Tofu Salad
Steamed Carrots with Dill
SuperFoodsRx Blueberry Oatmeal Muffin with
     Walnuts
SuperFoodsRx Pumpkin Walnut Muffins
SuperFoodsRx Salad Inspirations
SuperFoodsRx SoupBase
SuperFoodsRx Soup Options # 1 through # 12
SuperFoodsRx Spicy Pumpkin Butter
Sweet Potato Soup
Tangy Tomato Dressing
Tangy Tomato Vegetable Juice
Thanksgiving Open-Faced Sandwich
Toasted Nuts and Seeds
Tofu "Eggless" Salad
Tofu Herb Dressing
Turkey (Or Tofu) Meatballs
Turkey Meatball Soup
Turkey Meatloaf with Tomato Gravy
Turkey Sausage and Tortellini Soup
Tuscan Bean Soup
Vegetable Kabobs with Shrimp Or Tofu
Year Round Salsa
Yogurt Cheese
Yogurt & Fruit Smoothie

Additional Contributions from WNB and Others

"Eggsellent" Spinach, Mushroom & Onion
     Scramble
Bean and Veggie Burrito
Citrus Apricot Couscous
Corn Salsa
Egg Frittata with Cherry Tomatoes, Spinach &
     Cheese
Fruit Delight Smoothie
Grilled Salmon with Yogurt Dill Drizzle
Honey Ginger Carrots
Layered Turkey (or Chicken) Salad
Marvelous Mediterranean Salad
Modern Ambrosia for One
Pear, Feta and Pecan Stuffed Pita
SuperFoodsRx Salads: Small, Medium, Large,
     and Entrée
Tofu Stir Fry
Honey Mustard Salad Dressing

Acknowledgments

This book has been a real collaboration with significant contributions made by many people. We are all eager to thank the SuperFoodsRx Partners for their constant encouragement and enthusiastic support of this project. David Stern and Ray Sphire have been the driving force behind the Super-FoodsRx books and they, along with Dr. Hugh Greenway and Dr. Geoffrey Harris, have been steadfast and encouraging in all aspects of this project.

Nancy Hancock, with her infinite experience and sense of detail, and the entire team at Rodale have been truly extraordinary. Their insightful guidance, hard work, and attention to detail have precipitated a near miracle: the fast and professional production of this book. We'd particularly like also to thank Beth Davey, Blanca Oliviery, Marina Padakis, Chris Gaugler, Beth Lamb, and Liz Perl.

Many thanks to David Vigliano and Michael Harriott for their early championing of this project that led to our wonderful relationship with Rodale.

We are all extremely appreciative of the SuperFoodsRx Kitchen—Tammy Algood, who oversaw the recipe development process for *The SuperFoodsRx Diet*, as well as culinary wonders Barbara Seelig-Brown and Barbara Snow. They have worked tirelessly to create recipes that are extraordinarily delicious—super-nutritious and gourmet, sophisticated yet incredibly simple—while simultaneously complying with our ambitious nutritional goals.

We are extremely and personally grateful to all of the SuperFoodsRx dieters who so enthusiastically and successfully embraced the diet. Your shared insights, experiences, and successes gave a special dimension to this book and will inspire others to mirror your success.

As the "Father of SuperFoods," I'm proud to add yet another book to what we had always envisioned would be a nutrition revolution. I'm grateful to

Wendy Bazilian, the newest member of the SuperFoodsRx team, for her development of the specifics of this extraordinary diet. Her work with our test groups and her dedication to perfection have helped create a diet program that is as practical as it is effective. Kathy Matthews has, as always, helped to create a lively, readable, and engaging text. My family, friends, and also my patients have been, as always, a reliable and patient support group and I am grateful to them all.

—Steven Pratt, MD

I've been thrilled to be a part of this collaborative project. In addition to those we've expressed mutual thanks to above, I must again thank Steven Pratt, whose dedication to the science and to his clients and readers has brought us the SuperFoods story and its sequels. Special thanks to Kathy Matthews, whose artful word-weaving and rich experience helped create structure out of thought, files into form, and words into messages.

My mentors, colleagues, and friends at Tufts University, UC San Diego, and Loma Linda University have shaped and influenced my life both professionally and personally, and thanks to those colleagues and scientists whose contributions through their research are acknowledged in the references and many whom, nonetheless important, are not listed due to limitations of space. My work colleagues in my various interactions have been sounding boards and inspirations to my writing and professional practice. And many thanks are also extended to all inspiring members of my extended Golden Door family over the past five years.

In addition, I'd like to add a special thanks to my parents, siblings, and grandfather, and to Tammy Algood, Deborah Miller, Pearl and Wayne and crew, Nancy and Michael, Salah, and many others for their individual contributions and support. Also to Marsha, Martha, Barbara, Rebecca, Deborah, Elizabeth, Patty, and oh, so many more. And to my husband, partner, and best friend, Jason, I am forevermore grateful for your enduring patience, love, support, and unending assistance.

—Wendy Bazilian, DrPH, MA, RD

Index

Underscored page references indicate boxed text and tables.

SuperNutrient Booster Yogurt & Fruit
  Smoothie, 327
"2 for 1" choice, 142–43
Fruit snacks, buying, 111

G

Garlic
  Basil Garlic Dressing, 308
  Garlic Lover's Dip (and Sandwich
    Spread), 299
  Rosemary Garlic Dressing, 308
Ghrelin, 176
Ginger
  Ginger Grilled Turkey Tenderloin,
    269
  Ginger Lime Option (for Broiled
    Salmon), 267
  Ginger Orange Dressing, 309
  Honey Ginger Carrots, 246
Glucagon, soy increasing, 21
Grains. See also Side dishes, with grain; Side
    dishes, without grain; specific grains;
    Whole grains
  brand name, 334
  as Flex food, 138–39
  in restaurant meals, 181
  selecting, 211–13, 213
  "2 for 1" choice, 143–44
Granola
  SuperFoodsRx Granola, 222
Granola bars, caution with, 157
Grapes
  Chicken Salad with Thyme, Walnuts &
    Grapes, 226
Grapeseed oil, 109
Green beans
  Almond Green Beans, 242
  Tortellini Vegetable Soup, 287
Green tea. See also Tea
  antioxidants in, 12
  brand name, 339–40
  as coffee substitute, 60
  polyphenols in, 10
  for Prep & Practice Week, 123,
    125
  as SuperFood, 4, 10
  synergy of, with oranges, 6
  for weight loss, 10–11

Guilt
  absent from SuperFoodsRx Diet, 133
  avoiding, over food disposal, 59, 99
Gumbo
  Seafood Gumbo, 286–87

H

Hair, improved by SuperFoodsRx Diet, x,
    xi–xii
Health history, food diary revealing, 72
Height-weight tables, for weight assessment,
    43
Herbs. See also specific herbs
  buying, 110
  Lemon Herb Option (for Broiled
    Salmon), 266
  Tofu Herb Dressing, 312
High blood pressure. See Hypertension
High-fructose corn syrup (HFCS), 100–101,
    103, 109
High-protein diets
  problem with, 23–24
  weight loss from, 23–25
High-sodium foods, 101–2
Honey
  Honey Ginger Carrots, 246
  Honey Mustard Salad Dressing, 310
  as SuperFood, 4
Honeydew melon
  Cold Fruit Soup, 292
Hot entrées
  Asian Stuffed Salmon Fillet, 270–71
  Asian Stuffed Turkey, 273
  Broiled Salmon, 264–67
  Chicken Croquettes, 268
  Ginger Grilled Turkey Tenderloin, 269
  Great Northern Shrimp Salad, 275
  Grilled Salmon with Yogurt Dill Drizzle,
    284
  Lemon Roasted Turkey, 276
  Lentil Meatballs, 277
  Orange Flaxseed (or Sesame) Salmon,
    274
  Pan Roasted Stuffed Turkey Breast with
    White Bean Sauce, 271–72
  Papillote, 278–79
  Peanut Glazed Shrimp, 279
  selecting, 202–3, 205–7

Low-fat foods
    calories in, 102
    caution with, 160–61
Lunch
    selections for, 193–213
    when eating out, 179 (*see also* Eating out
        guidelines)
Lycopene
    healthy oil and, 63
    in tomatoes, 26

M

Mangoes
    Black Bean & Mango Salsa, 296
    Chicken Salad with Mango, Soy
        Nuts, Cilantro and Lime,
        226
    Salmon Taco with Mango and
        Avocado, 253
Marinade
    Asian Marinade Option (for Broiled
        Salmon), 265
Mayonnaise, caution with, 158
Meal selections. *See also* Menu plans
    breakfast, 188–93
    choosing, during Prep & Practice Week,
        107–8
    lunch and dinner, 193–213
    snacks, 213–15
Meal skipping, avoiding, 64, 169
Meatballs
    Lentil Meatballs, 277
    Turkey (or Tofu) Meatballs, 280
    Turkey Meatball Soup, 290
Meatloaf
    Turkey Meatloaf with Tomato Gravy,
        281
Melon
    Cold Fruit Soup, 292
Men
    FlexPlan guidelines for, 162
    SlimDown guidelines for, 91
Menu plans. *See also* Meal selections
    excessive variety in, 88
    for FlexPlan, 163, 164–65
    for SlimDown, 91–93, 94–95, 117,
        118–19, 125
    when and how to select, 134

Metabolic syndrome, 21
Metabolism
    of high-fructose corn syrup vs. glucose,
        100–101
    increasing, with
        afternoon snack, 67
        breakfast, 58
        fluids, 69
        green tea, 11
        regular meals, 64, 169
        snacks, 169
        strength training, 149–50
        water, 123–24
    omega-3 fatty acids and, 15, 16
    sleep and, 175, 176
    stress hormones and, 171
    SuperFoods and, 7, 168
Milk, soy
    brand name, 340
    buying, 110
Mindful eating
    for portion control, 38
    during SlimDown, 86–87
Mirror test, for weight assessment,
    48–49, 48
Moderation, in FlexPlan,
    128–29
Mood, recorded in food diary, 73
Mortality, healthy foods increasing,
    xiv
Motivation, 114, 187
    notes and photos for, 114
    from SuperFoodsRx Diet Prep &
        Practice Week, 97
Motivators, in SuperFoodsRx Diet, xiii,
    xiv
Mousse
    Chocolate Tofu Mousse, 317
Muffins, 191
    SuperFoodsRx Blueberry Muffin with
        Walnuts, 318–19
    SuperFoodsRx Pumpkin Walnut
        Muffins, 320–21
Muscle
    affecting scale weight, 44, 78
    calcium preserving, 18
    calorie burning from, 146, 150
    exercise building, 146
    loss of, 147, 150

Weigh-ins
  guidelines for, 44–45
  for long-term weight-loss success, 169
  during SlimDown, 86
Weight assessment methods, 43–50
Weight gain
  calcium preventing, 16–17
  diet soda and, 104
  sleep deprivation and, 175–76
Weight loss
  behavior change for, 37
  breakfast for, 58–59
  calories and, 26–27
  exercise for, 15–16, 146–47
  factors contributing to, 166
  food diary for, 69–71
  healthy fats for, 87
  from high-protein diets, 23–25
  plateaus in, 78, 185–87
  in postmenopausal women, 46
  salads for, 61, 62
  soups for, 62–63
  SuperFoods and SuperNutrients for, 1, 7,
    8, 9, 168–69
    beans, 21–23
    calcium, 17
    fiber, 30 31
    low-calorie, 25–26, 28–29
    nuts, 18 19
    oats, 31
    omega-3 fatty acids, 14–15
    pumpkin, 31
    salmon, 15
    soy, 20–21
    tea, 10–11
    turkey, 25
    vitamin C, 12–13
    whole grains, 31–32, 64–65
    yogurt, 16–18
Weight-loss goal, setting, 42, 51
Weight-loss maintenance, 166–68
  LifePlan for (see LifePlan)
Whole foods, synergy of nutrients in,
    5–6
Whole grains. See also Grains
  in bread, identifying, 106
  daily portions of, 41
  guidelines for, 66

with or without rule about, 65–67, 65
selecting, 211–13, 213
for weight loss, 31–32, 64–65
WHR, for weight assessment, 47, 47–48, 48
Wild rice
  Confetti Salad, 249
Willpower, xv, 35, 96–97, 124
With or without grains rule, 65–67, 65
Workplace, improving food options in, 117
Wraps, 195, 196, 197
  Cold Vegetable Tortillas, 256–57
  Greek Salad Roll-Ups, 258
  Poached Salmon in Spinach Tortillas,
    260–61

Y

Yogurt
  buying, 110
  Cucumber Yogurt Option (for Broiled
    Salmon), 266–67
  Cucumber Yogurt Sauce, 310–11
  Fruit on the Bottom Yogurt, 190
  Grilled Salmon with Yogurt Dill Drizzle,
    284
  health benefits of, 16
  live active cultures in, 16
  as mayonnaise substitute, 158
  Pumpkin Dessert Crepe with Yogurt
    Sauce, 315–16
  sidekick of, 4
  as SuperFood, 4
  SuperNutrient Booster Yogurt & Fruit
    Smoothie, 327
  for weight loss, 16–18
  Yogurt, Strawberry, and Chopped
    Walnut Breakfast Parfait, 189
  Yogurt Banana Strawberry Spread,
    298–99
  Yogurt Cheese, 217
Yo-yo dieting, xviii

Z

Zucchini
  Roasted Vegetable Pita Sandwiches, 261
  Vegetable Kabobs with Shrimp or Tofu,
    282–83

Page - 184
    - 23 - metabolic syndrom △

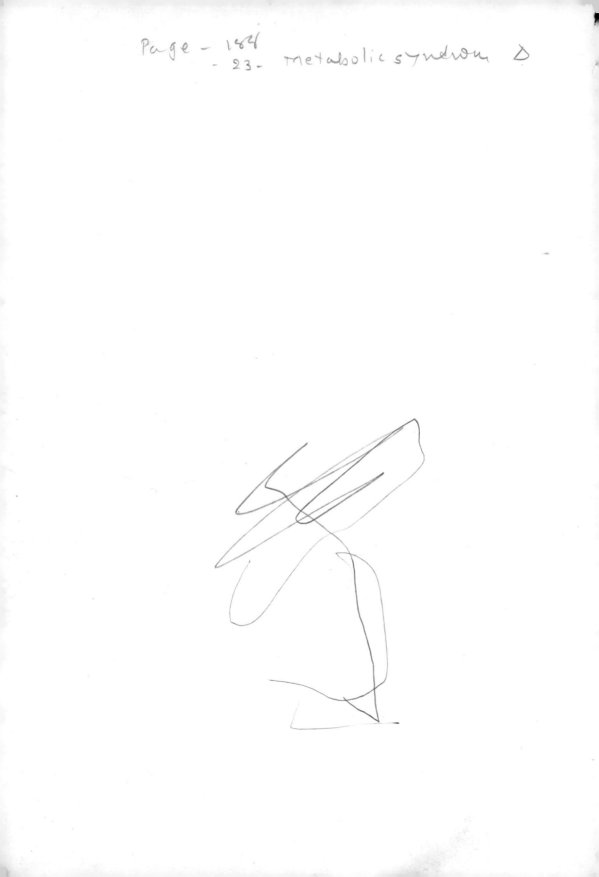